NUTRITION, LIFESTYLE FACTORS, AND BLOOD PRESSURE

NUTRITION, LIFESTYLE FACTORS, AND BLOOD PRESSURE

EDITED BY
PAO-HWA LIN, Ph.D.
LAURA P. SVETKEY, MD

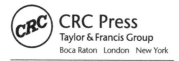

CRC Press
Taylor & Francis Group
Boca Raton London New York

CRC Press is an imprint of the
Taylor & Francis Group, an **informa** business

CRC Press
Taylor & Francis Group
6000 Broken Sound Parkway NW, Suite 300
Boca Raton, FL 33487-2742

First issued in paperback 2016

© 2012 by Taylor & Francis Group, LLC
CRC Press is an imprint of Taylor & Francis Group, an Informa business

No claim to original U.S. Government works

Version Date: 20120510

ISBN 13: 978-1-138-19919-4 (pbk)
ISBN 13: 978-1-4398-3075-8 (hbk)

Library of Congress Cataloging-in-Publication Data

Nutrition, lifestyle factors, and blood pressure / edited by Pao-Hwa Lin and Laura P. Svetkey.
   p. cm.
   Summary: "Aiming to increase awareness, this book covers measures to prevent health conditions and diseases that are associated with high blood pressure. The first section provides a comprehensive review of diet, nutrition, lifestyle, and blood pressure control. It also discusses the consequences of high blood pressure, including heart disease, kidney disease, diabetes, and stroke. The second section focuses on implementation of strategies to promote behavioral changes for blood pressure control. The final section addresses key subgroup populations and situations that require special considerations. Case studies demonstrate how lifestyle factors can be changed to control blood pressure"-- Provided by publisher.
   Includes bibliographical references and index.
   ISBN 978-1-4398-3075-8 (hardback)
   1. Hypertension--Diet therapy. 2. Exercise therapy. 3. Self-care, Health. I. Lin, Pao-Hwa. II. Svetkey, Laura P.

RC685.H8N87 2012
616.1'320654--dc23
2011052602

Visit the Taylor & Francis Web site at
http://www.taylorandfrancis.com

and the CRC Press Web site at
http://www.crcpress.com

Contents

SECTION I   Evidence on Lifestyle Factors and Blood Pressure

SECTION II   Implementation of Lifestyle Intervention for Blood Pressure Control

SECTION III   Special Considerations

SECTION IV   Putting It All Together: Practical Tools

Preface

Hypertension is a major risk factor for coronary heart disease, stroke, and premature death, and it affects approximately one-third of adults in the United States. Approximately, another one-third of the adults in the United States have prehypertension, which is also associated with a graded, increased risk of cardiovascular diseases and progression to hypertension. National surveys (NHANES 2007–2008) indicate that, despite steady progress, the awareness, detection, and treatment of hypertension remain unsatisfactory in the United States, that is, about 20% of all hypertensive individuals are unaware of their illness, 28% are not being treated, and only 69% of treated patients had controlled hypertension. The direct and indirect costs of hypertension in the United States were $63.5 billion in 2006, reflecting a public health challenge and a continuing need for effective health policy and practice to prevent and manage hypertension. In the face of the aging population and the growing epidemic of obesity, the challenges related to hypertension continue to rise.

Even though enormous advancement has been made in identifying evidence-based lifestyle strategies for hypertension prevention and management, little progress has been made in implementing these proven strategies. Accumulating evidence supports that hypertension is preventable and that it is closely related to modifiable factors such as dietary pattern and other lifestyle factors. The Joint National Committee (JNC) on Prevention, Detection, Evaluation and Treatment of High Blood Pressure was appointed by the National Heart, Lung, and Blood Institute to provide evidenced-based clinical guidelines for the prevention and management of hypertension. Current JNC guidelines (JNC7) recommend reduction in salt intake, moderate alcohol consumption, weight loss if overweight, aerobic exercise, increase in potassium intake, and following the DASH eating pattern to lower blood pressure (BP). JNC8 was in progress at the time this book was written, but it is unlikely to change these evidence-based recommendations. These lifestyle modifications are all recommended as part of the first-line therapy for low-risk individuals defined as those without diabetes or cardiovascular diseases and with systolic blood pressure or diastolic blood pressure < 160/100 mmHg (i.e., stage 1 hypertension). These lifestyle modifications are also recommended for individuals with prehypertension to prevent the development of high BP and for use in combination with pharmacotherapy for hypertension more severe than stage 1.

Most of these lifestyle recommendations, however, have fared poorly in the United States. Adherence to these recommendations by both the clinicians and the public has been less than satisfactory. In most of the cases, clinicians do not even mention about lifestyle modifications to patients during their clinic visit, perhaps due to lack of training and limited resources. At the population level, the amount of salt intake continues to stay above the recommended levels, and the obesity epidemic remains worrisome; only less than 5% of the adults in the United States meet the recommended physical activity level; and finally, Americans continue to consume far less than the recommended amounts of fruits, vegetables, fiber, calcium, magnesium, and potassium—all of which are key components of the DASH dietary pattern, which lowers BP.

Undoubtedly, implementing dietary and lifestyle modifications is challenging, and effective strategies for sustainable implementation are urgently needed. Thus, the main purpose of this book is to compile science-based practical information for health care providers to provide effective lifestyle interventions for controlling BP. The book is divided into four sections. Section I provides an overview of the scientific evidence relating nutrition and lifestyle to BP control and relevant considerations for real-life situations. Section II focuses on the different aspects of implementing the recommended lifestyle modifications. Section III discusses several special considerations in BP control and lifestyle modifications among children and adolescents, pregnant women, and those with diabetes. Section IV compiles simple practical tools that health care providers can put into practice in particular settings. At the end of each of the chapters, a summary table with existing key evidences and expert recommendations is also included.

We have collectively conducted many lifestyle intervention trials and observed the effect of nutrition and lifestyle interventions on BP and many other health indicators. It is our desire and sincere wish that this book may supplement the existing resources and shorten the gap between current understanding of the science about the relationship between lifestyle factors and BP and the actual implementation of the science. Ultimately, we hope that the trend in lifestyle interventions for hypertension prevention and treatment may be shifted. We sincerely appreciate all the authors for their contribution to this book. Without their help, this book would not have been completed.

Pao-Hwa Lin
Duke University Medical Center
Durham, North Carolina

Laura P. Svetkey
Duke Hypertension Center and Sarah W.
Stedman Center for Nutrition and Metabolism
Duke University Medical Center
Durham, North Carolina

Editors

Pao-Hwa Lin is an associate research professor in the Division of Nephrology at Duke University Medical Center and **Laura P. Svetkey** is a professor of medicine in the Division of Nephrology at Duke University Medical Center. Svetkey is also the director of Duke Hypertension Center and Director of Clinical Research of Sarah W. Stedman Nutrition and Metabolism Center. Together, they have conducted many clinical trials on nutrition, lifestyle, and BP control.

Contributors

Marlyn Allicock
Department of Nutrition
Gillings School of Global Public Health
University of North Carolina at Chapel
    Hill
Chapel Hill, North Carolina

Cheryl A.M. Anderson
Bloomberg School of Public Health
Welch Center for Prevention,
    Epidemiology, and Clinical Research
Johns Hopkins Medical Institutions
Baltimore, Maryland

Jamy D. Ard
Department of Nutrition Sciences
University of Alabama at Birmingham
Birmingham, Alabama

Sarah C. Armstrong
Department of Pediatrics
Duke University Medical Center
Durham, North Carolina

Carissa M. Baker-Smith
Division of Pediatric Cardiology
University of Maryland School of
    Medicine
Baltimore, Maryland

Jessica Bartfield
Loyola University Gottlieb Memorial
    Hospital
Melrose Park, Illinois

Bryan C. Batch
Department of Medicine
Duke University Medical Center
Durham, North Carolina

Hayden B. Bosworth
Veterans Affairs Medical Center
Durham, North Carolina
and
Department of Medicine, Department
    of Psychiatry and Behavioral
    Sciences, and School of Nursing
Duke University
Durham, North Carolina

George A. Bray
Pennington Biomedical Research Center
Louisiana State University System
Baton Rouge, Louisiana

Marci K. Campbell (Deceased)
Gillings School of Global Public Health
    and UNC Lineberger Comprehensive
    Cancer Center
University of North Carolina at Chapel
    Hill
Chapel Hill, North Carolina

Catherine M. Champagne
Pennington Biomedical Research Center
Louisiana State University System
Baton Rouge, Louisiana

Liwei Chen
School of Public Health
Louisiana State University Health
    Sciences Center
New Orleans, Louisiana

Paul R. Conlin
Harvard Medical School
Boston, Massachusetts
and
VA Boston Healthcare System
West Roxbury, Massachusetts

Anna E. Czinn
University of Maryland School of
    Medicine
Baltimore, Maryland

Deborah Day
Amity Regional High School
Woodbridge, Connecticut

Diana H. Dolinsky
Department of Pediatrics
Duke University Medical Center
Durham, North Carolina

Denise Ernst
Denise Ernst Training and Consultation
Portland, Oregon

Lauren Gratian
Department of Medicine
Duke University Medical Center
Durham, North Carolina

David W. Harsha
Pennington Biomedical Research Center
Louisiana State University System
Baton Rouge, Louisiana

S. Joseph Huang
Department of Obstetrics, Gynecology
    and Reproductive Sciences
Yale University
New Haven, Connecticut

Stephen P. Juraschek
Johns Hopkins University School of
    Medicine and
Johns Hopkins Bloomberg School of
    Public Health
Johns Hopkins Medical Institutions
Baltimore, Maryland

Pao-Hwa Lin
Department of Medicine
Duke University Medical Center
Durham, North Carolina

Angelo S. Milazzo
Division of Pediatric Cardiology
University of Maryland School of
    Medicine
Baltimore, Maryland

Edgar R. Miller III
Department of Medicine
Johns Hopkins Medical Institutions
Baltimore, Maryland

Ira Ockene
Division of Cardiovascular Medicine
University of Massachusetts Medical
    School
Worcester, Massachusetts

Elena Salmoirago-Blotcher
Division of Cardiovascular
    Medicine
University of Massachusetts Medical
    School
Worcester, Massachusetts

Bei Sun
Division of Endocrinology, Diabetes,
    and Hypertension
Brigham and Women's Hospital
Harvard Medical School
Boston, Massachusetts

Laura P. Svetkey
Duke Hypertension Center and
Sarah W. Stedman Center for Nutrition
    and Metabolism
Department of Medicine
Division of Nephrology
Duke University Medical Center
Durham, North Carolina

Jonathan S. Williams
Division of Endocrinology, Diabetes,
    and Hypertension
Brigham and Women's Hospital
Harvard Medical School
Boston, Massachusetts

Zhen-Ming Wu
Department of Obstetrics, Gynecology
    and Reproductive Sciences
Yale University
New Haven, Connecticut
and
Department of Obstetrics and Gynecology
Shanghai Jiao Tong University
Shanghai, China

Chang-Ching Yeh
Department of Obstetrics, Gynecology
    and Reproductive Sciences
Yale University
New Haven, Connecticut
and
Department of Obstetrics and Gynecology
Taipei Veterans General Hospital
Taipei, Taiwan

Deborah Rohm Young
Department of Epidemiology and
    Biostatistics
University of Maryland School of
    Public Health
College Park, Maryland

Section I

Evidence on Lifestyle Factors and Blood Pressure

OVERVIEW

Pao-Hwa Lin, Paul Conlin, and Laura P. Svetkey

Nonpharmacological interventions, including dietary modification, weight loss, sodium reduction, and physical activity, are a critical part in the prevention of high blood pressure (BP), and they serve as a cornerstone of treatment for those with hypertension. In individuals without hypertension, adopting a healthy lifestyle reduces BP and prevents hypertension. This is directly relevant to clinical outcomes as there is a continuum of risk between increases in BP and cardiovascular events, and more importantly, no threshold appears in this relationship. The risk of death from cardiovascular events increases linearly, beginning at BP levels of 115/75 mmHg. Therefore, reducing BP not only prevents or delays the incidence of hypertension but also lowers the risk of BP-related cardiovascular complications, producing a significant impact on public health. For those with stage 1 hypertension, dietary and lifestyle changes may be sufficient to control hypertension in the absence of medications. For those with higher levels of BP, lifestyle modifications help to enhance the efficacy of antihypertensive medications.

This section reviews the current evidence on the BP-related effects of dietary modifications, weight loss, reduction in sodium intake, and physical activity. Chapter 1 reviews the association of macronutrients and dietary patterns with BP. Many studies have attempted to dissect the effects of individual macronutrients or different combinations of macronutrients on BP. However, it is challenging to draw definitive conclusions from these studies due to various design difficulties. The Dietary Approaches to Stop Hypertension (DASH) was the first major clinical trial using controlled feeding protocol to test the effect of two dietary patterns on BP, with rigorous findings. The DASH study and another study with modified DASH dietary patterns are reviewed in this chapter.

In addition, many dietary factors including minerals and antioxidants have shown BP-lowering potentials. However, these micronutrients coexist in natural foods with many other nutrient factors that may also affect BP. Hence, it is impossible to test the effects of individual micronutrients by food or dietary manipulation without significant confounding. The contribution of antioxidants, minerals, and micronutrients to BP is best tested in the setting of placebo-controlled randomized trials because they can be concentrated in pills or capsules. Thus, Chapter 2 reviews the evidence on the effects of minerals, antioxidants, and flavonoid-containing supplements on BP.

Abundant evidences from animal studies, large-scale observational human studies, and intervention studies in humans have shown that high intake of dietary salt (sodium chloride) independently leads to higher BP, hypertension, and cardiovascular disease. In brief, a median reduction in dietary salt by approximately 4.5–6.9 g/day resulted in lowering systolic BP by 3.7–4.9 mmHg in hypertensive patients and by 1.0–2.0 mmHg in normotensive individuals. Furthermore, a dose–response relationship was reported in a Cochrane review of salt intake and BP. Every 6-g decrease in salt intake was associated with 7.1/3.9 mmHg reduction in systolic and diastolic BP among hypertensive individuals and 3.6/1.7 mmHg in normotensive individuals. Recent evidence also indicates that lower sodium intake reduces the long-term risk of cardiovascular disease events.

However, despite repeated campaigns encouraging reduced sodium intake, survey data continue to indicate that most people exceed the intake limits and that long-term adherence to sodium-restricted diets is low. Indeed, excessive consumption remains a major public health problem. Since at least 75% of the dietary salt consumed in the United States comes from processed foods, there have been numerous pleas directed to the food industry to reduce salt in the food supply. Chapter 3 reviews the existing evidence on the effect of sodium intake on BP and discusses the strategies that may help in reducing sodium intake at the population level.

Being overweight and obese are established risk factors for hypertension. Based on data from National Health and Nutrition Examination Survey (NHANES) studies conducted between 1988–1994 and 1999–2004, it was found that there was 4.5% increase in the age-standardized prevalence of hypertension, and nearly all of the increased prevalence was explained by increases in body mass index. Chapter 4 reviews various clinical trials in which the impact of weight loss on BP was examined. Overall, the results of the studies strongly support the concept that weight loss interventions are an effective approach to both preventing and treating hypertension, even without a significant amount of sustained weight loss.

Even though regular physical activity is known to confer a number of health benefits, including lower incidence of coronary heart disease, stroke, type 2 diabetes, some types of cancers, and obesity, only less than half of the U.S. population meets the federal guidelines for physical activity. Chapter 5 reviews the evidence linking regular physical activity to lowering of BP, provides an overview of potential mechanisms for this association, clarifies recommendations on physical activity to control BP, and identifies physical activity interventions and also policies to increase physical activity.

1 Macronutrients, Dietary Patterns, and Blood Pressure

Pao-Hwa Lin
Duke University Medical Center

Liwei Chen
Louisiana State University Health Sciences Center

CONTENTS

1.1 INTRODUCTION

Dietary intake is closely related to blood pressure (BP) control. Besides sodium, many nutrients and minerals have been examined for their relationship with BP. In this chapter, we review the epidemiologic and clinical trial evidences for the potential impact of the intake of macronutrients, including protein, fat, carbohydrate, fiber, and alcohol, and of dietary patterns on hypertension and BP control. Data from meta-analyses or well-designed randomized trials and prospective studies with a large sample size are included in this review. It should be noted that although meta-analyses are useful for evaluating consistency in the literature, they tend to weigh large studies more heavily [1,2], and it is rarely feasible to conduct subanalyses on potentially important modifying factors or to account for variable dietary adherence among studies.

Studies on macronutrients and BP are often subject to various limitations, and thus the interpretation of results is complicated. For example, when a study is designed to examine the effect of the amount of fat intake on BP, alteration in fat intake under isocaloric conditions will change the amount of intake of protein and/ or carbohydrate inevitably, and it may change the intake of other nutrients as well. As a result, it may be difficult to attribute the effect on BP to changes in fat intake alone. In addition, the effect of macronutrients on BP potentially is due to aspects of both absolute quantity and the type of macronutrients consumed. Both aspects can affect BP independently, but they are not always distinguishable in research designs.

1.2 MACRONUTRIENTS AND BP

1.2.1 DIETARY PROTEIN

Many observational studies have shown an inverse relationship between total dietary protein intake and BP [3]. Nevertheless, results have been mixed when animal and plant proteins were examined separately. Cross-sectional studies conducted in rural Japanese and Chinese populations found an inverse relationship between animal protein and BP [4,5]. In contrast, cohort studies conducted in the U.S. populations have shown mitigation of the increase in systolic BP (SBP) with aging and higher baseline intake of plant protein, but not animal protein [6,7]. Thus, there may be differential effects of animal and plant proteins on BP, but the exact relationship is not clear.

Evidence from randomized controlled trials suggests that an increased intake of protein, both from plant and animal sources, may lower BP. In a 6-week randomized 3-period crossover trial of subjects with diagnosed hypertension, substitution of protein for carbohydrate led to a decrease in SBP of 3.5 mmHg [8]. Recently, Hodgson et al. [9] demonstrated that replacing carbohydrate with lean red meat while keeping total calorie and fat intake constant reduced SBP by 1.9 mmHg, but not diastolic BP (DBP). Some peptides in fermented milk have also been shown to lower BP, probably through inhibition of the angiotensin-converting enzyme [10]. In contrast, in the PREMIER clinical trial of lifestyle intervention for BP lowering, dietary plant protein intake was inversely associated with both SBP and DBP in cross-sectional analyses at the 6-month follow-up ($p = .0009$ and $.0126$ for SBP and DPB, respectively) [11]. An increase in plant protein intake from baseline to month 6 was marginally associated with a reduction of both SBP and DBP ($p = .0516$ and $.082$, respectively), independent of the change in body weight. In the PREMIER trial, animal protein was not associated with BP or change in BP. Furthermore, among the PREMIER participants with prehypertension, increased intake of plant protein was significantly associated with a lower risk of developing hypertension at 6 months.

Soy protein has also been hypothesized to reduce BP because it is rich in arginine, a potential vasodilator and a precursor for the vasodilator nitric oxide [12]. The results of numerous randomized controlled trials that supplemented soy protein have been mixed. In a 12-week randomized double-blind controlled trial, He et al. [13] demonstrated a decrease in SBP/DBP of 4.31/2.76 mmHg in the soybean protein-supplemented group as compared to the placebo group. Further, Rivas et al. [14] demonstrated that soymilk supplement significantly reduced SBP by 18.4 mmHg in a 3-month randomized trial. In contrast, three randomized controlled trials [15–17] showed that there was no difference in SBP or DBP between the soybean protein–supplemented group and the placebo group. It should be noted that many intervention trials employ different types or amounts of protein, and the delivery mechanism may differ as well, all of which may contribute to variation in results. Most trials use protein supplements that include soy, plant protein, or animal protein and do not control for other nutrients that may also influence BP. Thus, the BP responses cannot be attributed to protein alone.

Although the exact mechanism(s) linking the amount or type of protein to BP is still unclear, possible explanations exist. First, an increase in protein intake may induce increases in renal plasma flow, renal size, glomerular filtration rate, and sodium excretion rate [4,18,19]. Second, certain amino acids such as arginine and glutamic acid may act as a vasodilator and have independent BP-lowering effects [20,21]. On the contrary, it should be noted that high protein intake might promote renal injury, especially in those with existing kidney diseases, which subsequently increases BP. A recent animal study showed that a high-protein diet increased the number of infiltrating immune cells in the kidneys, which may contribute to increased BP [22]. Further, a very low protein diet, examined during the long-term follow-up of the Modification of Diet in Renal Disease study, did not delay progression to kidney failure but appeared to increase the risk of death [23]. Thus, the ideal amount of protein intake for patients with chronic kidney disease is yet to be defined. Patients with kidney disease should follow protein-intake recommendations prescribed by their physicians.

Even though the overall effect of protein on BP may be beneficial, it is not clear if protein from food and from supplements affect BP similarly. In addition, the existing evidence does not seem to suggest using protein supplements as a dietary approach to treat hypertension. Ensuring an adequate protein intake from natural plant and lean animal sources, which is consistent with the current recommendation of 10%–35% of total calorie intake [24], on the basis of a healthy eating pattern may likely be beneficial for BP control.

1.2.2 DIETARY FAT

Numerous studies have investigated the relationship between dietary fat and BP. However, because of differences in the study design, lack of adequate sample size, and other limitations, the topic remains controversial. Both the total absolute intake of dietary fat and the relative fatty acid composition may independently relate to BP control.

Most observational studies have not found an association between total fat intake and BP [25–29]. Two large studies [28,29], but not others [26,30], show a positive relationship between saturated fatty acids and BP. In addition, Hajjar et al. examined the National Health and Nutrition Examination Survey (NHANES) III data and reported that the south region of the United States, which consumed the highest amounts of monounsaturated and polyunsaturated fats, had the highest SBP and

DBP when compared with other regions [31]. These findings imply that both the quantity and the type of fat intake may affect BP.

As discussed previously in this chapter, any change in the total fat intake often introduces changes in other dietary components as well, leading to the issue of confounding. Thus, BP responses may not be attributed solely to the change in fat intake. Nonetheless, in a crossover randomized study, consumption of a high-fat meal (42-g fat) was found to increase both SBP and DBP significantly more than consumption of a low-fat meal (1-g fat) did [32]. In a 6-month double-blind randomized crossover study on 23 hypertensive individuals, Ferrara et al. [33] found that monounsaturated (extra-virgin olive oil) fat diet significantly reduced SBP and DBP more than polyunsaturated fat (sunflower oil) diet did. In another randomized controlled trial, Appel et al. [8] reported that substituting monounsaturated fats for saturated fats significantly reduced SBP by 2.9 mmHg in a group of 191 participants with prehypertension or stage 1 hypertension. This study suggests that high fat intake (37% energy), mainly provided as monounsaturated fat, in combination with other beneficial dietary factors can lower BP effectively. In other words, this study suggests that a total fat intake contributing to as high as 37% energy may not negatively impact BP if the fat source is monounsaturated.

Fish oil supplement is a topic of much public interest, but the research on its impact on BP is inconclusive. Many short-term intervention trials have been undertaken to determine if supplementation of either fish or fish oil lowers BP. Because of the variations in the research design, participant criteria, dosage and type of the fish oil supplements, and the length of intervention, the results have been inconsistent. Recently, a meta-analysis of randomized controlled trials (36 of which included fish oil) explored the impact of fish oil intake on prevalence of hypertension in five populations (Finland, Italy, the Netherlands, the United Kingdom, and the United States) [34]. Meta-regression of pooled data from these trials showed that 4.1-g supplement of fish oil is associated with 2.1/1.6-mmHg decrease in SBP/DBP (both $p < .01$). Long-term studies are required to confirm the beneficial effects of fish oil on BP. Until such information is available, individuals are encouraged to consume fish as part of a healthy balanced diet rather than taking fish oil supplements for BP control. Even though the evidence that total fat intake and saturated fat intake negatively affect BP is weak, individuals are encouraged to follow the current recommendation for total fat intake (20%–35% of total calorie) and saturated fat intake (<10% of total calorie) for overall health.

1.2.3 DIETARY CARBOHYDRATES

Although not well understood, carbohydrate may contribute to the development of essential hypertension through its glycemic effect. Kopp [35] suggests that consumption of a diet with high glycemic index may create a chronic state of postprandial hyperinsulinemia, sympathetic nervous system overactivity, and vascular remodeling of renal vessels, leading to chronic activation of the renin–angiotensin–aldosterone system and development of essential hypertension. Although logical, available evidence on the relationship between a high-carbohydrate diet and high BP has been controversial and is challenging to interpret. It is possible that both the quantity and quality of carbohydrate will affect BP; however, very few studies have examined either or both aspects specifically. When studying the impact of carbohydrate on BP, simultaneous manipulation of fat, protein, and/or calories may confound interpretation.

Few observational studies have specifically reported the relationship between carbohydrate intake and BP. In a cross-sectional analysis using the NHANES III data, moderate carbohydrate intake (45.1%–50.7% of total energy intake) was associated with a decreased risk for high SBP (≥140 mmHg) after adjustment for potential confounders, that is, total sugar and fiber intake. This finding suggests that the beneficial effect may come only from nonsugar carbohydrates (i.e., complex carbohydrates) [36]. Recently, two cross-sectional studies, using NHANES continuous survey (1999–2004), reported positive associations between consumption of sugary drinks and SBP among adolescents [37,38]. Further, another cross-sectional study also found a positive association between fructose intake from added sugars and the odds of a higher BP in adults without a history of hypertension using NHANES 2003–2006 data [39]. In line with these cross-sectional studies, in a prospective analysis of the 810 PREMIER study participants, we found that reduction of intake of sugary drinks (regular soft drinks, fruit drinks, lemonade, fruit punch, and other sweetened beverages) by one serving per day (12 fluid oz) was associated with an average of 1.8/1.1 mmHg reduction in SBP/DBP (95% CI: 1.2–2.4/0.7–1.4, respectively) [40]. This effect was independent of age, gender, race, family history of hypertension, physical activity, alcohol intake, baseline BMI, and dietary factors such as sodium intake and consumption of the Dietary Approaches to Stop Hypertension (DASH) diet, and it may be attributed to the sugar content of these beverages. For every tablespoon per day of sugar intake, there was an association of an average of 0.60/0.45 mmHg increase in SBP/DBP (95% CI: 0.32–0.87; $p <$ .001 and CI: 0.27–0.63; $p <$ .001, respectively) [40]. In contrast, a prospective study by Forman et al. using data from the Nurses' Health Study I and II and the Health Professional Study [41] found no association between dietary fructose intake and incidence of hypertension. A possible explanation for the discrepancy between these studies could be that a large proportion of fructose intake was from fruits in the Forman's study, and thus high fructose was correlated with high fruit and/ or fiber intake in that study, whereas in the PREMIER study and NHANES study, high intake of fructose was associated with low fruit and fiber intake, both of which may benefit BP control.

Although studies on the relationship between intake of other types of carbohydrate and BP are limited, evidence from a few studies tends to suggest that consumption of whole grain may be protective for hypertension. In the Women's Health Study, high intake of whole grain (≥4 servings/day) was associated with 23% reduced risk of hypertension compared with low intake (<0.5 servings/day) in women [42]. In this study, intake of refined grain was not associated with hypertension. The inverse association between intake of whole grain and risk of developing hypertension was confirmed in men in the Health Professionals Follow-up Study [43]. In contrast to refined grains, whole grains contain bran and germ components, which provide a range of nutrients with potential BP-lowering effects, including potassium, magnesium, and cereal fiber.

Limited research has been designed to specifically examine the impact of the amount of carbohydrate alone on BP, which is likely due to the difficulty in manipulating the amount of carbohydrate without changing the intake of other macronutrients if total energy is to be kept constant. In the context of change in whole dietary pattern, both low and high carbohydrate intakes in combination with other dietary changes have been associated with BP lowering [8,44–46]. In a meta-analysis of 10 intervention studies that compared high-carbohydrate diets and high–monounsaturated fat diets isocalorically and kept study participants' weight stable during the interventions, it was found that the high-carbohydrate diet resulted in slightly higher SBP/DBP (2.6/1.8 mmHg) compared with the diet rich in monounsaturated fat [47]. The magnitude of difference in BP between the two diets is small and thus may not justify a public health recommendation of altering dietary carbohydrate and monounsaturated fat content to manage BP.

Although it has been well documented that diets high in glucose, fructose, or sucrose can induce hypertension in animal models [48–50], studies in humans regarding the effects of different types of carbohydrates on BP are limited in number and inconsistent in results. In the following section, we discuss the acute effects of different carbohydrates on BP separately, since acute and chronic effects may involve different mechanisms. In a randomized crossover study among 20 healthy nonhypertensive men [51], SBP rose significantly (9–10 mmHg) 1 hour after ingestion of glucose or sucrose solution (22% weight per volume). This acute BP-elevating effect lasted for 2 hours but did not affect DBP and was not observed from ingestion of fructose. Interestingly, in a recent study with the same design and in a similar population (15 healthy young men and women), ingestion of a fructose drink (500 ml, 60 g), but not glucose, significantly increased both SBP and DBP within 2 hours [52]. However, in an experiment conducted by Jansen et al., BP did not change after ingestion of fructose load (75 g, 300 ml) and even decreased after ingestion of the same amount of glucose load in elderly hypertensive and nonhypertensive individuals [53]. Two possible pathways have been proposed for the acute BP effect of sugar: one is through enhancing activity of the sympathetic nervous system and the other is through modifying sodium balance [54,55].

Effects of sugar on BP in interventions lasting from days to months are also mixed. In a study on patients with coronary artery disease, both SBP and DBP decreased after 4 days of a sucrose and fructose load (4 g/kg/day), but not glucose load [56]. However, this result likely does not reflect the effect of sugar alone since the study participants also lost weight (0.2–1.7 lbs) during the interventions. In another study designed to compare the metabolic effect between hypocaloric low-fat, high-sucrose diets and low-fat, low-sucrose diets (percent of energy from protein, fat, and carbohydrate are comparable in the two diets) in a group of overweight women, BP was not changed over 6 weeks and did not differ between low- and high-sucrose diets [57]. Again, since weight loss occurred during the intervention, the effects of sugar intake and weight loss on BP are not distinguishable. In a 5-week crossover study that examined the metabolic effects of high- or low-fructose diets with stable body weight [58], DBP was not affected by the diet type, but SBP was 4% greater when the participants consumed 0% fructose (starch diet) than when the participants consumed either of the high- or low-fructose diets (5% or 10% energy from fructose).

Thus, further research is needed to clarify the acute effect of the types of sugars on BP. Even though it is plausible that long-term high-sugar consumption may impact BP by promoting insulin resistance and/or hyperinsulinemia, the evidence for an effect is inconclusive, and the mechanisms are unclear [49].

Overall, we cannot conclude from existing data if the amount of carbohydrate alone or the type of carbohydrate affects BP. Future research designed specifically to examine these questions is needed to help clarify the role of carbohydrate on altering BP. However, the evidence for consuming whole grains for lowering BP and improving heart health is strong. In addition, individuals are encouraged to reduce the intake of simple sugars and to select whole grains for at least half of the total carbohydrate intake as often as possible for achieving weight control and maintaining overall health.

1.2.4 DIETARY FIBER

Dietary fiber is a special type of carbohydrate that is resistant to hydrolysis by the digestive enzymes of humans. It has been referred to as "nonstarch polysaccharides" and may indirectly lower BP through reduction of insulin levels, since hyperinsulinemia is often associated with obesity and impaired glucose tolerance, and it may be in the causal pathway to hypertension [59].

Both cross-sectional [26,59,60] and prospective analyses [61] have demonstrated inverse associations between fiber and BP; however, they have also noted a high correlation of fiber with other nutrients that can affect BP in a beneficial manner. In a prospective study on 12,741 participants followed for 8 years, the highest quintile of total dietary fiber and nonsoluble dietary fiber intakes was associated with 11.6% lower risk of hypertension as compared with the lowest quintile [62]. Among the few intervention studies that examined the effect of fiber on BP, most added cereal fiber to the diet. These studies suggest that an average supplementation of 14 g of fiber reduces SBP/DBP by about 1.6/2.0 mmHg, respectively [59]. Similarly, a meta-analysis of 25 randomized controlled trials between 1966 and 2003 demonstrates that an average of 11.5 g per day fiber supplementation leads to a reduction of BP by 1.13/1.26 mmHg (95% CI: −2.49 to 0.23/−2.04 to −0.48) [63].

Thus, available evidence suggests a consistent but small benefit of fiber intake on BP. Individuals should be encouraged to increase fiber intake to the currently recommended level (25 g/day for women and 38 g/day for men) not only for BP control but possibly for other benefits to cardiovascular health. This recommendation should be achieved by increasing fiber-rich fruits, vegetables, whole grains, and nuts/seeds/legumes based on the foundation of a healthy eating pattern, rather than using a supplement.

1.2.5 ALCOHOL

The exact mechanism through which alcohol can raise BP is not clear, but possibilities include stimulation of the sympathetic nervous system, inhibition of vascular relaxing substances, calcium or magnesium depletion, and increase of intracellular calcium in vascular smooth muscle [64–66].

While acute alcohol intake has vasodilatory effects, it is clear from observational studies that excessive, habitual alcohol consumption is associated with higher BP and higher prevalence of hypertension [65]. In addition, men who discontinue alcohol intake experience less age-related increase in BP than those who do not [67]. Men who consume ≥3 drinks per day [68] and women who consume ≥2 drinks per day [69] are at higher risk, but consumption below this level is not associated with increased risk of hypertension. There is no consistent relationship between BP and the type of alcohol consumed.

Fuchs et al. examined incident hypertension among 8334 participants of the Atherosclerosis Risk in Communities cohort study [70]. Participants were free of hypertension at baseline and were followed for 6 years. The risk of incident hypertension was increased by 20% (95% CI: 0.85–1.67) to 131% (95% CI: 1.11–4.86) in those who consumed greater than or equal to 210 g of alcohol (about 78-oz wine, 191-oz beer, or 21-oz liquor or 14–16 drinks) per week as compared to that in those who did not consume alcohol.

The relatively few intervention studies on alcohol and BP have tended to be small and of short duration. In nine of the ten studies examined in a review, SBP was significantly reduced after a reduction of 1–6 alcoholic beverages per day [64]. The Prevention and Treatment of Hypertension Study (PATHS) [71] was designed to evaluate the long-term BP-lowering effect of reducing alcohol consumption in nondependent moderate drinkers (those who consumed >3 drinks/day). The goal of intervention was either two or fewer drinks daily or a 50% reduction in intake (whichever was less). After 6 months, the intervention group experienced 1.2/0.7 mmHg greater reduction in BP than the control group did (NS), and this reduction was more modest among hypertensive individuals. In this study, the intervention group reduced their intake by 2 alcoholic drinks per day, but the control group also lowered their alcohol intake during the intervention so that the difference in intake between the groups was only 1.3 drinks per day. This small difference between the two groups may have limited the interpretation of the true effect of the intervention on BP. In addition, perhaps a greater reduction in alcohol consumption is necessary to see a significant effect on BP. Nevertheless, reduction from an average of 4.4 drinks per day to an average of 2.0 drinks per day appears realistic in moderate alcohol drinkers and is similar to the absolute reduction achieved in an earlier study [72].

In another study [73] of mainly heavier drinkers (>5 drinks/day), replacing alcohol with low-alcohol substitutes resulted in a reduction of approximately 5 drinks per week and a greater reduction in BP (−4.8/3.3 mmHg; both $p < .01$). Importantly, participants of this intervention also reduced body weight by an average of 2.1 kg, which may explain the larger BP reduction than that observed in the PATHS trial. However, in a meta-analysis [74] of 15 randomized controlled trials including a total of 2234 participants who drank an average of 3–6 drinks per day at baseline, reducing alcohol by 29%–100% from baseline was associated with a significant mean BP reduction of 3.31/2.04 mmHg (95% CI: −2.52 to −4.10/−1.49 to −2.58), while the body weight was minimally changed (mean change = −0.56 kg, NS). There was a dose–response relationship between the mean percentage of alcohol reduction and mean percentage of BP reduction.

Thus, limiting the alcohol consumption to the current recommendation of ≤2 drinks per day for men and ≤1 drink for women is supported by most of the research evidences and will likely improve BP control. Since moderate alcohol consumption (as compared to no alcohol intake) may benefit by reduction of the overall risk of cardiovascular disease (CVD), there is no strong evidence to recommend total abstinence [75,76].

1.3 DIETARY PATTERNS AND BP

The previous sections highlight the potential of individual macronutrients or foods/beverages that affect BP, but extensive confounding clouds the interpretation of studies targeting a single nutrient or food/beverage. It is difficult to control and study one component of the diet without affecting others. Thus, it may be more appropriate to focus on dietary patterns in which multiple nutrients naturally change together rather than focusing on individual macronutrients, and indeed there is extensive evidence that dietary patterns affect BP. In the following sections, we review several major dietary patterns that have been studied relatively extensively in relationship to BP.

1.3.1 VEGETARIAN DIETARY PATTERN

Vegetarian groups in the United States and other countries have been observed to have lower BP compared with their nonvegetarian counterparts in many [77,78], but not all, studies [79]. The term "vegetarian" comprises several heterogeneous groups [80], but in general, the diet tends to be high in whole grains, beans, vegetables, and sometimes fish, dairy products, eggs, and fruits [78]. Aspects of the vegetarian diet that have been suggested to benefit BP control include intake of ample amount of plant foods; low intake of animal products [78]; high intake of potassium, magnesium, fiber, and (sometimes) calcium [80,81]; high polyunsaturated fat–saturated fat ratio; and, often, low intake of sodium. However, as outlined previously, studies on individual nutrients often have shown inconsistent results. Explanations for such inconsistencies may include the following: (1) the effect of individual nutrients may be too small to be detected, particularly when trials do not contain sufficient sample size and thus statistical power; (2) most intervention studies employed supplements of nutrients that may function differently compared with nutrients naturally occurring in foods; (3) other dietary factors in foods, which are not hypothesized to affect BP, may also have an impact on BP; and (4) nutrients occurring in foods simultaneously may exert synergistic or antagonistic effects on BP. Differences in physical activity, stress, alcohol consumption, and other unmeasured factors may also contribute to a lower BP among vegetarians. But when research participants were counseled to follow the vegetarian diet pattern in intervention studies, significant reductions in BP in both nonhypertensive [82] and mildly hypertensive [81] participants were reported.

Despite the clear BP-lowering effect of a vegetarian diet, it is not realistic to expect a wide-scale adoption of such a dietary pattern. In addition, vegetarian diet does not include all dietary factors associated with lowering of BP. Thus, the DASH multicenter trials were designed to test the impact of nonvegetarian whole dietary patterns on BP while simultaneously controlling for multiple nutrients and body weight [83,84].

1.3.2 THE DASH DIETARY PATTERN

The original DASH trial [44] was an 11-week randomized controlled feeding trial of 459 individuals with prehypertension or unmedicated stage-1 hypertension. Three dietary patterns varying in amounts of fruits, vegetables, dairy products, meats, sweets, and nuts and seeds, and thus fats, cholesterol, fiber, calcium, potassium, and magnesium were tested (Table 1.1). In brief, the three dietary patterns tested in the

TABLE 1.1

Nutrient Target and the Associated Food Group Servings for the Three Dietary Patterns Tested in the DASH Trial

Item	Control Diet Nutrient Target	Fruits-and-Vegetables Diet Nutrient Target	DASH Diet Nutrient Target
Nutrients			
Fat (% kcal)	37	37	27
Saturated	16	16	6
Monounsaturated	13	13	13
Polyunsaturated	8	8	8
Carbohydrates (% kcal)	48	48	55
Protein (% kcal)	15	15	18
Cholesterol (mg/day)	300	300	150
Fiber (g/day)	9	31	31
Potassium (mg/day)	1700	4700	4700
Magnesium (mg/day)	165	500	500
Calcium (mg/day)	450	450	1240
Sodium (mg/day)	3000	3000	3000
Food groups (servings/day)			
Fruits and juices	1.6	5.2	5.2
Vegetables	2.0	3.3	4.4
Grains	8.2	6.9	7.5
Low-fat dairy	0.1	0.0	2.0
Regular-fat dairy	0.4	0.3	0.7
Nuts, seeds, and legumes	0.0	0.6	0.7
Beef, pork, and ham	1.5	1.8	0.5
Poultry	0.8	0.4	0.6
Fish	0.2	0.3	0.5
Fat, oils, and salad dressing	5.8	5.3	2.5
Snacks and sweets	4.1	1.4	0.7

study included (1) the control diet that mimicked what most Americans were consuming at the time of the trial, which was relatively high in total fats, saturated fats, and cholesterol and low in fruits, vegetables, and dairy products; (2) the "fruits-and-vegetables" diet, which contained a similar macronutrient profile as that of the control diet except for a higher amount of fruits and vegetables; and (3) the "DASH dietary pattern," which was higher in fruits, vegetables, and low-fat dairy products; lower in total fats, saturated fats, and cholesterol; and rich in fiber, potassium, magnesium, and calcium. In all three treatment groups, body weight and alcohol consumption were kept constant, and the level of sodium intake was similar to typical American intake (3000 mg/2000 kcal/day).

After 8 weeks of intervention, the DASH dietary pattern reduced BP by 5.5/3.0 mmHg more than the control group (for both SBP and DBP, $p < .001$). The fruits-and-vegetables diet reduced BP by 2.8/1.1 mmHg more than the control diet ($p < .001$ for SBP and $p = .07$ for DBP). The reductions in BP were significant after the participants consumed the diets for 2 weeks and sustained them for the following 6 weeks. These reductions occurred while body weight, alcohol consumption, and exercise patterns remained stable, and when there was no restriction in sodium intake. BP lowering with DASH was equally effective in men and women and in younger and older persons, and it was particularly effective among African Americans and those with stage-1 hypertension at baseline. Among the 133 participants with hypertension at baseline (SBP $\geq$ 140 mmHg and/or DBP $\geq$ 90 mmHg), the DASH dietary pattern lowered BP by 11.4/5.5 mmHg. These effects observed in the hypertensive participants are similar to reductions seen with single-drug therapy [85] and are more effective than most of the other lifestyle modifications for BP reduction [86]. Among African Americans with hypertension, DASH lowered BP by an average of 13.2/6.1 mmHg (95% CI: −18.2 to −8.1/−9.1 to −3.1).

Even though the DASH trial was not designed to identify specific nutrient(s) responsible for the BP-lowering effect, data from the fruits-and-vegetables diet group support the hypothesis that increasing potassium, magnesium, and dietary fiber intake reduces BP. However, these nutrients do not account for the entire DASH effect. By further lowering total fat, saturated fat, and cholesterol and by increasing low-fat dairy products, BP reduction was nearly double with the DASH dietary pattern compared with the fruits-and-vegetables diet. Since whole food items, rather than single nutrients, were manipulated in this trial, other nutrients that were not controlled for in the study and other beneficial factors as yet unrecognized may also have contributed to the BP responses. Further research is needed to analyze the specific nutrients or factors responsible for the effect on BP. More details on the DASH dietary pattern can be found on the National Heart, Lung, and Blood Institute's Web site: http://www.nhlbi.nih.gov/hbp/prevent/h_eating/h_eating.htm

Other feeding studies have confirmed the BP-lowering effect of the DASH dietary pattern [45,87]. In the DASH-Sodium study on 412 participants [45], reduction in sodium intake from high (3.3 g/day) to intermediate (2.5 g/day) while consuming the DASH diet further reduced SBP/DBP by 1.3/0.6 mmHg (95% CI: −2.6 to 0.0 and −1.5 to 0.2, respectively). Reducing sodium from the intermediate level (2.5 g/day) to low (1.5 g/day) level when consuming the DASH diet further decreased SBP/DBP by 1.7/1.0 mmHg (95% CI: −3.0 to −0.4 and −1.9 to −0.1, respectively). This study showed that combining sodium reduction and adopting the DASH diet yielded the greatest benefit with respect to BP. In another smaller trial of 55 participants with essential hypertension [87], the BP-lowering effect of the DASH diet was reconfirmed, and it was found that the DASH diet enhanced the ambulatory BP response to losartan significantly (–11.7/–6.9 mmHg, $p < .05$). In addition, other trials have confirmed the feasibility of individuals adopting this dietary pattern on their own [88,89]. Several behavioral intervention trials ranging from 18 months to 3 years have also examined the implementation of the DASH dietary pattern and shown the feasibility of adopting this eating pattern [86–88]. In these trials, behavioral lifestyle interventions that were designed to implement the DASH dietary pattern resulted in increased intake of fruits, vegetables, dairy products, and many vitamins and minerals; weight loss; and reduction in BP. Resources to facilitate implementation of the DASH dietary pattern are included at the end of this book.

1.3.3 Variation of DASH Dietary Pattern—OmniHeart Study

Even though the DASH trial provided strong evidence of the efficacy of the DASH dietary pattern in reducing BP, this trial alone was not able to test all hypotheses related to dietary pattern and BP. As discussed in the previous sections, research suggests that high intake of unsaturated fat and protein may benefit BP control. Thus, the OmniHeart study [8] was designed to further understand the impact of macronutrient variations of the DASH dietary pattern on BP, while keeping fiber, potassium, magnesium, calcium, and sodium constant (Table 1.2). The dietary patterns tested were (1) carbohydrate diet in which protein energy was reduced from 18% in the original DASH dietary pattern to 15% kcal, (2) the unsaturated diet in which 10% of the carbohydrate energy in the DASH dietary pattern was replaced with energy from

TABLE 1.2

Comparison of the Macronutrient Profiles of the Three Dietary Patterns Tested in the OmniHeart Study with the DASH Dietary Pattern

Item	DASH Diet Nutrient Target	Carbohydrate Diet Nutrient Target	Protein Diet Nutrient Target	Unsaturated Fat Diet Nutrient Target
Nutrients				
Fat (% kcal)	27	27	27	37
Saturated	6	6	6	6
Monounsaturated	13	13	13	21
Polyunsaturated	8	8	8	10
Carbohydrates (% kcal)	55	58	48	48
Protein (% kcal)	18	15	25	15
Cholesterol (mg/day)	150	140	140	140
Fiber (g/day)	31	30	30	30

mainly monounsaturated fats, and (3) the protein diet in which 10% of the carbohydrate energy in the DASH dietary pattern was replaced with energy from protein. A total of 164 adults with prehypertension or unmedicated stage-1 hypertension were randomized into the three diet groups in a crossover fashion for 6 weeks each. All three diets lowered BP significantly, but the protein and unsaturated fat diets significantly reduced SBP by 1.4 and 1.3 mmHg more than the carbohydrate diet did. Further reductions in BP were even greater among those who were hypertensive at baseline. In addition, the protein diet significantly reduced low-density lipoprotein cholesterol by 3.3 mg/dL (0.09 mmol/L; $p = .01$), high-density lipoprotein cholesterol by 1.3 mg/dL (0.03 mmol/L; $p = .02$), and triglycerides by 15.7 mg/dL (0.18 mmol/L; $p < .001$). The unsaturated fat diet had no significant effect on low-density lipoprotein cholesterol, but it increased high-density lipoprotein cholesterol by 1.1 mg/dL (0.03 mmol/L; $p = .03$) and lowered triglycerides by 9.6 mg/dL (0.11 mmol/L; $p = .02$).

Overall, these studies have vigorously and consistently proven that whole dietary patterns such as the DASH dietary pattern or the two modified DASH patterns in the OmniHeart study are effective strategies for BP control. In addition, both the DASH and the OmniHeart studies demonstrate that the benefits of adopting a whole dietary approach extend beyond BP to other health indicators such as lipids [8]. A nutritional approach to BP control that involves changes in overall dietary pattern appears to be superior to approaches that manipulate only a small number of nutritional factors. Thus, the DASH dietary pattern is recommended by many national and international organizations including the National Institute of Health (it is included in the seventh report of the Joint National Committee on Prevention, Detection, Evaluation, and Treatment of High Blood Pressure—JNC7) [90], the American Heart Association [91], the American Dietetic Association [92], the Canadian Hypertension Education Program [93], and the British Hypertension Society [94]. It is also recommended by the 2010 Dietary Guidelines for Americans [95].

1.3.4 THE MEDITERRANEAN DIET

The Mediterranean diet, which is characterized by high intake of fruits, vegetables, legumes, nuts, cereals, fish, and olive oil, is another dietary pattern that has been shown to benefit BP control and reduction of overall risk of CVD. Adherence to the Mediterranean diet has been associated with a reduced risk of CVD and mortality [96,97]. In a large prospective cohort that included 9408 men and women enrolled in the Seguimiento Universidad de Navarra Study, high adherence to the Mediterranean diet was associated with a moderate, but significant, reduction of 3.1/1.9 mmHg in SBP/DBP (95% CI: −5.4 to −0.8/−3.6 to −0.1) during a median follow-up of 4.2 years, independent of known risk factors for high BP [98]. In a recent randomized controlled trial that compared the Mediterranean diet versus low-fat diet (not particularly designed to meet the features of the Mediterranean diet) on coronary heart disease (CHD) risk factors among 772 asymptomatic, but at high cardiovascular risk, individuals, the Mediterranean diet supplemented with either olive oil (1 L/week) or nuts (30 g/week) resulted in a lower mean SBP than the low-fat diet did (−5.9 mmHg in the olive oil group and −7.1 mmHg in the nuts group) at 3 months [99]. This finding is consistent with that of the DASH and OmniHeart trials in suggesting that a plant-based dietary pattern that includes fruits, vegetables, and healthy oils benefits BP control.

1.4 SUMMARY

The evidence that diet modification involving macronutrients and/or a whole dietary pattern can prevent and treat hypertension is strong, and recommendations are summarized in Table 1.3. For some macronutrients, the effective intervention strategy and mechanisms involved are still being clarified. Owing to various design limitations, inadequate statistical power, and measurement issues, studies on single nutrients generally provided inconsistent results. However, when multiple nutrients or dietary factors are combined in a whole dietary strategy, as seen in the DASH and OmniHeart studies, BP is significantly and effectively reduced. Nutrients may have additive or interactive effects when provided together in whole foods. Thus, the current national guideline of lifestyle modification for BP control includes the DASH pattern, sodium reduction, weight loss, increased physical activity, and moderation of alcohol consumption. Concurrent adherence to several recommendations is likely to hold the greatest

---

TABLE 1.3
Summary: Take-Home Messages

Key Evidences	Recommendation for Health Care Providers
• Moderately strong evidence shows that intake of protein, particularly from plant or soy sources, may benefit BP control.	• Encourage adoption of dietary patterns similar to vegetarian, DASH, modified DASH, or Mediterranean patterns.
• There is weak evidence that total and saturated fats may be negatively associated with BP, while monounsaturated fat may benefit BP control.	• Increase intake of fruits, vegetables, whole grains, lean proteins, and nonfat dairy.
• The evidence for the impact of the amount and type of carbohydrate on BP is weak; however, the evidence that whole grains may benefit BP control and improve heart's health is moderately strong.	• Reduce intake of total and saturated fats. • Follow moderate alcohol consumption to less than 2 drinks per day for men and 1 drink per day for women.
• Moderately strong evidence shows that dietary fiber has a small but significant beneficial impact on BP.	
• Excessive alcohol is associated with higher BP, and there may be a dose–response relationship between lowering alcohol and BP reduction.	
• Dietary patterns, including the vegetarian, DASH, modified DASH, and Mediterranean, have all been shown to benefit BP control effectively. Some common features of these dietary patterns include intake of high amounts of fruits and vegetables, moderate amounts of animal products, low amounts of saturated fat, and high amounts of fiber, potassium, magnesium, and calcium.	

promise for preventing and treating hypertension and has been shown to be feasible [88,100,101]. Future research should focus on strategies to motivate and maintain lifestyle changes for BP control. At both the population and individual levels, success in dietary and lifestyle intervention relies on multiple levels of support ranging from clinicians to government agencies to private institutes and the food and beverage industry. In particular, partnering with the food industry to improve the nutritional quality of the food supply, such as reducing sodium and fat content of processed foods, making fruits and vegetables available and affordable, and promoting foods and nutrients consistent with the DASH dietary pattern, will play a critical role in implementing dietary and lifestyle modifications. Consistent efforts to educate and promote adherence to dietary and lifestyle guidelines by dietitians and other health care professionals are also instrumental to the prevention and management of hypertension.

REFERENCES

1. Birkett NJ. Comments on a meta-analysis of the relation between dietary calcium intake and blood pressure. *Am J Epidemiol.* 1998;148(3):223–228.
2. Stoto MA. Invited commentary on meta-analysis of epidemiologic data: The case of calcium intake and blood pressure. *Am J Epidemiol.* 1998;148(3):229–230.
3. Obarzanek E, Velletri PA, Cutler JA. Dietary protein and blood pressure. *JAMA.* 1996;275(20):1598–1603.
4. Yamori Y, Kihara M, Nara Y, et al. Hypertension and diet: Multiple regression analysis in a Japanese farming community. *Lancet.* 1981;1(8231):1204–1205.
5. Zhou B, Zhang X, Zhu A, et al. The relationship of dietary animal protein and electrolytes to blood pressure: A study on three Chinese populations. *Int J Epidemiol.* 1994;23(4):716–722.
6. Stamler J, Caggiula AW, Grandits GA. Relation of body mass and alcohol, nutrient, fiber, and caffeine intakes to blood pressure in the special intervention and usual care groups in the Multiple Risk Factor Intervention Trial. *Am J Clin Nutr.* 1997;65(1 Suppl):338S-365S.
7. Stamler J, Liu K, Ruth KJ, Pryer J, Greenland P. Eight-year blood pressure change in middle-aged men: Relationship to multiple nutrients. *Hypertension.* 2002;39(5):1000–1006.
8. Appel LJ, Sacks FM, Carey VJ, et al. Effects of protein, monounsaturated fat, and carbohydrate intake on blood pressure and serum lipids: Results of the OmniHeart randomized trial. *J Am Med Assoc.* 2005;294(19):2455–2464.
9. Hodgson JM, Burke V, Beilin LJ, Puddey IB. Partial substitution of carbohydrate intake with protein intake from lean red meat lowers blood pressure in hypertensive persons. *Am J Clin Nutr.* 2006;83(4):780–787.
10. Jauhiainen T, Korpela R. Milk peptides and blood pressure. *J Nutr.* Mar 2007;137(3 Suppl 2):825S–829S.
11. Wang YF, Yancy WS Jr., Yu D, Champagne C, Appel LJ, Lin PH. The relationship between dietary protein intake and blood pressure: Results from the PREMIER study. *J Hum Hypertens.* 2008;22(11):745–754.
12. Moncada S, Higgs A. The L-arginine-nitric oxide pathway. *N Engl J Med.* 1993;329:2002–2012.
13. He J, Gu D, Wu X, Chen J, Duan X, Whelton PK. Effect of soybean protein on blood pressure: A randomized, controlled trial. *Ann Intern Med.* 2005;143(1):1–9.
14. Rivas M, Garay RP, Escanero JF, Cia P Jr., Cia P, Alda JO. Soy milk lowers blood pressure in men and women with mild to moderate essential hypertension. *J Nutr.* 2002;132(7):1900–1902.

15. Kreijkamp-Kaspers S, Kok L, Bots ML, Grobbee DE, Lampe JW, van der Schouw YT. Randomized controlled trial of the effects of soy protein containing isoflavones on vascular function in postmenopausal women. *Am J Clin Nutr.* 2005;81(1):189–195.

16. Sagara M, Kanda T, Jelekera N, et al. Effects of dietary intake of soy protein and isoflavones on cardiovascular disease risk factors in high risk, middle-aged men in Scotland. *J Am Coll Nutr.* 2004;23(1):85–91.

17. Teede HJ, Dalais FS, Kotsopoulos D, Liang YL, Davis S, McGrath BP. Dietary soy has both beneficial and potentially adverse cardiovascular effects: A placebo-controlled study in men and postmenopausal women. *J Clin Endocrinol Metab.* 2001;86(7):3053–3060.

18. He J, Klag MJ, Whelton PK, Chen JY, Qian MC, He GQ. He J, Klag MJ, Whelton PK, Chen JY, Qian MC, He GQ. Dietary macronutrients and blood pressure in southwestern China. *J Hypertens.* 1995;13(11):1267–1274.

19. Henderson DG, Schierup J, Schodt T. Effect of magnesium supplementation on blood pressure and electrolyte concentrations in hypertensive patients receiving long term diuretic treatment. *BMJ.* 1986;293:664–665.

20. Palloshi A, Fragasso G, Piatti P, et al. Effect of oral L-arginine on blood pressure and symptoms and endothelial function in patients with systemic hypertension, positive exercise tests, and normal coronary arteries. *Am J Cardiol.* 2004;93(7):933–935.

21. Stamler J, Brown IJ, Daviglus ML, et al. Glutamic acid, the main dietary amino acid, and blood pressure: The INTERMAP Study (International Collaborative Study of Macronutrients, Micronutrients and Blood Pressure). *Circulation.* 2009;120(3):221–228.

22. De Miguel C, Lund H, Mattson DL. High dietary protein exacerbates hypertension and renal damage in Dahl SS rats by increasing infiltrating immune cells in the kidney. *Hypertension.* 2011;57(2):269–274.

23. Menon V, Kopple JD, Wang X, et al. Effect of a very low-protein diet on outcomes: Long-term follow-up of the modification of diet in renal disease (MDRD) study. *Am J Kidney Dis.* 2009;53(2):208–217.

24. Food and Nutrition Board, Institute of Medicine. Dietary reference intakes for energy, carbohydrate, fiber, fat, fatty acids, cholesterol, protein, and amino acids. Washington, DC: National Academy Press; 2002.

25. Elliott P, Fehily AM, Sweetnam PM, Yarnell JWG. Diet, alcohol, body mass, and social factors in relation to blood pressure: The Caerphilly heart study. *J Epidemiol Community Health.* 1987;41:37–43.

26. Reed D, McGee D, Yano K, Hankin J. Diet, blood pressure, and multicollinearity. *Hypertension.* 1985;7:405–410.

27. Salonen J, Tuomilehto J, Tanskanen A. Relation of blood pressure to reported intake of salt, saturated fats, and alcohol in healthy middle-aged population. *J Epidemiol Community Health.* 1983;37:32–37.

28. Salonen JT, Salonen R, Ihanainen M, et al. Blood pressure, dietary fats, and antioxidants. *Am J Clin Nutr.* 1988;48:1226–1232.

29. Stamler J, Caggiula A, Grandits GA, Kjelsberg M, Cutler JA. Relationship to blood pressure of combinations of dietary macronutrients. Findings of the Multiple Risk Factor Intervention Trial (MRFIT). *Circulation.* 1996;94(10):2417–2423.

30. Gruchow HW, Sobocinski KA, Barboriak JJ. Alcohol, nutrient intake and hypertension in U.S. adults. *JAMA.* 1985;253:1567–1570.

31. Hajjar I, Kotchen TA. Trends in prevalence, awareness, treatment, and control of hypertension in the United States, 1988–2000. *JAMA.* 2003;2003/07/10(2):199–206.

32. Jakulj F, Zernicke K, Bacon SL, et al. A high-fat meal increases cardiovascular reactivity to psychological stress in healthy young adults. *J Nutr.* 2007;137(4):935–939.

33. Ferrara A, Raimondi AS, d'Episcopo L, Guida L, dello Russo A, Marotta T. Olive oil and reduced need for antihypertensive medications. *Arch Int Med.* 2000;160(6):837–842.

34. Geleijnse JM, Kok FJ, Grobbee DE. Blood pressure response to changes in sodium and potassium intake: A metaregression analysis of randomised trials. *J Hum Hypertens.* 2003;17(7):471–480.

35. Kopp W. Pathogenesis and etiology of essential hypertension: Role of dietary carbohydrate. *Med Hypotheses.* 2005;64(4):782–787.

36. Yang EJ, Chung HK, Kim WY, Kerver JM, Song WO. Carbohydrate intake is associated with diet quality and risk factors for cardiovascular disease in U.S. adults: NHANES III. *J Am Coll Nutr.* 2003;22(1):71–79.

37. Bremer AA, Auinger P, Byrd RS. Relationship between insulin resistance-associated metabolic parameters and anthropometric measurements with sugar-sweetened beverage intake and physical activity levels in US adolescents: Findings from the 1999–2004 National Health and Nutrition Examination Survey. *Arch Pediatr Adolesc Med.* 2009;163(4):328–335.

38. Nguyen S, Choi HK, Lustig RH, Hsu CY. Sugar-sweetened beverages, serum uric acid, and blood pressure in adolescents. *J Pediatr.* 2009;154(6):807–813.

39. Jalal DI, Smits G, Johnson RJ, Chonchol M. Increased fructose associates with elevated blood pressure. *J Am Soc Nephrol.* 2010.

40. Chen L, Caballero B, Mitchell DC, et al. Reducing consumption of sugar-sweetened beverages is associated with reduced blood pressure: A prospective study among United States adults. *Circulation.* 2010;121(22):2398–2406.

41. Forman JP, Choi H, Curhan GC. Fructose and vitamin C intake do not influence risk for developing hypertension. *J Am Soc Nephrol.* 2009;20(4):863–871.

42. Wang L, Gaziano JM, Liu S, Manson JE, Buring JE, Sesso HD. Whole- and refined-grain intakes and the risk of hypertension in women. *Am J Clin Nutr.* 2007;86(2):472–479.

43. Flint AJ, Hu FB, Glynn RJ, et al. Whole grains and incident hypertension in men. *Am J Clin Nutr.* 2009;90(3):493–498.

44. Appel LJ, Moore TJ, Obarzanek E, et al. A clinical trial of the effects of dietary patterns on blood pressure. *N Engl J Med.* 1997;336:1117–1124.

45. Sacks FM, Svetkey LP, Vollmer WM, et al. Effects on blood pressure of reduced dietary sodium and the Dietary Approaches to Stop Hypertension (DASH) diet. DASH-sodium collaborative research group. *N Engl J Med.* 2001;344(1):3–10.

46. Wood RJ, Fernandez ML, Sharman MJ, et al. Effects of a carbohydrate-restricted diet with and without supplemental soluble fiber on plasma low-density lipoprotein cholesterol and other clinical markers of cardiovascular risk. *Metabolism.* 2007;56(1):58–67.

47. Shah M, Adams-Huet B, Garg A. Effect of high-carbohydrate or high-cis-monounsaturated fat diets on blood pressure: A meta-analysis of intervention trials. *Am J Clin Nutr.* 2007;85(5):1251–1256.

48. Hwang IS, Ho H, Hoffman BB, Reaven GM. Fructose-induced insulin resistance and hypertension in rats. *Hypertension.* 1987;10(5):512–516.

49. Preuss HG, Zein M, MacArthy P, Dipette D, Sabnis S, Knapka J. Sugar-induced blood pressure elevations over the lifespan of three substrains of Wistar rats. *J Am Coll Nutr.* 1998;17(1):36–47.

50. Reaven GM, Ho H. Sugar-induced hypertension in Sprague-Dawley rats. *Am J Hypertens.* 1991;4(7 Pt 1):610–614.

51. Hodges RE, Rebello T. Carbohydrates and blood pressure. *Ann Intern Med.* 1983;98(Part 2):838–841.

52. Brown CM, Dulloo AG, Yepuri G, Montani JP. Fructose ingestion acutely elevates blood pressure in healthy young humans. *Am J Physiol Regul Integr Comp Physiol.* 2008;294(3):R730–R737.

53. Jansen R, Penterman B, Van Lier H, Hoefnagels W. Blood pressure reduction after oral glucose loading and its relation to age, blood pressure and insulin. *Am J Cardiol.* 1987;60:1087–1091

54. Rebello T, Hodges RE, Smith JL. Short-term effects of various sugars on antinatri-uresis and blood pressure changes in normotensive young men. *Am J Clin Nutr.* 1983;38(1):84–94.

55. Rowe JW, Young JB, Minaker KL, Stevens AL, Pallotta J, Landsberg L. Effect of insulin and glucose infusions on sympathetic nervous system activity in normal man. *Diabetes.* 1981;30(3):219–225.

56. Palumbo PJ, Briones ER, Nelson RA, Kottke BA. Sucrose sensitivity of patients with coronary-artery disease. *Am J Clin Nutr.* 1977;30:394–401.

57. Surwit RS, Feinglos MN, McCaskill CC, et al. Metabolic and behavioral effects of a high-sucrose diet during weight loss. *Am J Clin Nutr.* 1997;65:908–915.

58. Hallfrisch J, Reiser S, Prather ES. Blood lipid distribution of hyperinsulinemic men consuming three levels of fructose. *Am J Clin Nutr.* 1983;37:740–748.

59. He J, Whelton PK. Effect of dietary fiber and protein intake on blood pressure: A review of epidemiologic evidence. *Clin Exp Hypertens.* 1999;21(5–6):785–796.

60. Ascerio A, Stampfer MJ, Colditz GA, Willett WC, McKinlay J. Nutrient intakes and blood pressure in normotensive males. *Int J Epidemiol.* 1991;20(4):886–891.

61. Ascherio A, Rimm E, Giovannucci EL, et al. A prospective study of nutritional factors and hypertension among U.S. men. *Circulation.* 1992;86:1475–1484.

62. Lairon D, Arnault N, Bertrais S, et al. Dietary fiber intake and risk factors for cardiovas-cular disease in French adults. *Am J Clin Nutr.* 2005;82(6):1185–1194.

63. Streppel MT, Arends LR, van 't Veer P, Grobbee DE, Geleijnse JM. Dietary fiber and blood pressure: A meta-analysis of randomized placebo-controlled trials. *Arch Intern Med.* 2005;165(2):150–156.

64. Cushman WC, Cutler JA, Bingham SF, et al. Prevention and treatment of hypertension study (PATHS). Rationale and design. *Am J Hypertens.* 1994;7:814–823.

65. MacMahon S. Alcohol consumption and hypertension. *Hypertension.* 1987;9:111–121.

66. Piano MR. The cardiovascular effects of alcohol: The good and the bad: How low-risk drinking differs from high-risk drinking. *Am J Nurs.* 2005;105(7):87, 89–91.

67. Gordon T, Doyle JT. Alcohol consumption and its relationship to smoking, weight, blood pressure, and blood lipids. *Arch Int Med.* 1986;146:262–265.

68. Klatsky AL, Friedman GD, Armstrong MA. The relationships between alcoholic bever-age use and other traits to blood pressure: A new Kaiser-Permanente study. *Circulation.* 1986;73:628–636.

69. Witteman JC, Willett WC, Stampfer MJ, et al. Relation of moderate alcohol consump-tion and risk of systemic hypertension in women. *Am J Cardiol.* 1990;65(9):633–637.

70. Fuchs FD, Chambless LE, Whelton PK, Nieto FJ, Heiss G. Alcohol consumption and the incidence of hypertension: The atherosclerosis risk in communities study. *Hypertension.* 2001;37(5):1242–1250.

71. Cushman WC, Cutler JA, Hanna E, et al. Prevention and treatment of hypertension study (PATHS): Effects of an alcohol treatment program on blood pressure. *Arch Intern Med.* 1998;158:1197–1207.

72. Wallace P, Cutler S, Haines A. Randomised controlled trial of general practitioner inter-vention in patients with excessive alcohol consumption. *BMJ.* 1988;297:663–668.

73. Puddey IB, Parker M, Beilin LJ, Vandongen R, Masarei JRL. Effects of alcohol and caloric restrictions on blood pressure and serum lipids in overweight men. *Hypertension.* 1992;20:533–541.

74. Xin X, He J, Frontini MG, Ogden LG, Motsamai OI, Whelton PK. Effects of alco-hol reduction on blood pressure: A meta-analysis of randomized controlled trials. *Hypertension.* 2001;38(5):1112–1117.

75. Beilin LJ. Alcohol, hypertension and cardiovascular disease. *J Hypertens.* 1995;13:939–942.

76. Rimm EB, Giovannucci EL, Willett WC, et al. A prospective study of alcohol consumption and the risk of coronary disease in men. *Lancet.* 1991;338:464–468.
77. Armstrong B, Van Merwyk AJ, Coates H. Blood pressure in seventh-day adventist vegetarians. *Am J Epidemiol.* 1977;105(5):444–449.
78. Sacks FM, Rosner B, Kass EH. Blood pressure in vegetarians. *Am J Epidemiol.* 1974;100(5):390–398.
79. Burr ML, Bates CJ, Fehily AM, St. Leger AS. Plasma cholesterol and blood pressure in vegetarians. *J Hum Nutr.* 1981;35:437–441.
80. Beilin LJ, Rouse IL, Armstrong BK, Oxon D, Margetts BM, Vandongen R. Vegetarian diet and blood pressure levels: Incidental or causal association? *Am J Clin Nutr.* 1988;48:806–810.
81. Margetts BM, Beilin LJ, Vandongen R, Armstrong BK. Vegetarian diet in mild hypertension: A randomised controlled trial. *BMJ.* 1986;293:1468–1471.
82. Rouse IL, Beilin LJ, Armstrong BK, Vandongen R. Blood-pressure-lowering effect of a vegetarian diet: Controlled trial in normotensive subjects. *Lancet.* 1983:i.
83. Sacks FM, Obarzanek E, Windhauser MM, et al. Rationale and design of the Dietary Approaches to Stop Hypertension trial. *Ann Epidemiol.* 1995;5:108–118.
84. Vogt TM, Appel LJ, Moore TJ, et al. Dietary Approaches to Stop Hypertension: Rationale, design, and methods. *J Am Diet Assoc.* 1999;99 (Suppl):S12–S18.
85. Materson BJ, Reda DJ, Cushman WC, et al. Single-drug therapy for hypertension in men. A comparison of six antihypertensive agents with placebo. The Department of Veterans Affairs Cooperative Study Group on Antihypertensive Agents. *N Engl J Med.* 1993;328(13):914–921.
86. Rosamond W, Flegal K, Friday G, et al. Heart disease and stroke statistics—2007 update: A report from the American Heart Association Statistics Committee and Stroke Statistics Subcommittee. *Circulation.* 2007;115(5):e69–171.
87. Conlin PR, Erlinger TP, Bohannon A, et al. The DASH diet enhances the blood pressure response to losartan in hypertensive patients. *Am J Hypertens.* 2003;16(5 Pt 1):337–342.
88. Svetkey LP, Pollak KI, Yancy WS Jr., et al. Hypertension improvement project: Randomized trial of quality improvement for physicians and lifestyle modification for patients. *Hypertension.* 2009;54(6):1226–1233.
89. Blumenthal JA, Babyak MA, Hinderliter A, et al. Effects of the DASH diet alone and in combination with exercise and weight loss on blood pressure and cardiovascular biomarkers in men and women with high blood pressure: The ENCORE study. *Arch Intern Med.* 25 2010;170(2):126–135.
90. Chobanian AV, Bakris GL, Black HR, et al. The seventh report of the joint national committee on prevention, detection, evaluation, and treatment of high blood pressure: The JNC 7 report. *JAMA.* 2003;289(19):2560–2572.
91. Appel LJ, Brands MW, Daniels SR, Karanja N, Elmer PJ, Sacks FM. Dietary approaches to prevent and treat hypertension: A scientific statement from the American Heart Association. *Hypertension.* 2006;47(2):296–308.
92. ADA. Hypertension evidence-based nutrition practice guideline. *ADA Evidence Analysis Library.* http://www.adaevidencelibrary.com/. Accessed September 13, 2011.
93. Khan NA, Hemmelgarn B, Herman RJ, et al. The 2009 Canadian Hypertension Education Program recommendations for the management of hypertension: Part 2—Therapy. *Can J Cardiol.* 2009;25(5):287–298.
94. Williams B, Poulter NR, Brown MJ, et al. Guidelines for management of hypertension: Report of the fourth working party of the British Hypertension Society, 2004-BHS IV. *J Hum Hypertens.* 2004;18(3):139–185.
95. USDA. Report of the Dietary Guidelines advisory Committee on the dietary guidelines for Americans, 2010. http://health.gov/DietaryGuidelines. Accessed September 13, 2011.

96. Trichopoulou A, Costacou T, Bamia C, Trichopoulos D. Adherence to a Mediterranean diet and survival in a Greek population. *N Engl J Med.* 2003;348(26):2599–2608.

97. Trichopoulou A, Bamia C, Norat T, et al. Modified Mediterranean diet and survival after myocardial infarction: The EPIC-Elderly study. *Eur J Epidemiol.* 2007;22(12):871–881.

98. Nunez-Cordoba JM, Valencia-Serrano F, Toledo E, Alonso A, Martinez-Gonzalez MA. The Mediterranean diet and incidence of hypertension: The Seguimiento Universidad de Navarra (SUN) Study. *Am J Epidemiol.* 2009;169(3):339–346.

99. Estruch R, Martinez-Gonzalez MA, Corella D, et al. Effects of a Mediterranean-style diet on cardiovascular risk factors: A randomized trial. *Ann Intern Med.* 2006;145(1):1–11.

100. Appel LJ, Champagne CM, Harsha DW, et al. Effects of comprehensive lifestyle modification on blood pressure control: Main results of the PREMIER clinical trial. *JAMA.* 2003;289(16):2083–2093.

101. Svetkey LP, Stevens VJ, Brantley PJ, et al. Comparison of strategies for sustaining weight loss: The weight loss maintenance randomized controlled trial. *JAMA.* 2008;299(10):1139–1148.

2 Effects of Minerals, Antioxidants, and Micronutrients on Blood Pressure

Edgar R. Miller III and Stephen P. Juraschek
Johns Hopkins Medical Institutions

CONTENTS

2.1 INTRODUCTION

Dietary recommendations for the prevention and treatment of hypertension are based on compelling evidence from clinical trials. Notably, the DASH and OmniHeart trials showed impressive blood pressure (BP) reductions with improved quality of diet [1,2]. These effects were seen in the setting of isocaloric feeding and fixed sodium intake. Many constituents of diets may account for the BP-lowering effects, yet minerals and antioxidants contained in diets high in fruits, vegetables, and low-fat dairy seem to be particularly relevant.

   These micronutrients coexist in natural foods with many other nutrient factors that may also affect BP. Hence, it is impossible to test the effects of individual micronutrients with food or dietary manipulation without significant confounding. The contribution of antioxidants, minerals, and micronutrients to BP is best tested in the setting of placebo-controlled randomized trials because they can be concentrated in pills or capsules. In this chapter, we review the effects of minerals, antioxidants, and fla-vonoid-containing supplements on BP, placing the greatest weight on peer-reviewed clinical trials, systematic reviews of trials, and meta-analyses of clinical trials.

2.2 MINERALS—CALCIUM, MAGNESIUM, AND POTASSIUM

Population-based epidemiological studies provide evidence that dietary calcium, magnesium, and potassium intake lowers the risk for hypertension. Laboratory and animal studies have established biological mechanisms and justification for clinical trials. These trials have provided the critical evidence for establishing the effects of diets on BP. Because of the large number of published trials, there is sufficient evidence to address questions of whether supplementation of diet with calcium, mag-nesium, or potassium can lower BP, whether there are safety concerns with supple-mentation, and whether supplementing minerals according to the deficiencies in diet is sufficient to lower BP or whether supraphysiological doses (i.e., doses greater than what can be achieved by dietary sources alone) are needed.

2.2.1 RECOMMENDED INTAKE OF CALCIUM, MAGNESIUM, AND POTASSIUM

Recommendations for dietary intake of calcium, magnesium, and potassium estab-lished by the Institute of Medicine (IOM) are based on clinical trials and epidemio-logical evidence [3]. Thresholds of "adequate intake" (AI) to prevent deficiencies and "upper tolerable limits" (UL) of daily mineral intake to avoid toxicities have been established. Population-based surveys suggest that dietary deficiencies of these minerals are common in adults, and these deficiencies may in some way contribute to hypertension or poor hypertension control (Table 2.1).

2.2.2 CALCIUM

2.2.2.1 Common Sources of Calcium

Dietary sources rich in calcium include milk, cheese, yogurt, broccoli, and kale [3]. The most common forms of dietary calcium supplements are calcium carbonate and calcium citrate; the latter is more readily absorbed. Other forms of calcium including calcium gluconate, calcium chloride, calcium acetate, and calcium glubionate are less commonly used.

2.2.2.2 Mechanism of Action

From epidemiological studies, there is only weak evidence of an association between dietary calcium intake and BP [4], yet there are a number of biological mechanisms that suggest an important role for calcium in BP regulation. According to Resnick's "Ionic hypothesis of hypertension," BP is regulated by reciprocating contributions of extracellular and intracellular calcium-dependent pressor mechanisms [5]. Reduced dietary calcium results in depletion of calcium membrane storage sites and increases intracellular free calcium. Elevated intracellular free calcium suppresses parathyroid

TABLE 2.1

Recommended Intake/Adequate Intake, Mean or Median Dietary Intake in the United States, Tolerable Upper Limit, and Common Dietary Sources of Calcium, Magnesium, and Potassium

Nutrient	Adult Recommended Daily Intake/Adequate Intake	U.S. Estimated Mean Intake (Diet + Supplement)	Upper Tolerable Limit	Common Dietary Sources	Typical Supplement Dose
Calcium	Male and female, 19–50 years: 1000 mg/day Male and female, >50 years: 1200 mg/day	Males, >19 years: 1087–1260 mg/day Females, >19 years: 945–1187 mg/day	Male and female, >19 years: 2500 mg/day	Milk, cheese, yogurt, corn tortillas, calcium-set tofu, Chinese cabbage, kale, and broccoli	500 mg, 600 mg, and 1000 mg
Magnesium	Male, 19–30 years: 400 mg/day Male, >30 years: 420 mg/day Female, 19–30 years: 310 mg/day Female, >30 years: 320 mg/day	Male, >19 years: 282–343 mg/day Female, >19 years: 209–239 mg/day	There is no UL for dietary intake of magnesium; only for magnesium supplements 350 mg/day	Green leafy vegetables, unpolished grains, nuts, meat, starches, milk, fish, and oatmeal	250 mg, 400 mg, and 500 mg
Potassium	Male and female, >19 years: 4.7 g/day	Male, >19 years: 2.9–3.4 g/day Female, >19 years: 2.2–2.5 g/day	No UL for dietary intake	Fruits and vegetables, dried peas, dairy products, meats, and nuts	Nonprescription supplements can be sold at a maximum dose of 99 mg/tablet

Source: Adapted from Institute of Medicine, Dietary reference intakes, http://fnic.nal.usda.gov/nal_display/index.php?info_center=4&tax_level=2&tax_subject=256&topic_id=1342.

Note: Conversion of mmol to mg: potassium mmol × 39.1 g/mol = mg; magnesium mmol × 24.31 g/mol = mg.

hormone (PTH) and production of 1,25 vitamin D hormones. Ultimately, calcium depletion will adversely affect vascular smooth muscle cell membranes and vascular reactivity, leading to a greater tendency toward vasoconstriction [6,7]. Calcium supplementation lowers serum PTH and 1,25 vitamin D concentrations through a counterregulatory mechanism, which may lower BP through several mechanisms [8–11]. It has also been observed that dietary calcium downregulates angiotensin-converting enzyme, which would decrease sodium retention and therefore may lower BP [12].

2.2.2.3   Clinical Trials of Calcium Supplementation

Trial of Hypertension Prevention (TOHP) was one of the earliest and largest trials that examined the effects of calcium supplementation on BP [13]. TOHP randomized 471 men and women with prehypertension and stage 1 hypertension to 1000 mg/day of calcium for 6 months or to placebo. Average age of the participants, among whom 68% were men and 86% were whites, was 43 years; their baseline BP was 126/84 mmHg. Calcium supplementation had the modest and nonsignificant effects on systolic blood pressure (SBP; −0.46 mmHg; 95% CI: −1.77, 0.86) and diastolic blood pressure (DBP; 0.20 mmHg; 95% CI: −0.71, 1.11).

A large number of smaller randomized trials have reported the effects of calcium supplementation on BP. Several meta-analyses that combine trials and report BP-regulation effects have been published over the past 20 years. A summary of the meta-analyses and the pooled effect sizes on BP is given in Table 2.2.

The first meta-analysis of calcium supplement trials on BP included 15 trials, 391 subjects with a median calcium dose of 1000 mg/day and a median trial duration of 6 weeks. This meta-analysis found nonsignificant reductions in SBP (−0.13 mmHg; 95% CI: −0.45, 0.19) and DBP (0.03 mmHg; 95% CI: −0.17, 0.22) [14]. A later meta-analysis

TABLE 2.2

Summary of Calcium Supplement Meta-analyses

Calcium	Meta-analyses	Number of Trials	SBP Summary Effect (mmHg, 95% CI)	DBP Summary Effect (mmHg, 95% CI)
Overall	Cappuccio et al. [14]	15	−0.13 (−0.45, 0.19)	0.03 (−0.17, 0.22)
	Allender et al. [15]	26	−0.89 (−1.74, −0.05)*	−0.18 (−0.75, 0.40)
	Bucher et al. [16]	33	−1.27 (−2.25, −0.29)*	−0.24 (−0.92, 0.44)
	Griffith et al. [17]	42	−1.44 (−2.20, −0.68)*	−0.84 (−1.44, −0.24)*
	van Mierlo et al. [18]	40	−1.86 (−2.91, −0.81)*	−0.99 (−1.61, −0.37)*
Baseline BP Status				
Hypertensive	Cappuccio et al. [14]	10	0.06 (−0.59, 0.72)	0.03 (−0.21, 0.27)
	Allender et al. [15]	13	−1.68 (−3.18, −0.18)*	0.02 (−0.96, 1.00)
	Bucher et al. [16]	6	−4.30 (−6.47, −2.13)*	−1.50 (−2.77, −0.23)*
	Dickinson et al. [19]	14	−3.2 (−6.2, −0.2)*	−2.4 (−4.8, 0.0)*
Normotensive	Allender et al. [15]	16	−0.53 (−1.56, 0.49)	−0.28 (−0.99, 0.42)
	Bucher et al. [16]	6	−0.27 (−1.80, 1.27)	−0.33 (−1.56, 0.90)

*$p < .05$

with additional trials ($N = 28$) and 1231 subjects reported a smaller pooled effect on SBP (−0.89 mmHg; 95% CI: −1.74, −0.05) and DBP (−0.18 mmHg; 95% CI: −0.75, 0.40) [15]. Trial sizes ranged from 14 to 471 participants, the mean age ranged from 21 to 48 years, the median duration was 8 weeks, and the median calcium dose was 1000 mg/day. In the same year, Bucher et al. (1996) reported pooled results from 33 trials with 2412 patients, showing similar small reduction in SBP (−1.27 mmHg; 95% CI: −2.25, −0.29) and DBP (−0.24 mmHg; 95% CI: −0.92, 0.44) [16]. Later, Griffith and colleagues (1999) included 44 trials confirming earlier findings: small reductions in SBP (−1.44 mmHg; 95% CI: −2.20, −0.68) and DBP (−0.84 mmHg; 95% CI: −1.44, −0.24) [17]. Then, van Mierlo et al. (2006) excluded several trials of inferior quality, yet included 40 trials with 2492 subjects in the meta-analysis [18]. The median dose was 1055 mg/day, the median age of participants was 45 years, and the median trial duration was 9.5 weeks. Overall, calcium supplementation was reported to reduce SBP (−1.86 mmHg; 95% CI: −2.91, −0.81) and DBP (−0.99 mmHg; 95% CI: −1.61, −0.37).

In 2006, the Cochrane Collaboration published a systematic review of calcium supplementation and BP, exclusively meta-analyzing trials that enrolled hypertensive participants and that had a minimum duration of 8 weeks [19]. Overall, pooled results from 13 randomized controlled trials resulted in a significant reduction in SBP (−2.5 mmHg; 95% CI: −4.5, −0.6), but not DBP (−0.8 mmHg; 95% CI: −2.1, 0.4). The trial size ranged from 9 to 90 subjects, the median duration was 8 weeks, the mean age was 45 years, and the mean dose was 1100 mg/day.

2.2.2.4 Practical Message to Providers

Most meta-analyses show significant heterogeneity across trials. Despite trial differences, meta-analyses have presented similar results—calcium supplementation only modestly lowers SBP by 1–2 mmHg with <1 mmHg reduction in DBP. Most trials examined short-term supplementation rather than long-term supplementation. Furthermore, two meta-analyses showed no benefit of calcium supplementation on cardiovascular disease events (relative risk [RR]: 1.14; 95% CI: 0.92–1.41) [20] or on clinical cardiovascular end points with or without vitamin D supplementation (hazard ratio [HR]: 1.17; 95% CI: 1.05–1.31; $p = .005$) [21]. No trials tested the effects of calcium on BP using exclusively dietary, as opposed to supplemental, sources of calcium, leaving open the possibility of an effect not detectable in the meta-analyses summarized above. In fact, the Dietary Approaches to Stop Hypertension (DASH) dietary pattern [1] described in Chapter 1 of this book includes increased dietary calcium compared with the usual U.S. intake, which is considered an integral component of this BP-lowering dietary pattern. Given the small beneficial effect of calcium on BP, other health benefits (e.g., preservation of bone), and the wide availability of dietary calcium (see Table 2.1), individuals should be encouraged to consume adequate amounts of dietary calcium.

2.2.3 Magnesium

2.2.3.1 Common Sources of Magnesium

Common dietary sources of magnesium include green leafy vegetables, unpolished grains, nuts, meat, starches, milk, fish, and oatmeal. The most common forms of magnesium supplements are magnesium oxide and magnesium citrate; the latter has better intestinal absorption. Other less common forms include magnesium sulfate, magnesium aspartate, magnesium chloride, magnesium oxide, magnesium diglyceride, magnesium lactate, magnesium pidolate, and magnesium hydroxide [3].

2.2.3.2 Mechanism of Action

In human observational studies, low dietary magnesium intake is associated with incident hypertension among middle-aged and older U.S. women [22]. Laboratory and clinical studies have helped define the role of magnesium in vascular function and vascular reactivity. Magnesium has been shown to alter permeability of the cell membrane to calcium and sodium and important mediators of BP [23]; it can induce direct vasodilation of coronary vessels [24]. Another proposed mechanism suggests that reduced intracellular magnesium levels due to concomitant elevations of cytosolic free calcium cause vasoconstriction, arterial stiffness, and hypertension [25]. Similar to calcium-channel blockers, magnesium inhibits calcium depolarizing effects and calcium-dependent excitation–contraction coupling, thus promoting vascular relaxation [26,27]. Magnesium may also reduce BP through effects on prostaglandin E1 synthesis. Magnesium is an essential cofactor in the rate-limiting step, converting linoleic acid to γ-linolenic acid, precursors of prostaglandin E1 [28,29]. Prostaglandin E1 is a vasodilator, and low concentrations of it promote vasoconstriction and elevation in BP [29].

2.2.3.3 Magnesium Supplementation Trials

Based on the strong biological plausibility for magnesium's effect on BP, a number of magnesium supplement trials have been performed. The largest trial, TOHP, was reported in 1992 [13]. In this trial, 461 subjects were randomized to 360 mg/day of magnesium diglycine or to placebo for 6 months. The mean age of participants was 43 years; 68% were men and 85% were whites. Baseline BP was 125/84 mmHg. The TOHP trial reported nonsignificant effects of magnesium supplementation on SBP (−0.20 mmHg; 95% CI: −1.47, 1.07) and DBP (−0.05 mmHg; 95% CI: −0.94, 0.84). Another large, well-conducted trial with 198 participants was reported in 1998 [30]. Ninety-five percent of the participants were whites; the participants had the mean age of 38 years and the mean BMI of 23 kg/m². The participants were randomized to 336 mg/day of magnesium lactate for 16 weeks or to placebo. Despite significant increases in urinary magnesium excretion (4.1–6.2 mmol/24 hours, $p < .01$), the effects on SBP (−0.9 mmHg; 95% CI: −2.6, 0.8) and DBP (−0.7 mmHg; 95% CI: −2.2, 0.8) were modest and nonsignificant.

These and other small trials were included in a meta-analysis to determine pooled trial effects. This meta-analysis included 20 trials of magnesium supplementation, 14 trials of hypertensive adults, and 6 trials of normotensive adults [31]. There were a total of 1220 participants, with the mean age ranging from 23 to 65 years, the median duration of 8.5 weeks, and the median dose of 365 mg (15 mmol)/day. The overall pooled effects showed nonsignificant effects on SBP (−0.6 mmHg; 95% CI: −2.2, 1.0) and DBP (−0.8 mmHg; 95% CI: −1.9, 0.4). However, a dose–response

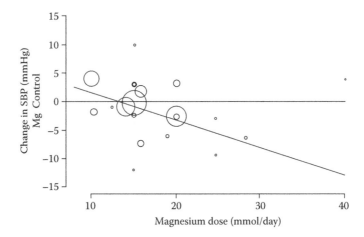

FIGURE 2.1 Dose–response effect of magnesium on SBP. Each circle represents a study, with the area of each circle inversely proportional to study variance. (From Jee, SH et al., *Am. J. Hypertens.*, 15, 691–696, 2002. With permission.)

relationship was noted, such that with each increase in 240 mg (10 mmol)/day of magnesium, there was a reduction of 4.3 mmHg SBP ($p < .001$) and 2.3 mmHg DBP ($p = .09$; Figure 2.1).

A subsequent meta-analysis conducted by a Cochrane review group utilized more stringent inclusion criteria, requiring an intervention period of at least 8 weeks and restricting the study population of the trials to hypertensive adults [32]. This meta-analysis included 12 randomized controlled trials with a total of 545 participants. The median duration of follow-up was 11 weeks, the mean age of participants was 54 years, and the mean dose of magnesium was 413 mg (17 mmol)/day. The summary effects were a nonsignificant reduction in SBP (−1.3 mmHg; 95% CI: −4.0, 1.5) but a significant reduction in DBP (−2.2 mmHg; 95% CI: −3.4, −0.9). This meta-analysis did not find a dose-dependent relationship between magnesium and BP.

2.2.3.4 Practical Message to Healthcare Providers

Meta-analyses have reported modest (1–2 mmHg) and mostly nonsignificant effects of magnesium supplementation on BP. One meta-analysis found a dose relationship between magnesium and SBP, but this association was not replicated in a second meta-analysis. At present, there are insufficient data to support clinical use of magnesium supplementation for the treatment of hypertension. However, as with calcium (see above), there are no trials testing the effect of dietary magnesium on BP. The DASH dietary pattern is rich in magnesium, and it is possible that this micronutrient contributes to the BP-lowering effect of DASH. Therefore, individuals should be encouraged to consume adequate magnesium (see Table 2.1) from dietary sources.

2.2.4 POTASSIUM

2.2.4.1 Common Sources of Potassium

Potassium exists at significant concentrations in fruits, green vegetables, and oil seeds [33]. One serving of tomatoes, potatoes, mango, black-eyed peas, or almonds, for example, contains more than 400 mg potassium. Supplements are available and are composed of a number of common salt forms, including potassium chloride, potassium gluconate, potassium acetate, potassium phosphate, potassium citrate, and potassium bicarbonate. The maximum dose of potassium allowed in over-the-counter supplements is 99 mg (~2.5 mmol) per dose, whereas prescription potassium doses are typically 390 mg (10 mmol) or 720 mg (20 mmol) [3].

2.2.4.2 Mechanism of Action

The effects of potassium on BP and cardiovascular disease risk may be mediated through BP-dependent and BP-independent pathways. Prospective studies have shown that high dietary potassium intake is associated with reduced risk of stroke mortality after adjustment for BP [34]. It has also been proposed that potassium inhibits proliferation of vascular arteriosclerosis and reduces vascular resistance through effects on endothelial function [33]. The endothelial effects of potassium may be mediated through hyperpolarization of vascular smooth muscle cells by stimulating electrogenic potassium pumps or potassium-rectifying channels. This hyperpolarization results in vasodilation [10,35]. It is also believed that potassium is one of the factors regulating synthesis of prostaglandin, a vasodilator, and platelet antiaggregator [29]. Other proposed mechanisms include natriuresis, reduced vascular responsiveness to norepinephrine and angiotensin II, blunted baroreceptor responsiveness, and increased sodium/potassium ATPase activity [10]. With regard to hypertensive patients, there is evidence that potassium supplementation promotes release of endothelial nitric oxide (NO) by inducing endogenous muscarinic agonists [36].

2.2.4.3 Potassium Supplement Trails

Because of strong biological plausibility of potassium as a mediator of BP regulation, a large number of clinical trials have been published. Several meta-analyses have been published, which report consistent, albeit modest, BP-lowering effects. The first meta-analysis, published in 1991, summarized 19 clinical trials of 586 patients, with the median age of 41 years, the median dose of 3.7 g/day (96 mmol), and the median trial duration of 28 days [37]. Potassium chloride was the predominant supplement formulation. Pooled trial effects of potassium supplementation showed significant reductions in SBP (−5.9 mmHg; 95% CI: −6.6, −5.2) and DBP (−3.4 mmHg; 95% CI: −4.0, 2.8). Larger effect sizes were reported in trials that enrolled hypertensive participants.

A subsequent meta-analysis by Whelton et al. (1997) pooled results from 32 randomized controlled trials with a total of 2661 participants: ages ranged from 18 to 79 years, the median dose was 2.9 g/day (75 mmol), and the median treatment duration was 5 weeks [38]. The most common formulation was potassium chloride. This meta-analysis reported a smaller, yet significant, effect size for SBP (−3.11 mmHg;

95% CI: −4.31, −1.91) and DBP (−1.97 mmHg; 95% CI: −3.42, −0.52). Results were greater in trials that enrolled African Americans and in subjects whose sodium intake was higher at baseline.

These findings were confirmed by a third meta-analysis of 27 trials that excluded trials lasting less than 2 weeks and trials that included participants with chronic diseases (renal disease, diabetes, etc.) [39]. The median duration of trials was 6 weeks and the mean age was 45 years. Potassium supplementation (trial doses unspecified) resulted in a mean increase in 24-hour urinary potassium excretion of 51 mmol. Overall, potassium supplementation significantly lowered both SBP (−2.42 mmHg; 95% CI: −3.75, −1.08) and DBP (−1.57 mmHg; 95% CI: −2.65, −0.50). BP-regulation effects were greater in trials of hypertensive participants compared with trials of normotensive participants (SBP/DBP: −3.20/−2.18 mmHg and −1.38/−0.78 mmHg, respectively; see Table 2.3).

The latest meta-analysis on potassium supplementation and BP was restricted to trials of hypertensive participants (SBP ≥ 140 mmHg or DBP ≥ 85 mmHg) [40]. This analysis included only five trials with a total of 425 participants, the potassium dose ranging from 1.9 (48 mmol) to 4.7 g (120 mmol)/day, and the median duration of 12 weeks. This analysis showed large yet nonsignificant reductions in SBP (−11.2 mmHg; 95% CI: −25.2, 2.7) and DBP (−5.0 mmHg; 95% CI: −12.5, 2.4).

In contrast to other micronutrients, there are randomized trials of potassium from dietary sources. A representative example is the DASH feeding trial [1] in which one treatment group received a diet that resembled a typical American diet except for increased intake of fruits and vegetables, which led to the average potassium intake of 4700 mg/2100 kcal/day. Although the BP-lowering effect of this intermediate diet was less than that of the DASH dietary pattern, its effects on BP were significant (2.8/1.1 mmHg) compared with a typical American diet. The fruits and vegetables added other nutrients (e.g., fiber and vitamin C), but the epidemiological and supplement data above suggest that the BP-lowering effect was at least in part due to increased potassium intake.

TABLE 2.3
Summary of Potassium Supplement Meta-analyses

Potassium	Meta-analysis	Number of Trials	SBP Summary Effect (mmHg, 95% CI)	DBP Summary Effect (mmHg, 95% CI)
Overall	Cappuccio et al. [37]	19	−5.9 (−6.6, −5.2)*	−3.4 (−4.0, 2.8)
	Whelton et al. [38]	32	−3.11 (−4.31, −1.91)*	−1.97 (−3.42, −0.52)*
Baseline BP Status				
Hypertensive	Cappuccio et al. [37]	13	−8.2 (−9.1, −7.3)*	−4.5 (−5.2, −3.8)*
	Whelton et al. [38]	20	−4.4 (−6.6, −2.2)*	−2.5 (−4.9, −0.1)*
	Geleijnse et al. [39]	19	−3.20 (−4.81, −1.60)*	−2.18 (−3.46, −0.90)*
	Dickinson et al. [40]	5	−11.2 (−25.2, 2.7)	−5.0 (−12.5, 2.4)
Normotensive	Whelton et al. [38]	12	−1.8 (−2.9, −0.6)*	−1.0 (−2.1, 0.0)*
	Geleijnse et al. [39]	11	−1.38 (−3.22, 0.46)	−0.78 (−2.25, 0.69)

*$p < .05$

2.2.4.4   Practical Message to Providers

There is a substantial heterogeneity among trials examining oral potassium supplementation and BP. Meta-analyses suggest that short-term, high-dose oral potassium supplementation results in significant SBP reduction in the 3–5 mmHg range. Greater effects were noted in trials that enrolled hypertensive participants. Long-term effects on clinical endpoints have not been established. Effects of supplements at lower doses typically consumed as a component of over-the-counter supplements have not been established. Other than to treat diuretic-induced hypokalemia, potassium supplements are not recommended for BP control. In contrast, several national guidelines (JNC-7, Dietary Guidelines for Americans, etc.) indicate that healthcare providers should encourage their patients to strive for adequate intake of potassium through consumption of fruits, vegetables, and other potassium-rich foods (see Table 2.1).

2.3   ANTIOXIDANTS, VITAMINS, AND OTHER DIETARY MICRONUTRIENTS

Although minerals contained in dietary patterns may account for much of the BP-lowering effects of diet, antioxidants, vitamins, and other micronutrients with biological activity contained in these diets may also have a role. Vitamin C, vitamin D, folate, vitamin B6, and vitamin B12 may affect biological mediators of BP regulation and are discussed in detail in the following section. Recommended intake, adequate intake, mean or median dietary intake, tolerable upper limit, common dietary sources, and typical supplement dose of vitamin C, vitamin D, folate, vitamin B6, and vitamin B12 are presented in Table 2.4. In this section, we review the evidence for the results of efficacy trials of these supplements and other dietary micronutrients on BP.

2.3.1   VITAMIN C

2.3.1.1   Common Sources of Vitamin C

Foods rich in vitamin C include citrus fruits, tomatoes, tomato juice, potatoes, brussel sprouts, cauliflower, broccoli, strawberries, cabbage, and spinach [3]. Supplements are available predominantly as ascorbic acid. Less common forms of vitamin C include ferrous ascorbate, dehydroascorbic acid, hybrin, L-ascorbic acid, magnesium ascorbicum, magnorbin, and sodium ascorbate.

2.3.1.2   Mechanism of Action

Vitamin C (ascorbic acid) is an essential micronutrient acquired primarily through the consumption of fruits, vegetables, and supplements. Vitamin C is a powerful aqueous-phase antioxidant that reduces oxidative stress [41] and enhances endothelial function through effects on NO production [42]. Antihypertensive effects of vitamin C were hypothesized as early as 1946 [43], and many laboratory [44,45] and human studies [46,47] have established biological plausibility. A number of mechanisms are believed to contribute to the antihypertensive effects of vitamin C.

TABLE 2.4

Recommended Intake/Adequate Intake, Mean or Median Dietary Intake, Tolerable Upper Limit, Common Dietary Sources, and Typical Supplement Dose of Vitamin C, Vitamin D, Folate, Vitamin B6, and Vitamin B12

Supplement	Adult Recommended Daily Intake/ Adequate Intake	U.S. Estimated Mean (Diet + Supplement) Intake	Tolerable Upper Limit	Common Dietary Sources	Typical Supplement Dose
Vitamin C	Male, >19 years: 90 mg/day Female, >19 years: 75 mg/day	Male, >19 years: 173–199 mg/day Female, >19 years: 122–202 mg/day	Male and female, >19 years: 2000 mg/day	Citrus fruits, tomatoes, tomato juice, potatoes, brussel sprouts, cauliflower, broccoli, strawberries, cabbage, and spinach	100 mg, 250 mg, 500 mg, and 1000 mg
Vitamin D	Male and female, 19–50 years: 5 µg/day Male and female, 50–70 years: 10 µg/day Male and female, >70 years: 15 µg/day	Males, >19 years: 6.6–10.7 µg/day Females, >19 years: 5.8–10 µg/day	Male and female, >19 years: 50 µg/day	Fish liver oils, flesh of fatty fish, liver, fortified milk products, and fortified cereals	10 mg (400 IU), 20 mg (800 IU), and 25 mg (1000 IU)
Folic acid	Male and female, >19 years: 400 µg/day	Male, > 19 years: 387–429 µg/day Female, >19 years: 369–413 µg/day	Male and female, >19 years: 1000 µg/day	Enriched cereal grains, dark leafy vegetables, enriched and whole-grain breads and bread products, and fortified ready-to-eat cereals	0.4 mg, 0.8 mg, 1 mg
Vitamin B6	Male, 19–50 years: 1.3 mg/ day Male, >50 years: 1.7 mg/day Female, 19–50 years: 1.3 mg/day Female, >50 years: 1.5 mg/day	Male, >19 years: 3.8–6.9 mg/day Female, > 19 years: 4.3–5.2 mg/day	Male and female, >19 years: 100 mg/day	Fortified cereals, organ meats, and fortified soy-based meat substitutes	25 mg, 50 mg, 100 mg, 250 mg, and 500 mg
Vitamin B12	Male and female, >19 years: 2.4 µg/day	Male, >19 years: 10.5–17.0 µg/day Female, >19 years: 9.6–14.4 µg/day	Not Determined	Fortified cereals, meat, fish, and poultry	50 µg, 100 µg, 250 µg, 500 µg, and 1000 µg

Source: Adapted from Institute of Medicine, Dietary reference intakes, http://fnic.nal.usda.gov/nal_display/index.php?info_center=4&tax_level=2&tax_subject=256&topic_id=1342.

Vitamin C is reported to have a mild diuretic effect. There is also some evidence that vitamin C has a uricosuric effect, that is, lowering serum uric acid, [48] which has been associated with hypertension risk [49]. In human studies, vitamin C can prevent endothelial dysfunction and reduce the vasoconstriction associated with consumption of a fatty meal by enhanced NO-mediated pathways [41,50–54]. Population-based observational studies have shown an inverse association between plasma vitamin C concentrations [55] and vitamin C intake, with BP levels [56] providing justification for trials evaluating vitamin C supplementation and BP reduction.

2.3.1.3 Vitamin C Supplement Trials

A large number of small, randomized controlled trials have evaluated the effect of vitamin C supplementation on BP, but the results are inconsistent, possibly because of heterogeneous methods and the small sample size of individual trials. Two reviews reported inconclusive results regarding vitamin C's ability to reduce BP [57–59]. A recent meta-analysis of the effects of vitamin C supplementations on BP included 29 trials [60] (see Table 2.5). Among the trials included in the meta-analysis, the median dose of vitamin C was 500 mg/day, the median duration was 6 weeks, and the trial size ranged from 10 to 111 participants. The authors concluded that oral vitamin C supplementation reduced SBP (−3.8 mmHg; 95% CI: −5.3, −2.4) and DBP (−1.5 mmHg; 95% CI: −2.9, −0.1). In a subgroup analysis, greater reductions in SBP were noted in trials with younger (<60 years old) participants.

2.3.1.4 Practical Message to Providers

Vitamin C is a supplement consumed by many adults despite little evidence to support its effects on BP or clinical end points. A large number of trials that report the effects of vitamin C supplementation on BP have been published, and pooled effects suggest that vitamin C supplementation may result in modest BP reduction (3.5–5 mmHg). Despite the BP-lowering effects demonstrated by the meta-analysis above, large long-term trials in which BP is a risk factor (e.g., stroke, heart failure, and cardiovascular events) do not provide evidence supporting benefit from vitamin C

TABLE 2.5
Vitamin C Supplement Trials by Hypertensive Status

	Systolic Blood Pressure		Diastolic Blood Pressure
	N^a	Mean (95% CI)	Mean (95% CI)
Primary analysis trials	29	−3.8 (−5.3, −2.4)*	−1.5 (−2.9, −0.1)*
Hypertensive	13	−4.9 (−7.5, −2.2)*	−1.7 (−4.1, 0.7)
Nonhypertensive	18	−3.1 (−4.5, −1.7)*	−1.4 (−3.1, 0.4)

[a] N is the number of trials. If a trial reported effects in two distinct subgroups, it was counted twice. As a result, the total number exceeds the 29 trials included in the primary analysis.

*$p < .05$

supplementation. A meta-analysis of 34 trials with 70,456 participants examining the pooled effect of vitamin C supplementation reported no benefit on mortality (RR: 0.97; 95% CI: 0.88, 1.06) [61]. Furthermore, two large trials, The Woman's Antioxidant Cardiovascular Study (WACS) and the Physicians Health Study II (PHS II) [62,63], corroborate no benefit of long-term vitamin C supplementation at reducing cardiovascular events, stroke, or mortality. Existing evidence does not support the recommendation to supplement vitamin C for BP control. However, consumption of recommended levels of fruits and vegetables will generally lead to adequate intake of vitamin C.

2.3.2 VITAMIN D SUPPLEMENTATION

2.3.2.1 Common Sources of Vitamin D

Vitamin D is primarily made during exposure to solar ultraviolet B radiation, where 7-deoxycholesterol in the skin is concerted to vitamin D3. However, dietary sources of vitamin D are important, and common sources of foods with high amounts of vitamin D include salmon, tuna, eggs, and fortified milk. Supplements are available as alphacalcidol, cholecalciferol (vitamin D3), ergocalciferol (vitamin D2), and 1,25-dihydroxycholecalciferol (active form) [64].

2.3.2.2 Mechanism of Action

Vitamin D status and supplementation are believed to contribute to a number of positive health effects [65]. Vitamin D3 (cholecalciferol), the most powerful form of vitamin D, is synthesized in the skin from 7-dehydrocholesterol by the action of sunlight (ultraviolet B radiation) [3]. Another major source of vitamin D is diet. Vitamin D is biologically inert and must be converted to the active hormone 1,25-dihydroxy vitamin D [1,25(OH)2D] (calcitriol). Vitamin D's pivotal role in regulating calcium homeostasis and bone metabolism has been long recognized [66,67]; however, mounting evidence suggests that vitamin D may also influence various nonskeletal medical conditions, including cardiovascular disease and hypertension [68–71]. There are several mechanisms that may explain vitamin D's effects on BP. Small clinical trials have demonstrated that vitamin D downregulates renin expression, leading to suppression of the renin–angiotensin system [72,73]. Vitamin D increases serum calcium concentration, suppresses PTH secretion, plays a role in calcium-phosphate metabolism [74], and improves endothelial cell–dependent vasodilatation [75,76].

2.3.2.3 Vitamin D Supplement Trials

In spite of broad enthusiasm for vitamin D supplementation, there is a relative paucity of trials examining vitamin D supplementation effects on BP. Two meta-analyses have reported pooled effects. Witham et al. (2009) pooled results from eight trials of hypertensive adults comprising 545 individuals. Trials lasted from 5 weeks to 12 months. The most common source of Vitamin D was alphacalcidol [77]. Overall, pooled results of vitamin D supplementation trials demonstrated a reduction in SBP (−3.6 mmHg; 95% CI −8.0, 0.7) and DBP (−3.1 mmHg; 95%

CI: −5.5, −0.6). One limitation of this meta-analysis, however, is its exclusion of trials that enrolled nonhypertensive participants. A second meta-analysis pooled results from 10 randomized clinical trials, which also included trials with nonhypertensive participants [78]. Doses of vitamin D ranged from 400 to 8571 IU/day, and the duration varied from 5 to 52 weeks. Pooled effects showed no significant effect of vitamin D on SBP (−1.9 mmHg; 95% CI: −4.2, 0.4) or DBP (−0.1 mmHg; 95% CI: −0.7, 0.5).

Two trials are noteworthy for reporting BP-lowering effects. The first trial randomized 148 ambulatory women aged 70 or older [76] to either 1200 mg calcium and 800 IU vitamin D3 or 1200 mg calcium/day for 8 weeks. Mean baseline SBP/DBP was 142/84 mmHg. This trial reported a significant decrease in SBP of 9.3% ($p = .02$). Furthermore, the trial compared vitamin D and calcium group with calcium-alone group and found that vitamin D and calcium in combination reduced SBP by 5 mmHg more than calcium alone did. The second trial reported BP-lowering effects in 34 patients with type 2 diabetes, mean age 64, who received 100,000 IU of ergocalciferol or placebo during winter. After 8 weeks, it was found that vitamin D significantly decreased SBP (−7.3 mmHg) when compared with placebo ($p = .001$) [75].

2.3.2.4 Practical Message to Providers

Results of meta-analyses of vitamin D supplementation on BP show inconsistent and modest effects in the 2–3 mmHg range. It is worth noting that a meta-analysis of four long-term trials examining vitamin D supplementation on clinical events found a nonsignificant risk reduction in cardiovascular events within trials of vitamin D alone (RR: 0.90; 95% CI: 0.77, 1.05) and in trials of vitamin D coadministered with calcium (RR: 1.04; 95% CI: 0.92, 1.18) [20]. In summary, there is only weak evidence from clinical trials for BP-regulation effects with vitamin D supplementation. In addition, no trials directly tested the effect of increasing vitamin D intake from dietary sources on BP. Providers should recommend adherence to recommended intake of vitamin D from dietary sources (see Table 2.4) for reasons unrelated to BP control (i.e., bone health).

2.3.3 FOLIC ACID, VITAMIN B6, AND VITAMIN B12

2.3.3.1 Common Sources of Folic Acid, Vitamin B6, and Vitamin B12

Folate, B12, and B6 are water-soluble vitamins important for normal cell metabolism—particularly during periods of rapid cell division. Leafy green vegetables (e.g., spinach and turnip greens), fruits (e.g., citrus fruits and juices), and dried beans and peas are all natural sources of folate [3]. Common forms of the folate include folic acid, folacin, folvite, pteroylglutamic acid, and vitamin M. Typically, folate supplements are in the form of folic acid—a synthetic form that is also used as an additive to fortify foods such as grains and breads. Vitamin B6 is a combination of six related compounds: pyridoxal, pyridoxine, pyridoxamine, pyridoxal 5′-phosphate, pyridoxine 5′-phosphate, and pyridoxamine 5′-phosphate; vitamin B12 is also referred to as cobalamin, cyanocobalamin, or eritron.

2.3.3.2 Mechanism of Action

There is reasonable biological plausibility for an antihypertensive effect of vitamin B supplementation (folic acid, B6, and B12) mediated through both homocysteine and homocysteine-independent effects. A number of epidemiological studies have described an association between hyperhomocysteinemia and elevated BP. Mechanisms suggested in support of a causal relationship between homocysteine and hypertension include increased arteriolar constriction, greater renal sodium reabsorption, overactive sympathetic nervous system, increased renin–angiotensin–aldosterone system activity, and reduced vascular compliance [79,80]. It is also believed that homocysteine lowers the bioactivity of NO and reduces the antioxidant enzymes responsible for detoxifying endothelial hydrogen peroxide [81] effects, which could promote lower BP. Supplementation with folic acid, B12, or B6 lowers homocysteine, which has made folic acid trials with clinical end points plentiful. Active folate (i.e., 5-methyltetrahydrofolate), converted in the liver from folic acid, functions with vitamin B12 as a cofactor to donate a methyl group for the conversion of homocysteine into methionine [81]. In an alternative pathway, vitamin B6 functions in the degradation to cysteine via cystathionine. Of these two pathways, serum folate shows a greater negative correlation with homocysteine than serum levels of either vitamin B12 or vitamin B6 [79]. Small clinical studies have demonstrated that in subjects with endothelial dysfunction, high dose of folic acid or its main circulating metabolite, 5-methyltetrahydrofolate (5-MTHF), can improve endothelial function independent of changes in homocysteine [82]. In vitro evidence suggests that stimulation of 5-MTHF can directly increase NO production, reduce superoxide production via endothelial NO synthase, and scavenge superoxide, all of which are potentially antiatherogenic processes and with BP-lowering effects.

In addition to its role in homocysteine metabolism, folic acid is reported to lower BP through other distinct mechanisms. Laboratory data suggest that circulating 5-methyltetrahydrofolate improves NO-mediated endothelial vasomotor response and reduces superoxides [83]. It has also been found that folic acid reduces generation of reactive oxygen species [84], thus having vasculoprotective effects [85].

2.3.3.3 Clinical Trials of B Vitamin Supplementation

There are a number of large clinical trials powered to detect the effects on clinical end points. There are very few trials of B vitamin supplementation on BP. One meta-analysis pooled results from eight small BP trials ($N = 293$ participants, total) [86]. The participants ranged in age from 32 to 59 years, the duration of trials ranged from 2 to 16 weeks, and the folic acid dose ranged from 5000 to 10,000 µg/day. Folic acid was not administered with other B vitamins in this meta-analysis. Pooled results showed that high dose of folic acid supplementation reduced SBP (−2.03 mmHg; 95% CI: −3.63, −0.43; $p = .04$) and had nonsignificant effects on DBP (0.01 mmHg; 95% CI: −1.12, 1.13).

Unlike the folic acid trials pooled in the meta-analysis above, vitamins B6 and B12 are rarely evaluated as individual interventions, but more often they are administered with folic acid to serve as cofactors in homocysteine metabolism. One trial evaluated the effect of 250 mg of vitamin B6 and 5 mg of folic acid on 130 patients with premature atherosclerosis or hyperhomocysteinemia over the course of 2 years. Utilizing a number of different models to adjust for various baseline characteristics (age, gender, serum homocysteine concentrations, cholesterol, etc.), the investigators reported significant reductions in BP. Depending on the adjustment model used, SBP reductions ranged from −3.7 to −6.6 mmHg (95% CI: −11.1, −2.1) and DBP ranged from −1.9 (95% CI: −3.7, −0.02) to −2.5 (95% CI: −5.4, 0.4) [87].

The Vitamin Intervention for Stroke Prevention study was one of the largest B vitamin supplement trials examining BP [88]. In this trial, investigators compared a high-dose formulation of B vitamins, containing 25 mg of vitamin B6, 0.4 mg of vitamin B12, and 2.5 mg of folic acid, with a low-dose formulation, containing 200 μg of vitamin B6, 6 μg of vitamin B12, and 20 μg of folic acid. The trial included 3689 adults with nondisabling cerebral infarction, who were recruited from hospitals throughout the United States. After 1 year, despite a significant mean reduction in total homocysteine (2 μmol/L greater in the high-dose group), there was no difference in SBP ($p = 0.91$) or in DBP ($p = 0.87$) between the groups.

2.3.3.4   Practical Message to Providers

There is mixed evidence from trials, suggesting BP-lowering effects of B vitamin supplementation in the 2–3 mmHg range. However, one meta-analysis of folic acid supplementation showed no benefit on clinical cardiovascular disease end points. Furthermore, there was a suggestion of a possible increase in the risk of cardiovascular events among individuals with elevated serum homocysteine levels before treatment [89]. Therefore, individuals are not advised to take vitamin B supplement for BP control.

2.3.4   FLAVONOID-RICH SUBSTANCES

2.3.4.1   Common Sources of Flavonoid-Rich Substances

Flavonoids are a class of plant metabolites that are proposed to have salutatory effects on human health, mediated through antioxidant and anti-inflammatory properties. There are a number of flavonoid classes including flavonols, flavones, flavanones, flavan-3-ols (also called flavanols, proanthocyanidins, and catechins), anthocyanidins (also called anthocyanins), and isoflavones. Significant food sources of flavonoids are cocoa or dark chocolate, black or green tea, soy products, and red wine [90]. Flavonoid supplements are available as concentrated extracts.

2.3.4.2   Mechanism of Action

Flavonoids are the largest group of plant polyphenols [91] that are common in many forms and in varying amounts depending on plant-based food sources. There are a number of proposed mechanisms by which flavonoids may lower BP. Laboratory data suggest that flavonoids have strong antioxidant properties that reduce reactive oxygen species and promote endogenous free radical scavenging processes [92]. Clinical trial evidence demonstrates that polyphenols promote NO-mediated endothelial relaxation and increase endothelial NO synthase activity by increasing free cytosolic calcium concentrations in endothelial cells, activating the PI3-kinase/Akt pathway, and enhancing NO synthase expression [93]. Another mechanism entails endothelium-derived hyperpolarizing factor, which causes endothelial relaxation independently of NO and is activated by flavonoids contained in red wine [93].

In addition to the shared polyphenol class mechanisms, common sources of dietary flavonoids express unique mechanisms of action on BP. It has been hypothesized that cocoa or chocolate may reduce BP through effects on NO production via stimulation of NO synthase, which enhances vasodilation, or through inhibition of angiotensin-converting enzyme activity [94]. Grape products (wines, juices, and extracts) are described as inhibitors of not only angiotensin-converting enzymes but also angiotensin II [95,96]. Black tea and wine polyphenols interact with estrogen receptors, activating endothelial NO synthase and promoting vasorelaxation [93]. Both green and black teas seem to increase aortic concentrations of catalase, which inhibits arterial smooth muscle contraction [97,98]. Green tea, different from black tea, is believed to downregulate caveolin-1, a protein that inhibits endothelial NO synthase expression [93]. Finally, soy products or phytoestrogens, with their similarity to mammalian estrogens, may evoke endogenous estrogen-derived responses by interacting with estrogen receptors [99].

2.3.4.3 Flavonoid Supplement Trials

Several meta-analyses of trials of flavonoid-containing products have been reported. The largest meta-analysis by Hooper et al. (2008) pooled together clinical trials on the effect of flavonoids and flavonoid-rich foods on BP [90]. This meta-analysis included 43 trials comprising 2804 participants. Overall, pooled results showed a nonsignificant reduction in SBP (−1.15 mmHg; 95% CI: −2.57, 0.28) and DBP (−0.90 mmHg; 95% CI: −1.84, 0.03). Subgroup analyses were performed to determine BP-regulation effects of common flavonoid-rich foods including red wine and grape, black tea, chocolate and cocoa, soy foods, soy protein isolates, and isoflavone (soy products) extract. A summary of these subgroup analyses is presented in Table 2.6.

There were three trials on 162 participants who received red wine or grape extract, which showed nonsignificant effects on SBP (0.59 mmHg; 95% CI: −0.88, 2.06) and DBP (0.38 mmHg; 95% CI: −0.71, 1.47). Similarly, black tea consumption did not have an effect on BP after pooling four trials that randomized 300 participants: SBP effects of −0.03 mmHg (95% CI: −2.78, 2.72) and DBP effects −0.57 mmHg (95% CI: −2.03, 0.89). Four trials with 194 participants tested the effects of cocoa and chocolate and reported significant reductions in SBP (−5.88 mmHg; 95% CI: −9.55, −2.21) and DBP (−3.30 mmHg; 95% CI: −5.77, −0.83). Significant heterogeneity was observed across cocoa and chocolate trials, which was associated with trial duration and cocoa dose. Trials of higher dose and shorter duration were associated with greater BP reductions. There appeared to be publication bias present in that small trials with large effects were seemingly overrepresented.

Two other meta-analyses pooled randomized trials examining cocoa supplements and BP. Taubert et al. (2007) pooled results from five trials that enrolled 173 subjects with the median duration of 2 weeks [100]. Cocoa was administered most commonly as dark chocolate with the median dose of 100 g/day. Compared with cocoa-free controls, cocoa significantly reduced SBP (−4.7 mmHg; 95% CI: −7.6, −1.8) and DBP (−2.8 mmHg; 95% CI: −4.8, −0.8). In a later meta-analysis of 10 trials with

TABLE 2.6

Summary of Meta-analyses of BP Trials of Flavonoid-Rich Foods

Supplement	Meta-analysis	Number of Trials (SBP/DBP)	SBP (Effect mmHg; 95% CI)	DBP (Effect mmHg; 95% CI)
All flavonoids	Hooper et al. [90]	44/43	−1.15 (−2.57, 0.28)	−0.90 (−1.84, 0.03)
Black tea	Hooper et al. [90]	4	−0.03 (−2.78, 2.72)	−0.57 (−2.03, 0.89)
Cocoa or	Taubert et al. [100]	5	−4.7 (−7.6, −1.8)*	−2.8 (−4.8, −0.8)*
chocolate	Hooper et al. [90]	5/4	−5.88 (−9.55, −2.21)*	−3.30 (−5.77, −0.83)*
	Desch et al. [94]	10	−4.5 (−5.9, −3.2)*	−2.5 (−3.9, −1.2)*
Red wine	Hooper et al. [90]	3	0.59 (−0.88, 2.06)	0.38 (−0.71, 1.47)
Soy foods	Hooper et al. [90]	5	−5.76 (−12.3, 0.77)	−4.04 (−8.30, 0.22)
Isoflavone extract	Hooper et al. [90]	7/8	−2.60 (−5.20, 0.00)*	0.05 (−1.66, 1.76)
Soy isoflavones	Liu et al. [101]	11	−2.5 (−5.35, 0,34)	−1.5 (−3.09, 0.17)
Soy isoflavones	Taku et al. [99]	14	−2.02 (−3.65, −0.39)*	−0.13 (−1.21, 0.96)
Soy protein isolate	Hooper et al. [90]	9	−1.60 (−3.62, 0.42)	−1.99 (−2.86, −1.12)*
Soy protein	Dong et al. [102]	27	−2.21 (−4.10, −0.33)*	−1.44 (−2.56, −0.31)*

*$p < .05$

297 participants, the effect size remained significant [94]. Treatment duration ranged from 2 to 18 weeks, and dose ranged from 5 to 174 mg/day. In order to be included in the meta-analysis, trials needed to use a cocoa intervention that was rich in flavonoid, that is, either dark chocolate or cocoa beverages. The pooled effects across all trials resulted in a significant reduction in SBP (−4.5 mmHg; 95% CI: −5.9, −3.2) and DBP (−2.5 mmHg; 95% CI: −3.9, −1.2).

Hooper et al. (2008) pooled results from soy trials (soy foods, soy protein isolate, and isoflavone extract) [90]. In five trials with 299 participants that measured the effects of soy food (tofu) on BP, they reported significant reductions in SBP (−5.76 mmHg; 95% CI: −12.3, 0.77) and DBP (−4.04 mmHg; 95% CI: −8.30, 0.22). In contrast, they reported nonsignificant effects of soy protein isolate on SBP (−1.60 mmHg; 95% CI: −3.62, 0.42) and DBP (−1.99 mmHg; 95% CI: −2.86, −1.12) from nine trials with 962 participants.

Isoflavone extract was examined in seven trials with 401 participants, which reported small effects on SBP (−2.60 mmHg; 95% CI: −5.20, 0.00) and DBP (0.05 mmHg; 95% CI: −1.66, 1.76) [90]. A later meta-analysis pooled the trial results of soy isoflavone extract supplements [99]. Fourteen trials with 789 participants were identified for analysis. The study durations ranged from 2 to 24 weeks, and the soy isoflavone dose ranged from 25 to 375 mg/day. Significant reductions in SBP (−2.02 mmHg; 95% CI: −3.65, −0.39) and nonsignificant effects on DBP (−0.13 mmHg; 95% CI: −1.21, 0.96) were observed. Another meta-analysis of soy isoflavone supplementation [101] pooled 11 trials that ranged in size from 18 to 302 participants, with the mean age ranging from 49 to 67 years, and BMI ranging from

25.5 to 32.2 kg/m^2. Isoflavone dosage ranged from 65 to 153 mg/day, and the intervention duration ranged from 1 to 12 months. The soy isoflavone group reportedly reduced SBP (−2.5 mmHg; 95% CI: −5.35, 0.34) and DBP (−1.5; 95% CI: −3.09, 0.17). When stratifying by hypertensive status, it was found that BP reductions were greater among hypertensive participants.

Finally, one meta-analysis did not differentiate trials by soy type, and it pooled 27 randomized controlled trials of soy protein. This meta-analysis showed a mean reduction in SBP (−2.21 mmHg; 95% CI: −4.10, −0.33) and DBP (−1.44 mmHg; 95% CI: −2.56, −0.31) [102]. Included studies comprised 1608 participants aged 18–75 years with baseline SBP ranging from 110 to 153 mmHg and baseline DBP ranging from 69 to 100 mmHg. The dose of soy ranged from 18 to 66 g/day, and the interventions lasted from 4 to 52 weeks.

Aside from evidence from these sources of flavonoids, there is insufficient evidence from human studies to report on the BP-regulation effects of flavonoid-rich fruits including pomegranate, cranberry, grapefruit, chokeberry, and marula [103].

2.3.4.4 Practical Message to Providers

Based on current evidence, it is inferred that pooled trials of flavonoid-containing foods or supplements were not associated with significant BP reduction. There is some suggestion that cocoa and chocolate could lower BP, but at high daily doses. There is substantial variation in terms of the form and the dosing of cocoa supplements, as well as evidence of publication bias. Additional trials are required to definitively guide regarding the clinical use of cocoa. In addition, it is necessary to consider possible weight gain from additional chocolate calories, which could offset BP lowering by chocolate itself. Similar to chocolate, trials of soy products provide inconclusive evidence of antihypertensive action. Individual trial results and the pooled effects from meta-analyses vary by the form of soy product and do not show consistent effects across types. Additional well-designed trials are necessary to elucidate whether flavonoids in foods or in supplements can result in meaningful effects on BP.

2.3.5 Coenzyme Q10

2.3.5.1 Common Sources of Coenzyme Q10

Coenzyme Q10 is an oil-soluble, vitamin-like substance present in most eukaryotic cells, primarily in the mitochondria. It is a component of the electron transport chain and participates in aerobic cellular respiration. Rich sources of dietary coenzyme Q10 mainly include meat, poultry, and fish. Other relatively rich sources include soybean, canola oils, and nuts. Coenzyme Q10 supplements are known as ubiquinone, Bio-Quinone Q10, ubidecarenone, ubiquinone 50, ubisemiquinone, and 2,3-dimethoxy-5-methyl-6-decaprenylenzoquinone.

2.3.5.2 Mechanism of Action

Interest in coenzyme Q10 (CoQ) is based on well-described biological functions as a component of the electron transport system and in aerobic cellular respiration.

There is both diet-derived and endogenous synthesis of CoQ. Its primary function is in generating energy (ATP); CoQ has been shown to reduce markers of oxidative stress [104,105]. CoQ may act as a free radical scavenger preventing depletion of NO directly [106,107] or by increasing endogenous antioxidant stores [23] and correcting provitamin deficiencies [108,109]. Coenzyme Q10 may also enhance prostacyclin (PGI_2) production or increase arterial smooth muscle sensitivity to PGI_2, both of which promote vasodilation [110]. Furthermore, it is believed that coenzyme Q10 reduces peripheral resistance by increasing endothelial concentrations of NO [111].

2.3.5.3   Coenzyme Q10 Supplement Trials

Observational studies suggest that coenzyme Q10 deficiency is associated with hypertension [112]. In spite of strong biological plausibility of benefit, only three randomized trials with clinical outcomes including BP have been reported. Two meta-analyses pooling results from these three trials comprising 120 participants have been published [105,113]. Trial lengths ranged from 8 to 12 weeks, and coenzyme Q10 dose ranged from 100 to 120 mg/day. Overall, it was found that compared with placebo, Q10 supplementation significantly reduced SBP (−10.72 mmHg; 95% CI: −13.77, −7.67) and DBP (−6.64 mmHg; 95% CI: −6.64, −5.17) [105].

2.3.5.4   Practical Message to Providers

Although meta-analyses of these three small trials report significant BP-lowering effects of coenzyme Q10 supplementation, these trials are of low methodological and reporting quality. Larger trials with longer duration and better assessment of the BP-regulation outcome are needed. Without additional clinical trial data, we do not currently recommend that individuals take coenzyme Q10 for BP control.

2.3.6   Garlic

2.3.6.1   Common Sources of Garlic

Garlic is a plant in the onion family that has been shown to have antiviral, anti-cholesterol, and antibacterial activity, with suggested effects on vascular activity. Garlic (*Allium sativum* or allicin) has been concentrated into pill or tablet form.

2.3.6.2   Mechanism of Action

Garlic is derived from the root of *Allium sativum*, which belongs to the onion family of plants. Garlic is believed to lower BP through several mechanisms [114]. Red blood cells catabolize garlic-derived organic polysulfides and produce hydrogen sulfide—a potent vasodilator [115]. Furthermore, garlic may activate kidney sodium–potassium pumps through unknown mechanisms and reduce BP through a sodium excretion pathway [116]. There is also laboratory evidence suggesting that garlic enhances endogenous production of antioxidants [114], promotes free-radical scavenging [117], and induces NO synthesis [118]. Other investigators posit that garlic's antihypertensive effect is through one of its constituents, allicin, which has angiotensin II inhibitory effects [119].

2.3.6.3   Garlic Supplement Trials

Based on biological plausibility, many trials testing the effects of garlic on BP have been conducted. There are a number of methodological challenges in designing trials of the effects of garlic on BP, for example, preparation, dose, and masking participants and investigators to treatment assignment. As such, there have been many trials, but only a handful of randomized controlled blind trials. Three meta-analyses of clinical trials studying the effect of garlic on BP report mixed findings. The earliest, published by Silagy et al. (1994), pooled 10 trials that enrolled 415 participants [120]. The trial duration ranged from 4 to 16 weeks with doses ranging from 600 to 900 mg/day of dried garlic powder, which is equivalent to 1.8–2.7 g/day of fresh garlic. Overall, it was reported that compared with placebo, garlic supplementation significantly lowered SBP (−7.7 mmHg; 95% CI: −11.0, −4.3) and DBP (−5.0 mmHg; 95% CI: −7.1, −2.9). However, the quality of the trials was considered methodologically poor. A later meta-analysis, published by Ried et al. (2008), pooled 11 trials that enrolled 565 participants for studying the effects on SBP and DBP [121]. Garlic powder dosage ranged from 600 to 900 mg/day, and the duration of the trials ranged from 12 to 23 weeks. In this meta-analysis, garlic supplementation lowered SBP (−4.6 mmHg; 95% CI: −7.4, −1.8) and DBP (−2.4 mmHg; 95% CI: −5.0, 0.1). A subgroup analysis in pooled trials that enrolled participants with hypertension showed greater effects on both SBP (−8.4 mmHg; 95% CI: −11.1, −5.6) and DBP (−7.3 mmHg; 95% CI: −8.8, −5.8). A third meta-analysis by Reinhart et al. (2008), including many of the same trials, reported similar effects [122].

The inconsistencies in the magnitude of BP-regulation effects of these meta-analyses (Sigaly and Ried) were examined in a systematic review that graded trial quality and methods as confounders in determining effect sizes [123]. In their review, Simons et al. found 32 trials that tested the effects of garlic on BP, of which only 14 had been included in meta-analyses by Sigaly or Ried. Of these 32 trials, they evaluated the quality of the trials' methodology and BP measurements. Of the five trials with the highest methodological quality, none concluded that garlic significantly reduced BP and only three of them had been included in the three meta-analyses above, suggesting that the large effect sizes reported may be biased by inclusion of trials of poor quality.

2.3.6.4   Practical Message to Providers

The results of these meta-analyses have important methodological limitations in terms of trial quality, thereby calling into question the pooled BP-regulation effects of garlic. Individual trials of the highest quality report null effects on BP. The fact that BP-lowering effects become apparent only with the inclusion of poor-quality trials suggests the need for additional high-quality trials. Currently, we do not recommend garlic for BP control.

2.3.7   L-Arginine

2.3.7.1   Common Sources of Arginine

Arginine is a nonessential amino acid that can be made by humans from common precursors, but it is mostly derived from diet. Dietary sources include dairy products, seafood, wheat germ, and nuts. L-arginine (isomer) has been synthesized and concentrated in the form of pills.

2.3.7.2 Mechanism of Action

Arginine is an amino acid that is classified as a semiessential or conditionally essential amino acid. The L-form of arginine (L-arginine) is a common natural amino acid found in a variety of food sources including dairy products, whole grains, and nuts, and it is a direct precursor of NO synthesis. L-arginine is believed to lower BP primarily through NO synthesis pathways that have direct effects on endothelial vasomotor function [124]. Furthermore, L-arginine has been shown to reduce angiotensin II synthesis [125,126] and modulate renal hemodynamics [124,126,127], and it has antioxidant properties, lowering the markers of oxidative stress [128].

2.3.7.3 Arginine Supplement Trials

In spite of well-established effects of arginine on NO pathways, few trials testing the effects on BP have been reported. One trial randomized 54 hypertensive and nonhypertensive outpatients in a double-blind trial to receive 2-g L-arginine, 4-g L-arginine, or placebo three times a day for 4 weeks [129]. Average ages ranged from 36 to 41 years, and BMI ranged from 23 to 28 kg/m^2. Twenty-four-hour ambulatory BP was recorded at baseline and at the end of follow-up. By the end of the trial, significant reductions in BP were noted among those given 4-g L-arginine supplement in both hypertensive and nonhypertensive groups. Within the hypertensive group, SBP lowered −5.6 mmHg (SD, 5.1) and DBP lowered −3.8 mmHg (SD, 3.4). Within the nonhypertensive group, SBP lowered −1.8 mmHg (SD, 1.7) and DBP lowered −1.8 mmHg (SD, 2.1). Significant reductions were not observed among the hypertensive and nonhypertensive patients treated with 2 g of L-arginine.

Another single-blind crossover trial evaluated the BP-regulation effects of L-arginine-enriched diet and L-arginine supplementation against a control group in six healthy volunteers [130]. The mean age of subjects was 39 years (SD, 10), and the mean BMI was 26 kg/m^2 (SD, 2). In both L-arginine interventions, decrease in BP was observed. Compared with the control group, the diet-based intervention resulted in a SBP reduction of −6.2 mmHg (95% CI: −11.8, −0.5) and a DBP reduction of −5.0 mmHg (95% CI: −7.2, −2.8). It should be noted that this intervention may be confounded by other dietary components that may lower BP. There was a similar magnitude of reductions noted in the L-arginine supplement group for both SBP (−6.2 mmHg; 95% CI: −10.5, −1.8) and DBP (−6.8 mmHg; 95% CI: −10.6, −3.0).

2.3.7.4 Practical Message to Providers

Evidence has been emerging that L-arginine plays a role in the reduction of human BP [131]. Furthermore, L-arginine, a substrate in NO synthesis, has well-established biologic plausibility. Despite promising results from several small trials, further trials of L-arginine supplementation are required to establish safety and efficacy. Increased dietary intake of L-arginine is consistent with current recommendations to consume dairy products, whole grains, and nuts—as in the DASH dietary pattern—but isolated effects of dietary L-arginine are unclear. At this time, healthcare providers should make no specific recommendations about L-arginine intake or supplementation for BP control.

2.4 SUPPLEMENTS WITH LIMITED OR NO EVIDENCE FOR BP REDUCTION

We performed a systematic review of the literature on a broad range of popular nutraceutical supplements to look for trials that examined BP-regulation effects. There were several supplements, with at least one clinical trial examining their effect on BP: bitter orange, carnitine, carotenoids (retinol, vitamin A, and beta carotene), chromium, cranberry, echinacea, ephedra/*Ephedra sinica*/Ma Huang, ginkgo, ginseng, grape seed extract, green tea, hawthorn or Crataegus berries, kava, lavender, melatonin, parsley (petroselinum), red clover, stevia (steviol, glycosides, and Rebaudisoside A), St. John's wort, saw palmetto, turmeric, valerian, vitamin E (alpha-tocopherol, beta-tocopherol, gamma-tocopherol, and tocotrienol), and zinc.

At this point, there is insufficient data to suggest that these nutrients should be recommended to lower BP. Literature review revealed no clinical trials examining the effects of the following agents on BP: aloe vera, astragalus, bilberry, black cohosh, black currant seed oil, bovine cartilage, bromelain, cat's claw, cayenne, chamomile, chasteberry, choline, chondroitin/structum, colloidal silver products, dandelion, dehydroepiandrosterone, Essiac/Flor-Essence, European elder, evening primrose oil, fennel, fenugreek, feverfew, ginger, glucosamine, goldenseal, Hoodia, hops, horse chestnut, inositol, inulin, iron, L-glutamic acid/L-glutamine, Lachesis, lecithin, milk thistle, mistletoe, noni, parsley (petroselinum), *Passiflora incarnata*, PC-SPES, peppermint oil, primrose oil, rosemary (aroma therapy), SAMe (S-adenosyl-L-methionine), selenium, Suma tea, thunder god vine, and yohimbe.

2.5 SUMMARY

In this chapter, we have summarized the evidence for the BP-lowering effects of mineral, antioxidant, and micronutrient supplements (Table 2.7). Overall, the BP effects examined in the setting of randomized trials and summarized by systematic reviews and meta-analyses, show, at best, modest effects of some supplements on BP. Oral potassium supplementation has the largest BP-lowering effect in the 3–5 mmHg range. Supplements of magnesium, vitamin D, or folic acid/B vitamins have minimal effects (1–2 mmHg range), whereas there was no clear and consistent evidence on BP reductions with the other supplements. The BP-lowering effects of supplements is far lower than those achieved with the whole dietary intervention or antihypertensive medication therapy. Adequate intake of these minerals, antioxidants, and micronutrients is best achieved by adoption of a dietary plan, for example, the DASH diet that contains sufficient amounts of these essential nutrients in combination.

TABLE 2.7
Summary: Take-Home Messages

Key Evidences	Recommendation for Health Care Providers
• Calcium, magnesium, vitamin D, or folic acid/B-vitamins supplementation only modestly lowers BP (1–2 mmHg)	• Evidence does not support a role for calcium, magnesium, vitamin D, or folic acid/B-vitamins supplementation as a therapy to lower BP • Adequate intakes, preferably from food sources, are recommended as part of the DASH dietary pattern and for other health benefits
• Oral potassium supplementation and dietary potassium lower SBP in the 3–5 mmHg range	• High potassium intake may lower BP and can be achieved with consumption of the DASH diet • High-dose potassium supplements (e.g., 40 meq/day) can lower BP but require prescription and may have side effects. Potassium supplements are therefore not recommended for BP control
• There is no clear and consistent evidence of BP-lowering effects of vitamin C, flavonoids, garlic, coenzyme Q10, or L-arginine	• There is insufficient evidence to support clinical use of supplements of vitamin C, flavonoids, garlic, coenzyme Q10, or L-arginine for the treatment of hypertension

REFERENCES

1. Appel LJ, Moore TJ, Obarzanek E, et al. A clinical trial of the effects of dietary patterns on blood pressure. DASH collaborative research group. *N Engl J Med.* 1997;336(16):1117–1124.
2. Appel LJ, Sacks FM, Carey VJ, et al. Effects of protein, monounsaturated fat, and carbohydrate intake on blood pressure and serum lipids: Results of the OmniHeart randomized trial. *JAMA.* 2005;294(19):2455–2464.
3. Institute of Medicine. Dietary reference intakes. http://fnic.nal.usda.gov/nal_display/index.php?info_center=4&tax_level=2&tax_subject=256&topic_id=1342. Accessed on October 24, 2011.
4. Cappuccio FP, Elliott P, Allender PS, Pryer J, Follman DA, Cutler JA. Epidemiologic association between dietary calcium intake and blood pressure: A meta-analysis of published data. *Am J Epidemiol.* 1995;142(9):935–945.
5. Resnick LM. Calcium metabolism in hypertension and allied metabolic disorders. *Diabetes Care.* 1991;14(6):505–520.
6. Resnick LM. Cellular ions in hypertension, insulin resistance, obesity, and diabetes: A unifying theme. *J Am Soc Nephrol.* 1992;3(4 Suppl):S78–85.
7. Hamet P. The evaluation of the scientific evidence for a relationship between calcium and hypertension. *J Nutr.* 1995;125(2 Suppl):311S–400S.
8. Resnick LM, Oparil S, Chait A, et al. Factors affecting blood pressure responses to diet: The vanguard study. *Am J Hypertens.* 2000;13(9):956–965.
9. Lijnen P, Petrov V. Dietary calcium, blood pressure, and cell membrane cation transport systems in males. *J Hypertens.* 1995;13(8):875–882.
10. Houston MC, Harper KJ. Potassium, magnesium, and calcium: Their role in both the cause and treatment of hypertension. *J Clin Hypertens (Greenwich).* 2008;10(7 Suppl 2):3–11.
11. Preuss HG. Diet, genetics and hypertension. *J Am Coll Nutr.* 1997;16(4):296–305.

12. Porsti I, Fan M, Koobi P, et al. High calcium diet down-regulates kidney angiotensin-converting enzyme in experimental renal failure. *Kidney Int.* 2004;66(6):2155–2166.
13. The effects of nonpharmacologic interventions on blood pressure of persons with high normal levels. Results of the trials of hypertension prevention, phase I. *JAMA.* 1992;267(9):1213–1220.
14. Cappuccio FP, Siani A, Strazzullo P. Oral calcium supplementation and blood pressure: An overview of randomized controlled trials. *J Hypertens.* 1989;7(12):941–946.
15. Allender PS, Cutler JA, Follmann D, Cappuccio FP, Pryer J, Elliott P. Dietary calcium and blood pressure: A meta-analysis of randomized clinical trials. *Ann Intern Med.* 1996;124(9):825–831.
16. Bucher HC, Cook RJ, Guyatt GH, et al. Effects of dietary calcium supplementation on blood pressure. A meta-analysis of randomized controlled trials. *JAMA.* 1996;275(13):1016–1022.
17. Griffith LE, Guyatt GH, Cook RJ, Bucher HC, Cook DJ. The influence of dietary and nondietary calcium supplementation on blood pressure: An updated meta-analysis of randomized controlled trials. *Am J Hypertens.* 1999;12(1 Part 1):84–92.
18. van Mierlo LA, Arends LR, Streppel MT, et al. Blood pressure response to calcium supplementation: A meta-analysis of randomized controlled trials. *J Hum Hypertens.* 2006;20(8):571–580.
19. Dickinson HO, Nicolson DJ, Cook JV, et al. Calcium supplementation for the management of primary hypertension in adults. *Cochrane Database Syst Rev.* 2006;(2):CD004639.
20. Wang L, Manson JE, Song Y, Sesso HD. Systematic review: Vitamin D and calcium supplementation in prevention of cardiovascular events. *Ann Intern Med.* 2010;152(5):315–323.
21. Bolland MJ, Avenell A, Baron JA, et al. Effect of calcium supplements on risk of myocardial infarction and cardiovascular events: Meta-analysis. *BMJ.* 2010;341:c3691.
22. Song Y, Sesso HD, Manson JE, Cook NR, Buring JE, Liu S. Dietary magnesium intake and risk of incident hypertension among middle-aged and older US women in a 10-year follow-up study. *Am J Cardiol.* 2006;98(12):1616–1621.
23. Singh RB, Rastogi SS, Mehta PJ, Cameron EA. Magnesium metabolism in essential hypertension. *Acta Cardiol.* 1989;44(4):313–322.
24. Teragawa H, Kato M, Yamagata T, Matsuura H, Kajiyama G. Magnesium causes nitric oxide independent coronary artery vasodilation in humans. *Heart.* 2001;86(2):212–216.
25. Resnick L. The cellular ionic basis of hypertension and allied clinical conditions. *Prog Cardiovasc Dis.* 1999;42(1):1–22.
26. Bo S, Pisu E. Role of dietary magnesium in cardiovascular disease prevention, insulin sensitivity and diabetes. *Curr Opin Lipidol.* 2008;19(1):50–56.
27. Paolisso G, Barbagallo M. Hypertension, diabetes mellitus, and insulin resistance: The role of intracellular magnesium. *Am J Hypertens.* 1997;10(3):346–355.
28. Das UN. Nutrients, essential fatty acids and prostaglandins interact to augment immune responses and prevent genetic damage and cancer. *Nutrition.* 1989;5(2):106–110.
29. Das UN. Nutritional factors in the pathobiology of human essential hypertension. *Nutrition.* 2001;17(4):337–346.
30. Sacks FM, Willett WC, Smith A, Brown LE, Rosner B, Moore TJ. Effect on blood pressure of potassium, calcium, and magnesium in women with low habitual intake. *Hypertension.* 1998;31(1):131–138.
31. Jee SH, Miller ER III, Guallar E, Singh VK, Appel LJ, Klag MJ. The effect of magnesium supplementation on blood pressure: A meta-analysis of randomized clinical trials. *Am J Hypertens.* 2002;15(8):691–696.
32. Dickinson HO, Nicolson DJ, Campbell F, et al. Magnesium supplementation for the management of essential hypertension in adults. *Cochrane Database Syst Rev.* 2006;3:CD004640.

33. Buemi M, Senatore M, Corica F, et al. Diet and arterial hypertension: Is the sodium ion alone important? *Med Res Rev.* 2002;22(4):419–428.

34. Fang J, Madhavan S, Alderman MH. Dietary potassium intake and stroke mortality. *Stroke.* 2000;31(7):1532–1537.

35. Haddy FJ, Vanhoutte PM, Feletou M. Role of potassium in regulating blood flow and blood pressure. *Am J Physiol Regul Integr Comp Physiol.* 2006;290(3):R546–52.

36. Taddei S, Mattei P, Virdis A, Sudano I, Ghiadoni L, Salvetti A. Effect of potassium on vaso-dilation to acetylcholine in essential hypertension. *Hypertension.* 1994;23(4):485–490.

37. Cappuccio FP, MacGregor GA. Does potassium supplementation lower blood pressure? A meta-analysis of published trials. *J Hypertens.* 1991;9(5):465–473.

38. Whelton PK, He J, Cutler JA, et al. Effects of oral potassium on blood pressure. Meta-analysis of randomized controlled clinical trials. *JAMA.* 1997;277(20):1624–1632.

39. Geleijnse JM, Kok FJ, Grobbee DE. Blood pressure response to changes in sodium and potassium intake: A metaregression analysis of randomised trials. *J Hum Hypertens.* 2003;17(7):471–480.

40. Dickinson HO, Nicolson DJ, Campbell F, Beyer FR, Mason J. Potassium supplementa-tion for the management of primary hypertension in adults. *Cochrane Database Syst Rev.* 2006;3:CD004641.

41. May JM. How does ascorbic acid prevent endothelial dysfunction? *Free Radic Biol Med.* 2000;28(9):1421–1429.

42. Jackson TS, Xu A, Vita JA, Keaney JF Jr. Ascorbate prevents the interaction of super-oxide and nitric oxide only at very high physiological concentrations. *Circ Res.* 1998;83(9):916–922.

43. Hoitink AWJH. [Researches on the influence of vitamin C administration on the human organism, in particular in connection with the working capacity]. *Verh Nederlands Inst Praevent.* 1946;4:1.

44. Yoshioka M, Aoyama K, Matsushita T. Effects of ascorbic acid on blood pressure and ascorbic acid metabolism in spontaneously hypertensive rats (SH rats). *Int J Vitam Nutr Res.* 1985;55(3):301–307.

45. Ettarh RR, Odigie IP, Adigun SA. Vitamin C lowers blood pressure and alters vas-cular responsiveness in salt-induced hypertension. *Can J Physiol Pharmacol.* 2002;80(12):1199–1202.

46. Koh ET. Effect of vitamin C on blood parameters of hypertensive subjects. *J Okla State Med Assoc.* 1984;77(6):177–182.

47. Feldman EB, Gold S, Greene J, et al. Ascorbic acid supplements and blood pressure. A four-week pilot study. *Ann N Y Acad Sci.* 1992;669:342–344.

48. Stein HB, Hasan A, Fox IH. Ascorbic acid-induced uricosuria. A consequence of mega-vitamin therapy. *Ann Intern Med.* 1976;84(4):385–388.

49. Feig DI, Kang DH, Johnson RJ. Uric acid and cardiovascular risk. *N Engl J Med.* 2008;359(17):1811–1821.

50. Levine M, Conry-Cantilena C, Wang Y, et al. Vitamin C pharmacokinetics in healthy volunteers: Evidence for a recommended dietary allowance. *Proc Natl Acad Sci U S A.* 1996;93(8):3704–3709.

51. Solzbach U, Hornig B, Jeserich M, Just H. Vitamin C improves endothelial dys-function of epicardial coronary arteries in hypertensive patients. *Circulation.* 1997;96(5):1513–1519.

52. Huang A, Vita JA, Venema RC, Keaney JF Jr. Ascorbic acid enhances endothelial nitric-oxide synthase activity by increasing intracellular tetrahydrobiopterin. *J Biol Chem.* 2000;275(23):17399–17406.

53. Baker TA, Milstien S, Katusic ZS. Effect of vitamin C on the availability of tetrahydrobiopterin in human endothelial cells. *J Cardiovasc Pharmacol.* 2001;37(3):333–338.

54. Carroll MF, Schade DS. Timing of antioxidant vitamin ingestion alters postprandial proatherogenic serum markers. *Circulation.* 2003;108(1):24–31.
55. Moran JP, Cohen L, Greene JM, et al. Plasma ascorbic acid concentrations relate inversely to blood pressure in human subjects. *Am J Clin Nutr.* 1993;57(2):213–217.
56. McCarron DA, Morris CD, Henry HJ, Stanton JL. Blood pressure and nutrient intake in the United States. *Science.* 1984;224(4656):1392–1398.
57. Svetkey LP, Loria CM. Blood pressure effects of vitamin C: What's the key question? *Hypertension.* 2002;40(6):789–791.
58. McRae MP. Is vitamin C an effective antihypertensive supplement? A review and analysis of the literature. *J Chiropr Med.* 2006;5(2):60–64.
59. Ness AR, Chee D, Elliott P. Vitamin C and blood pressure—an overview. *J Hum Hypertens.* 1997;11(6):343–350.
60. Juraschek SP, Guallar E, Appel LJ, Miller ER III. Effects of vitamin C supplementation on blood pressure: A meta-analysis of randomized controlled trials. American heart association: Nutrition, physical medicine, and metabolism conference 2010: San Francisco, CA, 2010.
61. Bjelakovic G, Nikolova D, Gluud LL, Simonetti RG, Gluud C. Mortality in randomized trials of antioxidant supplements for primary and secondary prevention: Systematic review and meta-analysis. *JAMA.* 2007;297(8):842–857.
62. Sesso HD, Buring JE, Christen WG, et al. Vitamins E and C in the prevention of cardiovascular disease in men: The physicians' health study II randomized controlled trial. *JAMA.* 2008;300(18):2123–2133.
63. Cook NR, Albert CM, Gaziano JM, et al. A randomized factorial trial of vitamins C and E and beta carotene in the secondary prevention of cardiovascular events in women: Results from the women's antioxidant cardiovascular study. *Arch Intern Med.* 2007;167(15):1610–1618.
64. Holick MF. Vitamin D deficiency. *N Engl J Med.* 2007;357(3):266–281.
65. Norman AW. From vitamin D to hormone D: Fundamentals of the vitamin D endocrine system essential for good health. *Am J Clin Nutr.* 2008;88(2):491S–499S.
66. Abrahamsen B, Masud T, Avenell A, et al. Patient level pooled analysis of 68 500 patients from seven major vitamin D fracture trials in U.S. and Europe. *BMJ.* 2010;340(7738):139.
67. Bischoff-Ferrari HA, Willett WC, Wong JB, Giovannucci E, Dietrich T, Dawson-Hughes B. Fracture prevention with vitamin D supplementation: A meta-analysis of randomized controlled trials. *J Am Med Assoc.* 2005;293(18):2257–2264.
68. Raiten DJ, Picciano MF. Vitamin D and health in the 21st century: Bone and beyond. executive summary. *Am J Clin Nutr.* 2004;80(6 Suppl):1673S–1677S.
69. Holick MF. Vitamin D: Importance in the prevention of cancers, type 1 diabetes, heart disease, and osteoporosis. *Am J Clin Nutr.* 2004;79(3):362–371.
70. Teegarden D, Donkin SS. Vitamin D: Emerging new roles in insulin sensitivity. *Nutr Res Rev.* 2009;22(1):82–92.
71. Autier P, Gandini S. Vitamin D supplementation and total mortality: A meta-analysis of randomized controlled trials. *Arch Intern Med.* 2007;167(16):1730–1737.
72. Li YC, Kong J, Wei M, Chen ZF, Liu SQ, Cao LP. 1,25-dihydroxyvitamin D(3) is a negative endocrine regulator of the renin-angiotensin system. *J Clin Invest.* 2002;110(2):229–238.
73. Yuan W, Pan W, Kong J, et al. 1,25-dihydroxyvitamin D3 suppresses renin gene transcription by blocking the activity of the cyclic AMP response element in the renin gene promoter. *J Biol Chem.* 2007;282(41):29821–29830.
74. Bednarski R, Donderski R, Manitius J. Role of vitamin D3 in arterial blood pressure control. *Pol Merkur Lekarski.* 2007;23(136):307–310.

75. Sugden JA, Davies JI, Witham MD, Morris AD, Struthers AD. Vitamin D improves endothelial function in patients with type 2 diabetes mellitus and low vitamin D levels. *Diabet Med.* 2008;25(3):320–325.
76. Pfeifer M, Begerow B, Minne HW, Nachtigall D, Hansen C. Effects of a short-term vitamin D(3) and calcium supplementation on blood pressure and parathyroid hormone levels in elderly women. *J Clin Endocrinol Metab.* 2001;86(4):1633–1637.
77. Witham MD, Nadir MA, Struthers AD. Effect of vitamin D on blood pressure: A systematic review and meta-analysis. *J Hypertens.* 2009;27(10):1948–1954.
78. Pittas AG, Chung M, Trikalinos T, et al. Systematic review: Vitamin D and cardiometabolic outcomes. *Ann Intern Med.* 2010;152(5):307–314.
79. van Guldener C, Nanayakkara PW, Stehouwer CD. Homocysteine and blood pressure. *Curr Hypertens Rep.* 2003;5(1):26–31.
80. Stehouwer CD, van Guldener C. Does homocysteine cause hypertension? *Clin Chem Lab Med.* 2003;41(11):1408–1411.
81. Rodrigo R, Passalacqua W, Araya J, Orellana M, Rivera G. Homocysteine and essential hypertension. *J Clin Pharmacol.* 2003;43(12):1299–1306.
82. Doshi SN, Moat SJ, McDowell IFW, Lewis MJ, Goodfellow J. Lowering plasma homocysteine with folic acid in cardiovascular disease: What will the trials tell us? *Atherosclerosis.* 2002;165(1):1–3.
83. Antoniades C, Shirodaria C, Warrick N, et al. 5-methyltetrahydrofolate rapidly improves endothelial function and decreases superoxide production in human vessels: Effects on vascular tetrahydrobiopterin availability and endothelial nitric oxide synthase coupling. *Circulation.* 2006;114(11):1193–1201.
84. Moens AL, Champion HC, Claeys MJ, et al. High-dose folic acid pretreatment blunts cardiac dysfunction during ischemia coupled to maintenance of high-energy phosphates and reduces postreperfusion injury. *Circulation.* 2008;117(14):1810–1819.
85. Wilmink HW, Stroes ES, Erkelens WD, et al. Influence of folic acid on postprandial endothelial dysfunction. *Arterioscler Thromb Vasc Biol.* 2000;20(1):185–188.
86. McRae MP. High-dose folic acid supplementation effects on endothelial function and blood pressure in hypertensive patients: A meta-analysis of randomized controlled clinical trials. *J Chiropr Med.* 2009;8(1):15–24.
87. van Dijk RA, Rauwerda JA, Steyn M, Twisk JW, Stehouwer CD. Long-term homocysteine-lowering treatment with folic acid plus pyridoxine is associated with decreased blood pressure but not with improved brachial artery endothelium-dependent vasodilation or carotid artery stiffness: A 2-year, randomized, placebo-controlled trial. *Arterioscler Thromb Vasc Biol.* 2001;21(12):2072–2079.
88. Toole JF, Malinow MR, Chambless LE, et al. Lowering homocysteine in patients with ischemic stroke to prevent recurrent stroke, myocardial infarction, and death: The vitamin intervention for stroke prevention (VISP) randomized controlled trial. *JAMA.* 2004;291(5):565–575.
89. Miller ER III, Juraschek S, Pastor-Barriuso R, Bazzano LA, Appel LJ, Guallar E. Meta-analysis of folic acid supplementation trials on risk of cardiovascular disease and risk interaction with baseline homocysteine levels. *Am J Cardiol.* 2010;106(4):517–527.
90. Hooper L, Kroon PA, Rimm EB, et al. Flavonoids, flavonoid-rich foods, and cardiovascular risk: A meta-analysis of randomized controlled trials. *Am J Clin Nutr.* 2008;88(1):38–50.
91. Grassi D, Desideri G, Croce G, Tiberti S, Aggio A, Ferri C. Flavonoids, vascular function, and cardiovascular protection. *Curr Pharm Des.* 2009;15(10):1072–1084.
92. Stoclet JC, Chataigneau T, Ndiaye M, et al. Vascular protection by dietary polyphenols. *Eur J Pharmacol.* 2004;500(1–3):299–313.

93. Schini-Kerth VB, Auger C, Etienne-Selloum N, Chaigneau T. Polyphenol-induced endothelium-dependent relaxations role of NO and EDHF. *Adv Pharmacol.* 2010;60:133–175.

94. Desch S, Schmidt J, Kobler D, et al. Effect of cocoa products on blood pressure: Systematic review and meta-analysis. *Am J Hypertens.* 2010;23(1):97–103.

95. Dohadwala MM, Vita JA. Grapes and cardiovascular disease. *J Nutr.* 2009;139(9):1788S–1793S.

96. Sarr M, Chataigneau M, Martins S, et al. Red wine polyphenols prevent angiotensin II-induced hypertension and endothelial dysfunction in rats: Role of NADPH oxidase. *Cardiovasc Res.* 2006;71(4):794–802.

97. Yung LM, Leung FP, Wong WT, et al. Tea polyphenols benefit vascular function. *Inflammopharmacology.* 2008;16(5):230–234.

98. Negishi H, Xu JW, Ikeda K, Njelekela M, Nara Y, Yamori Y. Black and green tea polyphenols attenuate blood pressure increases in stroke-prone spontaneously hypertensive rats. *J Nutr.* 2004;134(1):38–42.

99. Taku K, Lin N, Cai D, et al. Effects of soy isoflavone extract supplements on blood pressure in adult humans: Systematic review and meta-analysis of randomized placebo-controlled trials. *J Hypertens.* 2010;28(10):1971–1982.

100. Taubert D, Roesen R, Schomig E. Effect of cocoa and tea intake on blood pressure: A meta-analysis. *Arch Intern Med.* 2007;167(7):626–634.

101. Liu XX, Li SH, Chen JZ, et al. Effect of soy isoflavones on blood pressure: A meta-analysis of randomized controlled trials. *Nutr Metab Cardiovasc Dis.* 2011 Feb 8. [Epub ahead of print]

102. Dong JY, Tong X, Wu ZW, Xun PC, He K, Qin LQ. Effect of soya protein on blood pressure: A meta-analysis of randomised controlled trials. *Br J Nutr.* 2011:1–10.

103. Chong MF, Macdonald R, Lovegrove JA. Fruit polyphenols and CVD risk: A review of human intervention studies. *Br J Nutr.* 2010;104 (3 Suppl):S28–S39.

104. Niklowitz P, Sonnenschein A, Janetzky B, Andler W, Menke T. Enrichment of coenzyme Q10 in plasma and blood cells: Defense against oxidative damage. *Int J Biol Sci.* 2007;3(4):257–262.

105. Ho MJ, Bellusci A, Wright JM. Blood pressure lowering efficacy of coenzyme Q10 for primary hypertension. *Cochrane Database Syst Rev.* 2009;(4):CD007435.

106. Wyman M, Leonard M, Morledge T. Coenzyme Q10: A therapy for hypertension and statin-induced myalgia? *Cleve Clin J Med.* 2010;77(7):435–442.

107. Pepe S, Marasco SF, Haas SJ, Sheeran FL, Krum H, Rosenfeldt FL. Coenzyme Q10 in cardiovascular disease. *Mitochondrion.* 2007;(7 Suppl):S154–S167.

108. Tran MT, Mitchell TM, Kennedy DT, Giles JT. Role of coenzyme Q10 in chronic heart failure, angina, and hypertension. *Pharmacotherapy.* 2001;21(7):797–806.

109. Yamagami T, Shibata N, Folkers K. Bioenergetics in clinical medicine. Studies on coenzyme Q10 and essential hypertension. *Res Commun Chem Pathol Pharmacol.* 1975;11(2):273–288.

110. Lonnrot K, Porsti I, Alho H, Wu X, Hervonen A, Tolvanen JP. Control of arterial tone after long-term coenzyme Q10 supplementation in senescent rats. *Br J Pharmacol.* 1998;124(7):1500–1506.

111. McCarty MF. Coenzyme Q versus hypertension: Does CoQ decrease endothelial superoxide generation? *Med Hypotheses.* 1999;53(4):300–304.

112. Burke BE, Neuenschwander R, Olson RD. Randomized, double-blind, placebo-controlled trial of coenzyme Q10 in isolated systolic hypertension. *South Med J.* 2001;94(11):1112–1117.

113. Rosenfeldt FL, Haas SJ, Krum H, et al. Coenzyme Q10 in the treatment of hypertension: A meta-analysis of the clinical trials. *J Hum Hypertens.* 2007;21(4):297–306.

114. Banerjee SK, Mukherjee PK, Maulik SK. Garlic as an antioxidant: The good, the bad, and the ugly. *Phytother Res.* 2003;17(2):97–106.

115. Benavides GA, Squadrito GL, Mills RW, et al. Hydrogen sulfide mediates the vasoactivity of garlic. *Proc Natl Acad Sci U S A*. 2007;104(46):17977–17982.
116. Al-Qattan KK, Khan I, Alnaqeeb MA, Ali M. Mechanism of garlic (*Allium sativum*) induced reduction of hypertension in 2K-1C rats: A possible mediation of Na/H exchanger isoform-1. *Prostaglandins Leukot Essent Fatty Acids*. 2003;69(4):217–222.117. Prasad K, Laxdal VA, Yu M, Raney BL. Evaluation of hydroxyl radical-scavenging property of garlic. *Mol Cell Biochem*. 1996;154(1):55–63.
118. Maslin DJ, Brown CA, Das I, Zhang XH. Nitric oxide—a mediator of the effects of garlic? *Biochem Soc Trans*. 1997;25(3):408S.
119. Sharifi AM, Darabi R, Akbarloo N. Investigation of antihypertensive mechanism of garlic in 2K1C hypertensive rat. *J Ethnopharmacol*. 2003;86(2–3):219–224.
120. Silagy CA, Neil HA. A meta-analysis of the effect of garlic on blood pressure. *J Hypertens*. 1994;12(4):463–468.
121. Ried K, Frank OR, Stocks NP, Fakler P, Sullivan T. Effect of garlic on blood pressure: A systematic review and meta-analysis. *BMC Cardiovasc Disord*. 2008;8:13.
122. Reinhart KM, Coleman CI, Teevan C, Vachhani P, White CM. Effects of garlic on blood pressure in patients with and without systolic hypertension: A meta-analysis. *Ann Pharmacother*. 2008;42(12):1766–1771.
123. Simons S, Wollersheim H, Thien T. A systematic review on the influence of trial quality on the effect of garlic on blood pressure. *Neth J Med*. 2009;67(6):212–219.
124. Gokce N. L-arginine and hypertension. *J Nutr*. 2004;134(10 Suppl):2807S–2811S; discussion 2818S–2819S.
125. Rajapakse NW, De Miguel C, Das S, Mattson DL. Exogenous L-arginine ameliorates angiotensin II-induced hypertension and renal damage in rats. *Hypertension*. 2008;52(6):1084–1090.
126. Higashi Y, Oshima T, Ono N, et al. Intravenous administration of L-arginine inhibits angiotensin-converting enzyme in humans. *J Clin Endocrinol Metab*. 1995;80(7):2198–2202.
127. Chen PY, Sanders PW. L-arginine abrogates salt-sensitive hypertension in Dahl/Rapp rats. *J Clin Invest*. 1991;88(5):1559–1567.
128. Lin CC, Tsai WC, Chen JY, Li YH, Lin LJ, Chen JH. Supplements of L-arginine attenuate the effects of high-fat meal on endothelial function and oxidative stress. *Int J Cardiol*. 2008;127(3):337–341.
129. Ast J, Jablecka A, Bogdanski P, Smolarek I, Krauss H, Chmara E. Evaluation of the antihypertensive effect of L-arginine supplementation in patients with mild hypertension assessed with ambulatory blood pressure monitoring. *Med Sci Monit*. 2010;16(5):CR266–CR271.
130. Siani A, Pagano E, Iacone R, Iacoviello L, Scopacasa F, Strazzullo P. Blood pressure and metabolic changes during dietary L-arginine supplementation in humans. *Am J Hypertens*. 2000;13(5 Pt 1):547–551.
131. Cylwik D, Mogielnicki A, Buczko W. L-arginine and cardiovascular system. *Pharmacol Rep*. 2005;57(1):14–22.

3 Sodium and Blood Pressure

Cheryl A.M. Anderson
Johns Hopkins Medical Institutions

CONTENTS

3.1 INTRODUCTION

A substantial body of research has been conducted to examine the relationship between dietary sodium intake and blood pressure (BP). These research studies have employed various study designs and approaches including animal studies [1–3], human genetic studies [4,5], observational epidemiologic studies [6–14], controlled interventions [15–24], and meta-analyses [25–27]. The resulting evidence largely supports the conclusion that excessive sodium intake increases BP in human populations.

In this chapter, we review published literature on the relationship between dietary sodium intake and BP and provide recommendations for practitioners. In making recommendations, we consider the strength of the evidence, giving greater emphasis to results from data generated in prospective studies or controlled interventions in which there is little evidence to the contrary.

3.2 DIETARY SODIUM INTAKE

3.2.1 INTAKE OF SODIUM IS REQUIRED FOR PHYSIOLOGIC FUNCTIONS

Sodium has important physiologic roles in mammals, including determination of the membrane potential of cells and active transport of molecules across cell membranes. As the principal cation of the extracellular fluid, sodium is important in the regulation of extracellular fluid volume and, as a result, is also important in the regulation of plasma volume. Of the total sodium content of the body, about 95% is found in the extracellular fluid. The concentration of sodium within the cell is usually less than 10% of that found outside cell membranes. To maintain this concentration gradient, an active energy-dependent process is required. In association with sodium, chloride is the principal osmotically active anion in the extracellular fluid (sodium chloride). Sodium chloride is important for maintaining fluid and electrolyte balance.

Although sodium is required for physiologic functions, the amount of dietary sodium needed for growth and for adult humans is low: estimated at 500 mg/day [28]. In fact, human populations have survived with sodium intakes as low as 200 mg/day (10 mmol/day) as observed in Yanomamo Indians in Brazil, whose exposure to sodium comes mostly from that occurring naturally in foods and water [29]. In contrast, human populations have also survived with intakes as high as 10,300 mg/day (450 mmol/day) as observed in populations in northern Japan, whose exposure to sodium comes mostly from salting of meats, fish, vegetables, and dairy products [30,31]. It has been suggested that the adverse effects of high dietary sodium intake result from human kidneys not being adapted to excrete excessively large quantities of sodium [31,32].

3.2.2 SOURCES OF DIETARY SODIUM

Very little sodium occurs naturally in foods comprising human diets. It has been estimated that approximately 90% of dietary sodium, in contemporary diets of developed and urban populations, is consumed as salt (sodium chloride) that is largely added in commercially processed foods [33–38]. Processed foods also provide sodium in forms such as sodium bicarbonate, monosodium glutamate, sodium phosphate, sodium carbonate, and sodium benzoate. Data relevant to the twenty-first century suggest that foods and food groups supplying the most dietary sodium in the diets of populations in Japan, United Kingdom, and the United States are commercially processed foods such as breads, grains, cereals, soups, sauces, and cured meats [33]. Discretionary sodium intake, that is, sodium chloride added to foods during home preparation or at the table, is a modest contributor to overall intake. These findings are similar to earlier reports showing that excessive salt intake in modern diets in these countries is mainly a result of salting in commercial food processing [34–38].

In contrast, data from rural population samples from the People's Republic of China (PRC) suggest that discretionary sodium use accounts for most sodium intake. Only a small proportion of sodium in foods consumed in PRC population samples is intrinsic (e.g., sodium in milk), and the majority is added by individuals while cooking or at the table [33]. This observation has been reported in other studies as well [9].

3.2.3 Sodium Intake Levels in Different Populations

There are striking differences among populations across the world regarding dietary sodium intake. One of the most recognizable early reports of the differences in sodium intake across populations was published by Louis Dahl in 1960 [13]. Daily sodium intake was reported to be as high as 10,600 mg/day (460 mmol/day) in Akita prefecture in northeast Japan and as low as 1560 mg/day (68 mmol/day) in Alaskan Eskimos. As populations become more industrialized, their dietary sodium intake increases [33]. Moreover, there is evidence that the current average sodium intake, for many countries, is well above the current World Health Organization recommendation of <2000 mg/day [39]. Still notably high, sodium intake in northern Japan approaches 5000 mg/day [33,40–43]. While data suggest that sodium intake of Japanese declined from the 1950s to the 1980s [44], data from International Study of Salt and Blood Pressure (INTERSALT) (1980s) and International Population Study on Macronutrients and BP (INTERMAP) (1990s) show only small differences in intakes [10,33], suggesting that the decline has stopped and that intake levels remain in excess of recommendations.

In the United States and other developed countries, high sodium intake is evident from contemporary surveillance systems [40–48]. Several authoritative medical bodies in the United States recommend sodium intakes that are lower than the current levels being consumed. The U.S. Department of Agriculture's Dietary Guidelines for Americans recommends sodium intake of <2300 mg/day for persons 2 years of age or older and <1500 mg/day for persons who have hypertension or prehypertension, diabetes, or kidney disease; adults over age 50; and African Americans of any age—groups that account for 69% of the total U.S. population [49]. The recommendation of <1500 mg/day is also supported by the Institute of Medicine [50] and the American Heart Association [51].

U.S. adults exceed recommended intake levels regardless of sex, age, race/ethnicity, income, or health conditions. The mean dietary sodium intake of the U.S. population has been estimated to be over 3600 mg/day [52,53]. These estimates are derived from 24-h urinary sodium excretion data, as well as self-reported dietary intake data. An analysis of 38 studies conducted in the United States between 1957 and 2003 suggested that the mean 24-h urinary sodium excretion per person was 3526 mg (95% CI: 3380, 3672 mg). When accounting for the fact that 95% of daily dietary sodium intake is excreted in the urine [54], this excretion amount corresponds to an intake of 3712 mg/day. The National Health and Nutrition Examination Survey regularly estimates the sodium intake of the U.S. population by using 24-h dietary recalls, which requires individuals to report intake over the past 24-h period. A challenge in the assessment of sodium intake is measurement errors. Dietary recall data may be biased because of errors in self-reporting and inaccurate or incomplete food databases [54]. Also, 24-h collections of urinary sodium excretions are subject to error and bias because of individual sodium losses through sweat and feces, as well as potential laboratory errors [54]. However, national estimates derived from both methods align and indicate that the consumption of sodium exceeds recommendations.

In the United States, sodium intake has been in excess of what is recommended, as per findings in the 40 years that sodium intake has been monitored, and trends persist across age and gender groups [53,55]. The general pattern of increased intake of sodium over time resembles the general pattern of increased intake of total kilocalories over the same period of time [56]. When kilocalorie intake is taken into account, the differences seen among children and adult men and women disappear to a large degree, suggesting that on a calorie-per-calorie basis, children, men, and women in the United States are eating equivalent amounts of sodium [57]. More specifically, higher intake of sodium in men than in women is primarily a function of consuming more food, not necessarily different foods. Sodium intake in the U.S. adult population appears to be well above current guidelines and does not appear to have decreased with time [53].

Given the excessive consumption of sodium in most populations, efforts to better understand the role of sodium in health, particularly in BP regulation, have been taken.

3.3   RELATIONSHIP BETWEEN SODIUM AND BLOOD PRESSURE

Extensive concordant research evidence from every research method is the foundation for the repeated conclusion by independent expert groups that high dietary sodium intake is etiologically related to the worldwide epidemics of prehypertension and hypertension and other cardiovascular diseases (CVDs) [21,31,33,58–66]. A large number of studies have been done in basic science laboratories, in observational epidemiologic settings, and with controlled intervention designs.

Excess sodium intake is one of several etiologic factors important in the development of hypertension. It has been suggested that the largest population-attributable risks for hypertension are due to overweight and obesity, regular nonnarcotic analgesic use, physical inactivity, poor dietary pattern, and nonadherence to a low-sodium diet [67]. However, others argue that the evidence for sodium's role in high BP, particularly in the age-related rise in BP, is much greater than that for other lifestyle factors such as overweight, low consumption of fruits and vegetables, and physical inactivity [68,69].

3.3.1   Key Evidence from Animal Research

The role of sodium in regulating BP has been studied in numerous animal models, including rats, dogs, chickens, rabbits, baboons, and chimpanzees [1–3,70]. Notably, in all forms of animal models, a high intake of sodium chloride is essential for BP to rise. Meneely et al. conducted a study in rats by varying the dietary sodium chloride given to rats for 9 months and observed its effect on BP [3]. Data suggested that increase in salt intake in rats was associated with an increase in the systolic BP. A study by Denton et al. investigated the long-term effect of adding sodium chloride supplements to the usual diet of chimpanzees [1]. Although the systolic BP of the two groups of chimpanzees, that is, the group on a diet with increased sodium chloride and the group on normal diet, was comparable at baseline, the BP of the chimpanzees on the diet with increased sodium chloride was significantly higher at 14 and 20 months, compared with the group on normal diet. The investigators stopped the intervention at 20 months and noticed that BP in both groups returned to baseline after 3–6 months. Chimpanzees have over 98% genetic homology with humans, and studies by Denton et al. suggest that there is a direct and progressive rise in the BP of chimpanzees with gradual increases in sodium chloride intake on levels comparable to levels of human sodium chloride intake (500 to over 10,000 mg/day).

3.3.2 KEY EVIDENCE IN HUMAN RESEARCH

3.3.2.1 Human Genetic Studies

There are several rare genetic causes of both high BP and low BP. Researchers have identified genetic variants in novel pathways that influence BP, pulse pressure, and mean arterial pressure [71,72]. Studies that have examined the rare genetic syndromes, such as glucocorticoid-remediable aldosteronism and Gitelman's syndrome that cause high BP, suggest that sodium chloride intake is important in regulating BP in humans. Furthermore, these genetic conditions all result in interference with the kidney's ability to excrete sodium chloride, thereby leading to high BP [4,5]. In genetic hypertension, BP is considerably affected if sodium chloride intake is altered, and there is evidence that genetic factors influence BP response to sodium intake in essential hypertension. However, to date, evidence of the genetic influence on sodium needs has been limited, and sodium intake guidelines do not take genotype into account [50].

3.3.2.2 Epidemiologic Studies

3.3.2.2.1 Ecologic Studies of Isolated Populations, Regions, and Migration

Isolated populations: There have been studies on isolated populations where circumstances have exposed specific communities to increased sodium chloride while others in the population remain unexposed. One such example is a rural community in Nigeria, which used a salt lake as its primary source of water. It was noted that the BP of those drinking the salt water was higher than the BP of those who had other sources of water [6]. A similar observation was made in the Solomon Islands where islanders using seawater as a source of water had significantly higher BP than those using fresh water [7]. Additionally, the Qash'qai tribe in Iran, which had access to salt deposits on the ground, developed high BP and an age-related rise in BP similar to that seen in Western populations, although all other aspects of their lifestyle were similar to those of other underdeveloped communities that did not have access to salt [8]. These three examples illustrate the possible association between increased salt intake and BP. Though the communities being compared were similar in other aspects of lifestyle and diet, it cannot be ruled out that other factors might possibly account for the observed association.

Regional studies: Observational studies have been conducted within populations of similar ancestry, aiming to compare whether groups with higher average sodium intake have greater prevalence of high BP. For example, studies comparing northern Chinese populations with southern Chinese populations [9] and northern Japanese populations with southern Japanese populations [10,13,73] have been conducted. In these studies, a twofold or greater difference in sodium intake correlated with similar differences in hypertension prevalence. The influence of high potassium intake in those populations with low sodium intake and low BP was not evaluated in these studies.

Migration studies: There have been two well-documented migration studies on BP. Jiang He et al. studied the effect of rural–urban migration among a remote Chinese tribe, Yi [11]. The Yi people had been isolated for many generations due to political and geographical reasons. In recent times, some of the Yi people migrated to urban areas. He et al. observed that the prevalence of high BP was low among the older rural Yi population. In contrast, the Yi migrants had a BP distribution similar to that in the Han population in the urban areas. Among the many contributing factors, a difference in diet intake has been proposed to explain BP differences. It has been postulated that the Yi rural people consumed a diet low in sodium and high in potassium, whereas urban populations consumed a diet high in sodium and low in potassium.

A similar conclusion was drawn by a study on rural tribes in Kenya [12]. Members of the tribe who migrated to urban centers had a right shift in the BP distribution compared with those practicing a native lifestyle. The specific relationship between sodium intake and BP in both of these studies is speculative, but the observations suggest that environmental factors may be important determinants of BP levels.

Other population studies: Population studies among various ethnic groups have been informative about the relationship between dietary sodium intake and BP. In the 1950s and 1960s, Louis Dahl conducted a cross-sectional study on daily salt intake and the prevalence of hypertension among four distinct ethnic groups. Dahl explored differences in populations with different hypertension rates and included Alaskan Eskimos, Marshall Islanders, Americans from Brookhaven, and Japanese from Hiroshima (South) and Akita (North). Large differences in the average daily salt intake between populations and within populations were reported. Communities with higher daily sodium chloride intakes had higher levels of BP. Dahl also noted that the populations of southern Japan had lower salt intakes and lower prevalence of hypertension than the populations of northern Japan.

Early observations of the relationship between sodium intake in humans and BP suggested that the age-related rise in BP is generally observed among populations in which the average sodium intake is greater than 2300 mg/day (100 mmol/day) and not among populations with lower sodium intake. These findings challenged the notion that BP inevitably rose with age as a function of normal physiologic occurrence. However, the findings of these early studies were challenged by some in the scientific community with counterarguments being based on the possibility that measurement error in BP or sodium intake accounted for the observed relationships. Counterarguments were also based on the notion that the populations studied were culturally isolated, had key lifestyle differences, were genetically homogeneous and that the studies did not adequately address the influence of high potassium intake in those groups with lower levels of BP.

In 1996, the design details and implications of the International Study of Salt and Blood Pressure (INTERSALT) were published [14]. INTERSALT was an ecological study that included over 10,000 study participants in 52 population samples and used more precise measurements of BP and sodium intake than those used in earlier human studies. Data from INTERSALT suggested a very significant relationship between sodium intake and BP ($r = 0.57$, $p < .001$), and an age-related rise in BP [69]. Adjusted for age and sex, every 100-mmol/dL increase in salt intake resulted in a 7-mmHg increase in the median systolic BP. INTERSALT and other ecological studies have limited utility in drawing causal inferences. However, since the INTERSALT data were published, there has been extensive concordant epidemiologic evidence that high dietary sodium intake is related to the epidemics of prehypertension and hypertension and to CVDs.

3.3.2.3 Intervention Studies

Metabolic balance to evaluate salt sensitivity: Since the 1970s, there has been evidence suggesting a difference in susceptibility to the BP-raising effects of sodium on the basis of ancestry [15]. This evidence comes from a series of metabolic ward studies including men of African American ancestry and white men. Participants in these controlled studies on dietary sodium, potassium, and calcium were healthy and young, with normal BP. BP and 24-h urinary excretion of electrolytes were measured before and after intervention. The protocol provided diets of 300 mmol/day sodium for 3 days, followed by 600–800 mmol/day for another 3 days, and then 1200–1500 mmol/day for final 3 days. After ingestion of these diets, a progressive and significant drop in BP was seen in comparison to the BPs observed before the intervention. The rise in BP was statistically significant in all participants, but the range was wide, with change in mean arterial pressure being as small as 5 mmHg or as large as 35 mmHg in some individuals. In African American participants, a significant rise in BP occurred at lower levels of sodium intake, whereas white participants demonstrated a significant rise in BP only at the highest level of sodium intake [15].

To further investigate and refine the concept of "salt sensitivity," studies have used protocols designed to evaluate BP responses to intravenous administration of 2 L of normal saline, sodium and volume depletion by a low-salt diet, and oral doses of furosemide in individuals who have high BP or normal BP [16,17]. In studies by Weinberger et al., salt sensitivity has been shown to be influenced by baseline BP, age, ancestry, and the renin and aldosterone response to sodium or volume depletion. Although salt sensitivity can occur in those with normal BP, individuals with high BP are significantly more salt sensitive than those with normal BP [16]. The long-term effects on mortality for individuals who are salt sensitive do not depend on whether salt sensitivity occurs in the context of normal BP or in the context of high BP. In terms of age, the magnitude of salt sensitivity of BP has been shown to increase progressively with decades of age among individuals with high BP. In individuals with normal BP, salt sensitivity was only observed in those older than 59 years [17]. In terms of ancestry, it has been observed that people with high BP who are of African American ancestry are often more salt sensitive than whites. However, the frequencies of salt sensitivity are same in those with normal BP, regardless of whether they are African Americans or whites. Lastly, salt sensitivity is enhanced by the failure of renin to respond to sodium or volume depletion, and response of renin affects the magnitude of decline in BP in response to low-sodium diets.

It has been suggested that the benefits of sodium reduction will be greater in individuals who are salt sensitive than in those who are not salt sensitive. However, there is a common misperception that only certain people should reduce their salt intake and that for the vast majority of the population salt reduction is unnecessary [74]. We believe that the opposite is true. Elevated BP is a huge public health problem. Approximately, one-third of adults have hypertension, and another third have prehypertension. For adults who reach the age of 50 years, the lifetime risk that hypertension will develop is 90% [75].

Population-based interventions worldwide: Numerous population-based interventions (not controlled trials) have aimed at reducing the salt intake of populations worldwide. One such effort was by the Japanese government in the 1950s in response to high incidence of stroke mortality [13]. Data suggested that the variation within the country was ecologically linked to local salt consumption. The Japanese government targeted a reduction in salt intake within a larger campaign promoting a healthier lifestyle. The population's sodium intake lowered from 13.5 to 12.1 g/day and was associated with BP reduction and 80% reduction in stroke mortality [13].

Similarly, Finland had high incidence of stroke and coronary heart disease in the 1970s. This led the Finnish government to implement broad interventions aimed at promoting healthy lifestyles. Laatikainen et al. analyzed Finnish data over 20 years and noted that salt intake had reduced by approximately 20%–30% during this period [18]. At the same time, the mean systolic and diastolic BP decreased by 10 mmHg. The causal inferences that can be made about the role of reduced sodium intake in lowering BP and stroke incidence are limited as other lifestyle behaviors were also modified and could have played a role in the observed health changes.

There have also been efforts in the United Kingdom to reduce sodium intake on a population level [19]. The goal of the current government-supported effort is to reduce salt consumption by 40% over 5 years. Sodium chloride in processed foods is being gradually reduced to achieve this result. Thus far, most manufacturers have reduced their salt usage by 10%–15% with no adverse complaints by the consumers [76].

Controlled trials and intervention studies: The magnitude of decrease in BP seen across controlled intervention studies varies according to the level of baseline sodium intake of the population studied, amount of reduction of sodium in the study, degree of adherence to sodium-reduction intervention, and length of the study.

Although there are several well-designed trials, particularly strong evidence of the effects of sodium on BP comes from the Dietary Approaches to Stop Hypertension—Sodium (DASH-sodium) study [21]. DASH-Sodium study tested the effect on BP of three levels of sodium intake in the context of either a typical American diet or the DASH dietary pattern on BP. As noted in Chapter 1, DASH emphasizes intake of fruits, vegetables, low-fat dairy foods; inclusion of whole grains, nuts, poultry, and fish; and reduction of fats, red meats, sugars, and sugar-sweetened beverages; it lowers BP at typical American levels of sodium intake [20].

The DASH-Sodium study [21] was a randomized controlled feeding study conducted in the United States in adult African Americans and whites with prehypertension or unmedicated stage 1 hypertension. All foods and beverages were prepared in a metabolic kitchen; participants ate only foods provided in the study, and the nutrient content of foods was confirmed by chemical analysis, thus allowing for precise determination of dietary sodium intake. In addition, weight was monitored daily and kept stable by adjusting energy intake, thus eliminating the potential confounding effect of weight change.

Over 400 participants were randomly assigned to the DASH or typical American dietary pattern for 3 months. Within this parallel design was a randomized crossover design in which each participant consumed sodium of three different levels for 30 days. The sodium levels tested were high (150 mmol/day), intermediate (100 mmol/day), and low (50 mmol/day).

The DASH-Sodium trial [21] demonstrated conclusively that reduced sodium intake lowers BP, but the effects were modest. In the context of a typical American diet, without concomitant weight loss, reducing sodium intake from the high to the intermediate level reduced systolic BP by an average of 2.1 mmHg ($p < .001$ compared with high sodium intake). Reducing sodium intake from the intermediate to the low level reduced SBP by 4.6 mmHg more ($p < .001$ intermediate vs. low). The effect of reducing sodium intake from high to low levels was a decrease in BP level of 6.7 mmHg Reduced sodium intake lowered BP more at each level when consumed in the context of the DASH dietary pattern, reducing BP by 7.2/3.5 mmHg with DASH and 100 mmol/day sodium intake and by 8.9/4.5 mmHg with DASH and 50 mmol/day sodium intake. Significant effects were seen in both prehypertension and hypertension, with greater effects in those with hypertension, approaching levels that might be anticipated with the use of one pharmacologic agent (i.e., mean reduction of 11.5 mmHg systolic BP) [21].

There have been other studies focused on sodium as a part of lifestyle approaches to preventing and treating hypertension. One such study was the Trials of Hypertension Prevention (TOHP) [22]. TOHP was a multicenter study with a Phase I component that tested seven different nonpharmacologic interventions for preventing high BP. Only weight and sodium were effective and were further tested in Phase II of the study. Participants were aged 30–54 years, had prehypertension, and were overweight. Two interventions were weight loss using group counseling sessions and sodium reduction using education and behavioral counseling. Participants were followed up for 3 years for the primary outcome of BP. These interventions were successful in reducing the incidence of hypertension. TOHP participants underwent additional observational follow-up for 10–15 years after the trial ended [24]. The goal of follow-up was to determine the long-term effect of sodium reduction (which was achieved by education and behavioral counseling) on cardiovascular events. The hazard of developing a CVD event in the intervention group was 0.75 (95% CI: 0.57, 0.99) times that of the control group after stratifying by trial and adjusting for clinic, age, race, sex, and weight loss intervention. The authors concluded that there was a possible "memory effect" of sodium reduction and that there were long-term benefits associated with an intervention to reduce sodium intake. Two published computer simulation models support the role of sodium reduction in CVD reduction and suggest that even modest population-wide reduction in sodium intake would decrease CVD and death and associated healthcare costs [9,11].

The trials of nonpharmacologic interventions in the elderly (TONE) also examined the role of sodium reduction in hypertension and CVD. An important result from the TONE study was that the percent of TONE participants with controlled BP after withdrawal of an antihypertensive medication was higher in those practicing sodium reduction than in those who did not.

Although sodium is one of several etiologic factors important in the development of high BP, the reduction in systolic BP that can be expected when following the DASH diet with sodium reduction is between 8 and 14 mmHg [77].

3.3.2.4   Meta-analyses, Systematic Reviews, and Pooled Analyses

There are published meta-analyses on the effects of salt reduction on BP [25–27]. The effects of drastic salt reduction have shown ambiguous or even harmful results in these analyses. However, population interventions aim at modest reductions, and as such, the meta-analysis of randomized trials by He et al. shows that modest reductions in sodium intake are associated with a decrease in BP [26]. The benefits of modest sodium reduction were more pronounced among those with hypertension than among those without hypertension. The pooled analysis of individuals without hypertension included 11 trials with a total of 2220 study participants. There was a median net reduction in 24-h urinary sodium of 74 mmol corresponding to 4.4 g of sodium chloride/day. The pooled estimates of systolic BP reduced by 2.0 mmHg (95% CI: 1.5, 2.6) and diastolic BP decreased by 1.0 mmHg (95% CI: 0.6, 1.4). In a weighted linear regression analysis, a reduction in sodium chloride intake of 100 mmol/day predicted a decrease in systolic BP of 3.6 mmHg and a decrease in diastolic BP of 1.7 mmHg. The analysis of individuals with hypertension included 17 trials with a total of 734 study participants. There was a median net reduction in 24-h urinary sodium excretion of 78 mmol corresponding to 4.6 g of sodium chloride/day. The pooled estimates of systolic BP decreased by 5.0 mmHg (4.2, 5.8) and of diastolic BP decreased by 2.7 mm Hg (95% CI: 2.2, 3.2). Assuming a linear relationship, a reduction of 100 mmol/day predicted a reduction in systolic BP of 7.1 mmHg and in diastolic BP of 3.9 mmHg.

In a systematic review by Hooper et al., advice to reduce dietary salt in adults produced larger short-term effects that became attenuated as the trials became longer [27]. The pooled estimates of urinary sodium excretion in these studies showed a reduction of 48.9 mmol/day (32.5, 65.4) at 6–12 months. For trials of 13–60 months duration, the net reduction was 35.5 mmol/day (23.8, 47.2), suggesting that reduced sodium intake may be difficult to sustain.

3.4   STRATEGIES TO DECREASE POPULATION SODIUM INTAKE

Lowering sodium intake can reduce BP and prevent hypertension, which is a major risk factor for heart disease and stroke. However, achieving success with sodium reduction is not straightforward due to the unique challenges associated with sodium use in the food supply. Under ideal circumstances, sodium in the food supply could be immediately reduced to levels that would translate to diets that meet recommended sodium intake for the average American. However, it is recommended that a gradual process be used, given the ubiquity of sodium in the food supply and its varied functions including improving food taste and flavor, maintaining food safety and shelf life, and impacting the texture of food [57].

In an effort to create a viable population strategy to reduce sodium intake in the United States, in 2010, a committee of the Institute of Medicine made the primary recommendation for the establishment of a coordinated approach to set standards for safe levels of sodium in foods [57]. The committee recommended that standards be set using existing U.S. Food and Drug Administration authorities to modify the "generally recognized as safe" (GRAS) status of salt and other sodium-containing compounds. GRAS status and food additive approvals are the two ways in which substances can gain approval for addition to food. Sodium chloride, commonly known as salt and the greatest contributor to sodium intake in the American diet, is currently considered GRAS at any level of use. In the report, the committee recommended that maximum levels be established for salt and other sodium-containing compounds so as to allow persons to consume a normal diet with a reasonable likelihood of keeping their sodium intake to recommended levels.

Population sodium intake will not be affected for some years by this recommendation as the implementation of proposed GRAS modifications will take time. For this reason, the committee also recommended that voluntary approaches aimed at population sodium reduction be implemented or continued until GRAS modifications can be completed. Examples of voluntary approaches include initiatives by food companies to reduce the sodium in their individual products and the well-known National Salt Reduction Initiative developed initially by the New York City Health Department. The recommended approach to gradually reduce sodium creates a level playing field for food manufacturers and restaurant and foodservice operations. This should lead to more successful adoption of products that are reformulated to help consumers meet current sodium intake recommendations. A summary of the key evidence on sodium and blood pressure and recommendations for health care providers are provided in Table 3.1.

3.5 SUMMARY

Excessive sodium intake in the American population has been long recognized as directly related to high BP. Risks for developing high BP can begin in early childhood. Once Americans reach their fifties, the risk of developing high BP over the remainder of the lifespan is estimated to be 90% even for those with normal BPs. It has been estimated that reducing sodium intakes could prevent more than 100,000 deaths annually and save billions in medical costs. Given the large excess of usual sodium intake above physiologic needs among individuals living in industrialized societies across the world, numerous agencies and policy-making bodies have issued guidelines that address sodium reduction. A population-wide reduction in sodium intake could be predicted to produce a significant BP reduction, which would result in a decreased risk for CVD in populations where CVD is likely [78]. It is generally agreed that even small, sustained reductions in population-wide BP can result in dramatic health benefits [79]. Achieving and maintaining a low-sodium diet is challenging in today's food environment. If populations are to follow guidelines of choosing and preparing foods that are low in sodium, there must be extensive efforts to educate the consumer as well as efforts to decrease sodium in the food supply. These steps are critical to the prevention and control of prehypertension and hypertension.

TABLE 3.1
Summary: Take-Home Messages

Key Evidences	Recommendation for Health Care Providers
• The vast majority of the U.S. population has excessive sodium intake • There is extensive concordant epidemiologic evidence that high dietary sodium intake is related to the epidemics of prehypertension and hypertension and to CVDs • There is convincing clinical trial evidence that lowering sodium intake will lower BP • Patient counseling should include recommendations to follow the DASH dietary pattern as this diet has been shown to lower BP • Innovative public health strategies are underway to reduce population sodium intake to levels within those set in the guidelines. However, until strategies are implemented, counseling on dietary sodium intake can enable patients to reduce sodium intake	• Review and evaluate the evidence on sodium and BP • Improve skills to effectively communicate with patients about reducing dietary sodium intake • Adequately counsel patients on approaches to reduce dietary sodium intake in a food environment where sodium is ubiquitous • Include recommendations to reduce sodium intake in the context of the DASH dietary pattern for increased BP-lowering effect

REFERENCES

1. Denton, D., Weisinger, R., Mundy, N.I., et al. The effect of increased salt intake on blood pressure of chimpanzees. *Nat Med*, 1995;1:1009–1016.
2. Elliott, P., Walker, L.L., Little, M.P., et al. Change in salt intake affects blood pressure of chimpanzees: Implications for human populations. *Circulation*, 2007;116:1563–1568.
3. Meneely, G.R., Ball, O.T. Experimental epidemiology of chronic sodium chloride toxicity and the protective effect of potassium chloride. *Am J Med*, 1958;25(5):713–725.
4. Lifton, R.P. Molecular genetics of human blood pressure variation. *Science*, 1996;272:676–680.
5. Lifton, R.P., Gharavi, A.G., Geller, D.S. Molecular mechanisms of human hypertension. *Cell*, 2001;104:545–556.
6. Uzodike, V.O. Epidemiological studies of arterial blood pressure and hypertension in relation to electrolyte excretion in three Igbo communities in Nigeria. Thesis (MD), University of London, London, 1993.
7. Page, L.B., Damon, A., Moellering, R.C. Jr. Antecedents of cardiovascular disease in six Solomon Islands societies. *Circulation*, 1974;49:1132–1146.
8. Page, L.B., Vandevert, D.E., Nader, K., Lubin, N.K., Page, J.R. Blood pressure of Qash'qai pastoral nomads in Iran in relation to culture, diet, and body form. *Am J Clin Nutr*, 1981;34:527–538.
9. Kesteloot, H., Huang, D.X., Li, Y.L., Geboers, J., Joossens, J.V. The relationship between cations and blood pressure in the People's Republic of China. *Hypertension*, 1987;9:654–659.

10. Sasaki, N. High blood pressure and the salt intake of the Japanese. *Jpn Heart J*, 1962;3:313–324.

11. He, J., Klag, M.J., Whelton, P.K., et al. Migration, blood pressure pattern, and hypertension: The Yi Migrant Study. *Am J Epidemiol*, 1991;134(10):1085–1101.

12. Poulter, N.R., Khaw, K.T., Hopwood, B.E.C., Mugambi, M., Peart, W.S., Rose, G., Sever, P.S. The Kenyan Luo migration study: Observations on the initiation of a rise in blood pressure. *BMJ*, 1990;300(6730):967–972.

13. Dahl, L.K. Possible role of salt intake in the development of essential hypertension. In: P. Cottier, D. Bock, eds. *Essential Hypertension—An International Symposium* (pp. 52–65). Springer-Verlag, Berlin, 1960.

14. Stamler, J. The INTERSALT study: Background, methods, findings, and implications. *Am J Clin Nutr*, 1997;65:626S–642S.

15. Luft, F.C, Rankin, L.I., Bloch, R., et al. Cardiovascular and humoral responses to extremes of sodium intake in normal white and black men. *Circulation*, 1979;60:697–703.

16. Weinberger, M.H. Salt sensitivity of blood pressure in humans. *Hypertension*, 1996;27:II481–II490.

17. Weinberger, M.H. Salt sensitivity, pulse pressure and death in normal and hypertensive humans. *Hypertension*, 2001;37(Part 2):429–432.

18. Laatikainen, T., Pietinen, P., Valsta, L., et al. Sodium in the Finnish diet-20-year trends in urinary sodium excretion among the adult population. *Eur J Clin Nutr*, 2006;60:965–970.

19. Laatikainen, T., Pietinen, P., Valsta, L., et al. Consensus Action on Salt and Health. Available at http://www.actiononsalt.org.uk/ (Last accessed September 19, 2011.)

20. Appel, L.J., Moore, T.J., Obarzanek, E., et al. for the DASH Collaborative Research Group. A clinical trial of the effects of dietary patterns on blood pressure. *N Engl J Med*, 1997;336:1117–1124.

21. Sacks, F.M., Svetkey, L.P., Vollmer, E.M., et al. for the DASH-Sodium Collaborative Research Group. Effects on blood pressure of reduced dietary sodium and the Dietary Approaches to Stop Hypertension (DASH) diet. *N Engl J Med*, 2001;344:3–10.

22. Whelton, P.K. on behalf of the Trials of Hypertension Prevention Collaborative Research Group. The effects of nonpharmacologic interventions on blood pressure of persons with high normal levels. *JAMA*, 1992;267(9):1213–1220.

23. Whelton, P.K., Lawrence, L.J., Espeland, M., et al. Sodium reduction and weight loss in the treatment of hypertension in older persons. *JAMA*, 1998;279(11):839–846.

24. Cook, N.R., Cutler, J.A., Obarzanek, E., et al. 2007. Long term effects of dietary sodium reduction on cardiovascular disease outcomes-observational follow-up of the trials of hypertension prevention (TOHP). *BMJ*, 2007;334:885–888.

25. Midgley, J.P., Matthew, A.G., Greenwood, C.M., Logan, A.G. Effect of reduced dietary sodium on blood pressure: A meta-analysis of randomized controlled trials. *JAMA*, 1996;275:1590–1597.

26. He, F.J., MacGregor, G.A. Effect of modest salt reduction on blood pressure: A meta-analysis of randomized trials. Implications for public health. *J Hum Hypertens*, 2002;16:761–770.

27. Hooper, L., Batlett, C., Smith, G.D., Ebrahim, S. Systematic review of long term effects of advice to reduce dietary salt in adults. *BMJ*, 2002;325:628–634.

28. Dahl, L.K. Salt and hypertension. *Am J Clin Nutr*, 1972;25:231–244.

29. Oliver, W.J., Cohen, E.L., Neel, J.V. Blood pressure, sodium intake, and sodium related hormones in the Yanomamo Indians, a "no salt" culture. *Circulation*, 1975;52:146–151.

30. Sasaki, N. The relationship of salt intake to hypertension in the Japanese. *Geriatrics*, 1964;19:735–744.

31. Stamler, J. Dietary salt and blood pressure. *Ann N Y Acad Sci*, 1993;676:122–156.

32. Denton, D. *The Hunger for Salt: An Anthropological, Physiological and Medical Analysis*. Springer-Verlag, Berlin, 1982.

33. Anderson, C.A., Appel, L.J., Okuda, N., et al. Dietary sources of sodium in China, Japan, the United Kingdom, and the United States, women and men aged 40 to 59 years: The INTERMAP Study. *J Am Diet Assoc*, 2010;110:736–745.

34. Sanchez-Castillo, C.P., Warrender, S., Whitehead, T.P., James, W.P. An assessment of the sources of dietary salt in a British population. *Clin Sci (Lond)*, 1987;72:95–102.

35. Mattes, R.D., Donnelly, D. Relative contributions of dietary sodium sources. *J Am Coll Nutr*, 1991;10:383–393.

36. Jacobson, M.F. Sodium content of processed foods: 1983–2004. *Am J Clin Nutr*, 2005;81:941–942.

37. Bull, N.L., Buss, D.H. Contributions of foods to sodium intakes. *Proc Nutr Soc*, 1980;39:30A.

38. James, W.P., Ralph, A., Sanchez-Castillo, C.P. The dominance of salt in manufactured food in the sodium intake of affluent societies. *Lancet*, 1987;1(8530):426–429.

39. World Health Organization Forum. Reducing salt intake in populations: Report of a WHO forum and technical meeting. Available at www.who.int/dietphysicalactivity/SaltReport-VC-April07.pdf (Last accessed September 1, 2011.)

40. Shimbo, S., Hatai, I., Saito, T., et al. Shift in sodium chloride sources in past 10 years of salt reduction campaign in Japan. *Tohoku J Exp Med*, 1996;180: 249–259.

41. The Resources Council, Science and Technology Agency, Japan. Standard Tables of Food Composition in Japan, 5th revised edition (Printed in Japanese, translation provided by Nagako Okuda). Printing Bureau, Ministry of Finance, Tokyo, 2000.

42. Kimira, M., Kudo, Y., Takachi, R., Haba, R., Watanabe, S. Associations between dietary intake and urinary excretion of sodium, potassium, phosphorus, magnesium and calcium. *Jpn J Hyg*, 2004;59(1): 23–30.

43. Ministry of Health, Labour and Welfare. The National Health and Nutrition Survey in Japan, 2005. (Printed in Japanese, translation provided by Nagako Okuda), Daiichi Shuppan, Tokyo, 2008.

44. Brown, I.J., Tzoulaki, I., Candelas, V., Elliott, P. Salt intakes around the world: Implications for public health. *Int J Epidemiol*, 2009;38(3):791–813.

45. Zhai, F.Y., Yang, X.G.. China National Health and Nutrition Survey—Report two: Food and nutrients intake in 2002 (Printed in Chinese, translation provided by Liancheng Zhao) (P. 100, 254). People's Medical Publishing House, Beijing, 2006.

46. Guansheng, M.A., Qin, Z., Yanping, L.I., et al. The salt consumption of residents in China. *Chn J Prev Control Chronic Non-Communicable Dis* (printed in Chinese, translation provided by Liancheng Zhao), 2008;16(4):331–333.

47. National Centre for Social Research. An assessment of dietary sodium levels among adults (aged 19–64) in the general UK population in 2008, based on the analysis of sodium in 24-hour urine excretion. June 2008:3. Available at www.food.gov.uk/multimedia/pdfs/08sodiumreport.pdf (Last accessed February 15, 2012)

48. World Action on Salt and Health. Survey of over 260 food products around the world from KFC, McDonalds, Kellogg's, Nestle, Burger King and Subway. Available at http://www.worldactiononsalt.com/media/international_products_survey_2009.xls (Last accessed September 20, 2011.)

49. United States Dietary Guidelines for Americans. Available at www.dietaryguidelines.gov (Last accessed September 20, 2011.)

50. Institute of Medicine. Dietary reference intakes: the essential guide to nutrient requirements (sodium and potassium). National Academies Press, Washington DC, 2006.

51. Appel, L.J., Brands, M.W., Daniels, S.R., Karanja, N., Elmer, P.J., Sacks, F.M., American Heart Association. Dietary approaches to prevent and treat hypertension. A scientific statement from the American Heart Association. *Hypertension*, 2006;47:296–308.

52. U.S. Department of Agriculture, Agricultural Research Service (2008). Nutrient intakes from food: Mean amounts consumed per individual, one day, 2005–2006. Available at www.ars.usda.gov/ba/bhnrc/fsrg (Last accessed September 20, 2011.)

53. Bernstein, A., Willett, W.C. Trends in 24-h urinary sodium excretion in the United States, 1957–2003: A systematic review. *Am J Clin Nutr*, 2010;92: 1172–1180.

54. Espeland, M.A., Kumanyika, S., Wilson, A.C., et al. Statistical issues in analyzing 24-hour dietary recall and 24-hour urine collection data for sodium and potassium intakes. *Am J Epidemiol*, 2001;153:996–1006.

55. Briefel, R.R., Johnson, C.L. Secular trends in dietary intake in the United States. *Annu Rev Nutr*, 2004;24:401–431.

56. Smiciklas-Wright, H., Mitchell, D.C., Mickle, S.J., Goldman, J.D., Cook, A. Foods commonly eaten in the United States, 1989–1991 and 1994–1996: Are portion sizes changing? *J Am Diet Assoc*, 2003;103(1):41–47.

57. IOM (Institute of Medicine). *Strategies to Reduce Sodium Intake in the United States.* The National Academies Press, Washington, DC, 2010.

58. Stamler, J., Stamler, R., Neaton, J.D. Blood pressure, systolic and diastolic, and cardiovascular risks: U.S. population data. *Arch Intern Med*, 1993;153:598–615.

59. Sasaki, S., Zhang, X.H., Kesteloot, H. Dietary sodium, potassium, saturated fat, alcohol, and stroke mortality. *Stroke*, 1995;26:783–789.

60. Khaw, K.T., Barrett-Connor, E. The association between blood pressure, age, and dietary sodium and potassium: A population study. *Circulation*, 1988;77:53–61.

61. Perry, I.J., Beevers, D.G. Salt intake and stroke: A possible direct effect. *J Hum Hypertens*, 1992;6:23–25.

62. Cutler, J.A., Roccella, E.J. Salt reduction for preventing hypertension and cardiovascular disease: A population approach should include children. *Hypertension*, 2006;48:818–819.

63. He, J., Ogden, L.G., Vupputuri, S., Bazzano, L.A., Loria, C., Whelton, P.K. Dietary sodium intake and subsequent risk of cardiovascular disease in overweight adults. *JAMA*, 1999;282:2027–2034.

64. Tuomilehto, J., Jousilahti, P., Rastenyte, D., et al. Urinary sodium excretion and cardiovascular mortality in Finland: A prospective study. *Lancet*, 2001;357:848–851.

65. Appel, L.J., Espeland, M.A., Easter, L., Wilson, A.C., Folmar, S., Lacy, C.R. Effects of reduced sodium intake on hypertension control in older individuals: Results from the Trial of Nonpharmacologic Interventions in the Elderly (TONE). *Arch Intern Med*, 2001;161:685–693.

66. Appel, L.J., Brands, M.W., Daniels, S.R., Karanja, N., Elmer, P.J., Sacks, F.M. American Heart Association. Dietary approaches to prevent and treat hypertension. A scientific statement from the American Heart Association. *Hypertension*, 2006;47:296–308.

67. Forman, J.P., Stampfer, M.J., Curhan, G.C. Diet and lifestyle risk factors associated with incident hypertension in women. *JAMA*, 2009;302:401–411.

68. He, F.J., MacGregor, G. A. Effect of modest salt reduction on blood pressure: A meta-analysis of randomized trials. Implications for public health. *J Hum Hypertens*, 2002;16:761–770.

69. INTERSALT Cooperative Research Group. INTERSALT: An international study of electrolyte excretion and blood pressure. Results for 24 h urinary sodium and potassium excretion. *BMJ*, 1988;297:319–328.

70. Tobian, L. Salt and Hypertension: Lessons from animal models that relate to human hypertension. *Hypertension*, 1991;17(S1):152–158.

71. The International Consortium for Blood Pressure Genome-Wide Association Studies. Genetic variants in novel pathways influence blood pressure and cardiovascular disease risk. *Nature*, epub ahead of print September 11, 2011. DOI: 10.1038/nature10405.

72. Wain, L.V, Verwoert, G.C., O'Reilly, P.F., Shi, G., Johnson, T., Johnson, A.D., et al. Genome-wide association study identifies six new loci influencing pulse pressure and mean arterial pressure. *Nature Genetics*, epub ahead of print September 11, 2011. DOI: 10.1038/ng.922.

73. Nakagawa, H., Morikawa, Y., Okayama, A., et al. Trends in blood pressure and urinary sodium and potassium excretion in Japan: Reinvestigation in the 8th year after the INTERSALT study. *J Hum Hypertens*, 1999;13:735–741.

74. Appel, L.J., Anderson, C.A. Compelling evidence for public health action to reduce sodium intake. *N Engl J Med*, 2010;362:650–652.

75. Vasan, R.S., Beiser, A., Seshadri, S., et al. Residual lifetime risk for developing hypertension in middle-aged women and men: The Framingham Heart Study. *JAMA*, 2002;287:1003–10.

76. Girgis, S., Neal, B., Prescott, J., et al. A one-quarter reduction in the salt content of bread can be made without detection. *Eur J Clin Nutr*, 2003;57: 616–620.

77. Chobanian, A.V., Bakris, G.L., Black, H.R., et al. Seventh report of the Joint National Committee on prevention, detection, evaluation, and treatment of high blood pressure. *Hypertension*, 2003;42(6):1206–1252.

78. Bibbins-Domingo, K., Chertow, G.M., Coxson, P.G., et al. Projected effect of dietary salt reductions on future cardiovascular disease. *N Engl J Med*, 2010;362:590–599.

79. Smith-Spangler, C.M., Juusola, J.L., Enns, E.A., Owens, D.K., Garber, A.M. Population strategies to decrease sodium intake and the burden of cardiovascular disease: A cost-effectiveness analysis. *Ann Intern Med*, 2010;152:481–487, W170–W173.

4 Body Weight and Blood Pressure

David W. Harsha, Catherine M. Champagne, and George A. Bray
Pennington Biomedical Research Center

CONTENTS

4.1 OVERVIEW

Overweight is an increasingly prevalent condition throughout the world. Recent, probably conservative, estimates indicate that at least 500,000,000 people worldwide are overweight as defined by a body mass index (BMI) between 25.0 and 29.9 kg/m^2, and an additional 250,000,000 are obese with a BMI of 30.0 kg/m^2 or higher [1]. In the United States, current indications are that as much as 66% of the adult population is overweight or obese [2,3].

Overweight and obesity are established risk factors for cardiovascular disease (CVD), stroke, non-insulin-dependent diabetes, certain cancers, and numerous other disorders [4–8]. They are also major risk factors for hypertension [9]. Hypertension, defined as a systolic blood pressure (SBP) in excess of 140 mmHg or a diastolic blood pressure (DBP) higher than 90 mmHg, is also an increasing public health issue internationally. Approximately one billion individuals worldwide are thought to exhibit medically important elevated blood pressure (BP), with about 50 million of those residing in the United States [8]. Hypertension itself is associated with increased risk for CVD, stroke, renal disease, and mortality from all causes [10–13].

The seventh report of the Joint National Committee on Prevention, Detection, Evaluation, and Treatment of High Blood Pressure (JNC VII) defines stage 1 hypertension as the condition in which BP levels are between 140 and 159 mmHg systolic or 90 and 99 mmHg diastolic. Additionally, the report establishes a category of pre-hypertension (SBP between 120 and 139 mmHg or DBP between 80 and 89 mmHg). Both stage 1 hypertension and prehypertension are deemed appropriate primary targets for lifestyle modification interventions, including weight loss. Although higher levels of BP or stage 1 hypertension, which persists despite efforts at lifestyle modification, should be treated with medications, lifestyle modification, including weight loss, remains relevant for BP control with or without concomitant medication treatment.

4.2   WEIGHT AND BP

Overweight and obesity are associated with higher BP and increased risk of hypertension. As early as the 1920s, a noteworthy association between body weight and BP was noted in men [14,15]. More recent epidemiological studies have confirmed this association. The Framingham Study found that hypertension is roughly twice more prevalent in obese individuals than in nonobese individuals of both sexes [16]. Stamler and colleagues [17] reported an odds ratio for hypertension of obese individuals relative to nonobese individuals (BMI < 25 kg/m^2) of 2.42 for younger adults and 1.54 for older ones. The Nurses Health Study [18] compared women with BMI less than 22 kg/m^2 and those with BMI above 29 kg/m^2 and found twofold to sixfold greater prevalence of hypertension among those in the higher BMI category.

More recent data from the Framingham Study further corroborated this relationship. After division into BMI quintiles, participants of both sexes in the Framingham study showed increasing BP with increasing overweight. In this instance, those in the highest BMI quintile exhibited 16 mmHg higher SBP and 9 mmHg higher DBP than those in the lowest quintile. This translates into an increase in SBP of 4 mmHg for each 4.5-kg increased weight [19]. In young Canadian adults, Rabkin et al. [20] noted a fivefold greater incidence of hypertension in both men and women with BMI more than 30 kg/m^2 relative to those with BMI less than 20 kg/m^2.

4.3   WEIGHT LOSS AND BP CONTROL

BP lowering with antihypertensive medication results in reduced cardiovascular risk [21]. Although there have been no weight-loss trials with hard clinical outcomes to date, it is reasonable to expect similar reductions in cardiovascular risk when BP is lowered through weight loss. In addition, it is known that weight loss prevents the onset of hypertension in individuals with prehypertension [22–24].

Numerous clinical interventions in humans have examined the relationship of weight loss and change in BP. Although weight-loss studies do not uniformly demonstrate a BP-lowering effect [25], a meta-analysis of 25 studies suggested a fairly consistent effect [24]. In this meta-analysis, Neter et al. estimated that 1-kg loss of body weight was associated with approximately 1-mmHg drop in BP [26]. A systematic review reached similar conclusions [27].

Importantly, this BP reduction was accomplished without the necessity to attain normal body weight. The Trial of Hypertension Prevention (TOHP), one of the largest of these studies, included a weight-loss intervention arm [28]. Here, 2-kg loss in weight over a 6-month period resulted in 3.7-mmHg decline in SBP and 2.7-mmHg decline in DBP. Moreover, 4.4-kg and 2-kg weight losses were associated with 42% and 20% decline in incident hypertension at 6 and 18 months, respectively [24].

Given such an association between weight change and BP levels, the question arises as to how this interaction functions physiologically. Rocchini [29] identified numerous potential biological mechanisms by which weight loss or fat loss might lead to a decline in BP. Among them are reduction in insulin resistance [30] and its effects on enhanced sodium retention [31,32], alterations in vascular structure and function [33], changes in ion transport [34], enhanced stimulation of the renin–aldo-sterone–angiotensin system [32], increased activation of the sympathetic nervous system [35], and changes in natriuretic peptide [32]. This wide range of potential mechanisms may also be a major factor in accounting for the apparent heterogeneity in BP response to any one treatment. Weight loss may variably and simultaneously affect several of these proposed routes of action. Since weight status itself is a result of multiple causes, the fashion in which it induces BP change would not surprisingly be variable.

Studies demonstrating the effect of weight loss on BP often involve other dietary changes that affect BP. In an early study, Dahl et al. [36] found that sodium restric-tion in low-calorie diets was the primary cause for BP reduction. This is also the finding of Fagerberg et al. [37]. However, a number of more recent studies have sided with the view that weight loss has an independent effect on BP reduction. Reisen et al. [38] found BP reductions in the order of 3 mmHg for each kilogram of weight loss in a sample of hypertensive men with no sodium restriction. Others have also reported independent effects of weight loss on BP [39,40].

Similarly, since weight loss cannot be accomplished in the absence of some combination of change in dietary pattern or physical activity behaviors, separating independent effects of each component on BP is extremely challenging. It is clear, however, that weight loss, regardless of how it is achieved, is associated with clini-cally significant reductions in BP.

A related issue is the extent to which maintained weight loss continues to influ-ence BP status. The vast majority of studies that link weight loss to BP reduction do so only in the short term, usually examining the impact of weight loss on BP over less than a year. The effect of long-term weight loss has predictably been much less examined. Nevertheless, a small number of clinical trials have examined the issue for more than 1 year of follow-up time.

The PREMIER clinical trial evaluated BP-regulation effects for 18 months. In this study, 810 individuals who had prehypertension or unmedicated stage 1 hypertension were randomized to a control group or to either of the two putatively heart-healthy active interventions [41]. Both the active interventions counseled the participants for an increase in physical activity and either a reduced fat and calorie diet or a diet high in fruits, vegetables, and low-fat dairy servings using the Dietary Approaches to Stop Hypertension (DASH) dietary pattern [23]. These active interventions also counseled a reduction in sodium intake and weight loss for the vast majority of par-ticipants who were overweight or obese. Weight and BP were monitored at baseline, at interim periods, and at the end of 18 months of intervention. At the end of the trial, both the active interventions resulted in sustained weight loss and BP reduction.

The active intervention without the DASH diet resulted in an average weight loss of 3.8 kg and that with the DASH diet, 4.3 kg. Mean BP reductions (systolic/diastolic) were 8.6/6.0 and 9.5/6.2 mmHg for the same intervention arms, respectively. Urinary sodium reductions were 18.4 and 24.5 mmol/day, respectively, for each arm. In sum, the PREMIER study demonstrated that free-living populations can make multiple lifestyle changes in physical activity and dietary patterns. Improvements in BP and body-weight profiles occurred simultaneously as did reduction in sodium intake. It appears that these lifestyle alterations mutually reinforced beneficial changes in both BP and body weight.

The TOHP reported 7 years of follow-up in 181 prehypertensive participants divided into three groups, that is, a group treated for weight loss, a group treated with sodium reduction, or a group that received no treatment [42]. The active phase of the intervention lasted for 18 months, but individuals were further monitored for BP, weight, and dietary status for 7 years. Incident hypertension was the outcome variable of interest. The group treated for weight loss in the absence of sodium restriction, which had an average weight reduction of 5 kg at 18 months [28], demonstrated after 7 years the incidence of new hypertension of 18.9% compared with that of 40.5% in the control group. This contrasts with the group treated with sodium reduction in the absence of weight loss, which had an incidence of hypertension of 22.4% compared with that of 32.9% in the control group over the same period. The impressive reduction in the incidence of hypertension with weight loss occurred in spite of the fact that much of the weight had been regained at year 7.

The Hypertension Prevention Trial followed up 841 prehypertensive individuals for up to 3 years after randomization to four intervention groups: caloric restriction/weight loss, sodium reduction, caloric restriction and sodium reduction, and sodium reduction with increased potassium intake [43]. At 3 years of follow-up, it was found that the caloric restriction group had maintained weight loss at about 4% of baseline and demonstrated 5.1/2.4 mmHg reduction in BP. The other dietary interventions resulted in less BP reduction relative to controls. The authors recommend caloric restriction and accompanying weight loss as the strategy of choice in regulating BP.

In the Weight Loss Maintenance trial [44], 1032 participants who had previously lost 4 kg or more were randomized to one of three weight-maintenance strategies: a self-directed control group, monthly personal contact, or an internet-based intervention. The maintenance phase lasted for 30 months. Although all three groups exhibited some regain of weight over this time, all maintained an average of at least 3 kg of weight loss, with the greatest weight loss maintenance (4.2 kg, $p < .001$ compared with that in the control group) in the monthly personal contact group. Three or more kilograms of maintained weight loss would result in significant reduction of BP in the general population.

A few other small-scale studies have documented a positive association between weight loss maintained for periods of up to 2 years and reduction in BP [45–47]. In sum, it is clear that nonsurgical intentional weight loss reduces BP and that the BP-lowering benefits are retained over at least the short- to mid-term, particularly in those who maintain the weight loss [24].

4.4 BARIATRIC SURGERY AND BP CONTROL

In the more specialized arena of bariatric surgery, the effects of this surgery on BP in the short- to mid-term are clear. Buchwald et al. [48] conducted a meta-analysis of the effect of bariatric surgery on CVD risk factors. An overall reduction of 61.2% in excess weight was associated with resolution of hypertension in 61.7% and significant improvement of the BP status in 78.5% of individuals treated with bariatric surgery.

The effects of surgery over longer periods are less clear. Sjostrom et al. [49] reported 8 years of follow-up on the relationship of weight loss and BP in a group of 1157 obese participants who underwent bariatric surgery. Initial weight losses of 38% of presurgical body weight were associated with a decline in BP of about 12 mmHg systolic and 8 mmHg diastolic. Over a 6- to 8-year period, weights increased only very slightly in this group, while BP levels rebounded and, at the end of the study, were similar to or higher than that in untreated control groups. The authors were unable to explain this phenomenon but were skeptical that this is a generalizable finding pointing to methodological and analytic inconsistencies in their sample [50]. However, Sjostrom and colleagues [51] suggest that surgically induced weight loss maintained over 10 years has a more complicated effect on BP, with mean SBP increasing by 2.5 mmHg and mean DBP decreasing by 2.4 mmHg. Even nonsurgical approaches to weight control may have mixed effects on BP over the long term: at 5 years of follow-up in the Weight Loss Maintenance study, there was a suggestion that BP-regulation effects were not sustained despite sustained weight loss [52]. Clearly, this is an area for further investigation.

4.5 CHALLENGES TO ACHIEVING WEIGHT LOSS AND BP CONTROL

Overall, it is clear that weight loss is associated with a decline in BP, at least in the short- and mid-term. These findings extend even to those who are initially in the nonhypertensive range and hold for both genders and virtually all racial/ethnic groups [29]. This conclusion was endorsed by the JNC VII expert panel and has become a part of the suggested lifestyle armamentarium in combating hypertension [9]. Undoubtedly, much of the attractiveness of weight loss stems from its multiple health benefits. Weight reduction is not only associated with lowering of BP but also confers benefits in the prevention and treatment of many other disorders including type 2 diabetes and musculoskeletal disorders. Although outcomes in trials are lacking, epidemiologic evidence suggests that weight loss may also prevent some cancers and CVD events and may reduce CVD and all-cause mortality [4–8].

Nevertheless, pursuing weight loss as the sole means to accomplish BP control is not without challenges. Chief among these is the difficulty involved in achieving and maintaining weight loss. Many who attempt weight loss achieve little in this regard, and many who are initially successful rebound to their earlier status or higher [53–55]. In the grimmest scenarios, the net result is not only a population that is at increased biomedical risk but also that suffers from a number of psychosocial insults that result from these failures [56]. Nevertheless, weight loss is successfully accomplished by many and is maintained by a significant percentage of those who are initially successful [44,57]. The methods and strategies employed for achieving sustained weight loss are still developing, and if careful attention is paid to refining them, the result will undoubtedly be improvement in those achieving weight loss and a decline in recidivism [58].

Maintenance of weight loss remains the challenge. Wing and Phelan [57] report that approximately 20% of those attempting weight reduction via lifestyle modification are successful at long-term weight control. Research into the mechanisms by which these results are obtained should increase these success rates. It appears that the strongest predictor of long-term weight loss maintenance is the amount of weight that was initially lost [59].

It should be noted that the impact of weight loss on BP does not require that optimal weight should be achieved (BMI 18.5–24.9 kg/m^2). Smaller decrements of weight loss clearly are of clinical significance in influencing BP levels. Likewise, maintenance of all of the lost weight is not necessary. Some recidivism in weight loss is common, but as long as the weight is at least 5%–10% below the baseline level, there is likely to be an impact on BP [60,61]. Nevertheless, greater initial weight losses would perforce result in larger BP declines and greater weight loss maintenance; therefore, we believe that achievement and maintenance of ideal weight would be an appropriate goal.

4.6 CONCLUSION

Current guidelines recommend weight loss intervention in overweight/obese individuals with prehypertension and all stages of hypertension [9]. In those with prehypertension, weight loss may prevent hypertension. In those with stage 1 hypertension, it may preclude the need for antihypertensive medications. In those with hypertension at any stage who are taking antihypertensive medication, weight loss may reduce medication needs and increase the chance of achieving BP control. Thus, weight loss may be appropriate for lowering of BP in the vast majority of adult Americans (i.e.,

TABLE 4.1

Summary: Take-Home Messages

Key Evidences	Recommendations for Health Care Providers
1. In most studies, it has been found that weight loss reduces BP	1. Evaluate your patient for body mass index and weight status. If these are found abnormal, advise them on the benefits of weight loss to improving health
2. Maintaining a lower weight can facilitate maintaining a lower BP	
3. Lifestyle modification is the preferred strategy for weight loss and should be included in all BP treatment plans	2. Provide in-office or referral options for patients who are ready to lose weight
	3. Encourage sustainable lifestyle modification for weight loss and overall BP management
	4. Educate that weight loss may be appropriate for BP control in those with prehypertension and all stages of hypertension

about 40% of the adult population with hypertension and 31% with prehypertension) [62,63]. This very large target for weight loss intervention has the potential for considerable impact on public health.

In conclusion, weight loss is clearly associated with a decrease in BP and numerous other improvements in biomedical status. For most people, weight loss is best achieved through appropriate lifestyle modification. Strategies for achieving long-term weight loss are emerging, and the proportion of those who are successful is growing. As a major public health issue, the management of overweight is of the highest priority and is receiving major support from the federal government and other institutions. Successfully accomplishing national goals for weight management can provide additional benefits in the reduction of BP and the associated biomedical burden of risk for CVD and stroke (Table 4.1).

REFERENCES

1. Seidell JC. Obesity, insulin resistance, and diabetes—A worldwide epidemic. *Br J Nutr.* 2000;83(Suppl): S5–S8.
2. Ogden CL, Carroll MD, Curtin LR, McDowell MA, Tabak CJ, Flegal KM. Prevalence of overweight and obesity in the United States, 1999–2004. *JAMA.* 2006;295: 1549–1555.
3. Flegal KM, Carroll MD, Odgen CL, Curtin LR. Prevalence and trends in obesity among US adults, 1999–2008. *JAMA.* 2010;303: 235–241.
4. Manson JE, Colditz GA, Stampfer MJ, et al. A prospective study of obesity and risk of coronary heart disease in women. *NEJM.* 1990;322: 882–889.
5. Huang Z, Hankinson SE, Colditz GA, et al. Dual effects of weight and weight gain on breast cancer risk. *JAMA.* 1997;278: 1407–1411.
6. Shoff SM, Newcomb PA. Diabetes, body size, and risk of endometrial cancer. *Am J Epidemiol.* 1998;148: 234–240.
7. Colditz GA, Willett WC, Stampfer MJ, et al. Weight as a risk factor for clinical diabetes in women. *Am J Epidemiol.* 1990;132: 501–513.
8. Field AE, Coakley EH, Must A, et al. Impact of overweight on the risk of developing common chronic diseases during a 10-year period. *Arch Intern Med.* 2001;161: 1581–1586.
9. JNC VII Express. *The Seventh Report of the Joint National Committee on Prevention, Detection, Evaluation, and Treatment of High Blood Pressure.* Bethesda, MD: National Institutes of Health, 2003. Publication No. 03-5233.
10. MacMahon S, Peto R, Cutler J, et al. Blood pressure, stroke, and coronary heart disease. Part 1, prolonged differences in blood pressure: prospective observational studies corrected for regression dilution bias. *Lancet.* 1990; 335: 765–774.
11. Kannel WB, Wilson PW, Zhang TJ. The epidemiology of impaired glucose tolerance and hypertension. *Am Heart J.* 1991;12 (4, Part 2): 1268–1273.
12. Whelton PK. Epidemiology of hypertension. *Lancet.* 1994;344(8915): 101–106.
13. Klag MJ, Whelton PK, Randall BL, et al. Blood pressure and end-stage renal disease in men. *NEJM.* 1996;334: 13–18.
14. Symonds B. Blood pressure of healthy men and women. *JAMA.* 1923;8: 232–236.
15. Dublin LI. *Report of the Joint Committee on Mortality of the Association of Life Insurance Medical Directors.* New York: Actuarial Society of America, 1925.
16. Hubert HB, Feinleib M, McNamara PM, Castelli WP. Obesity as an independent risk factor for cardiovascular disease: A 26-year follow-up of participants in the Framingham Heart Study. *Circulation.* 1983;67: 968–977.

17. Stamler R, Stamler J, Riedlinger WF, Algera G, Roberts R. Weight and blood pressure: Findings in hypertension screening of 1 million Americans. *JAMA.* 1978;240: 1607–1609.
18. Manson JE, Willett WC, Stampfer MJ, et al. Body weight and mortality among women. *NEJM.* 1995;333(11): 677–685.
19. Higgins M, Kamel W, Garrison R, Pinsky J, Stokes J. Hazards of obesity-the Framingham experience. *Acta Med Scand.* 1998;723(Suppl): 23–26.
20. Rabkin SW, Chen Y, Leiter L, Liu L, Reeder BA. Canadian Heart Health Surveys Research Group. Risk factor correlates of body mass index. *CMAJ.* 1997;157(1 Suppl): S26–S31.
21. Neal B, MacMahon S, Chapman N. Effects of ACE inhibitors, calcium antagonists, and other blood-pressure-lowering drugs: results of prospectively designed overviews of randomised trials. Blood pressure lowering treatment trialists' collaboration. *Lancet.* 2000;356 (9246): 1955–1964.
22. Cutler JA, Follman D, Allender PS. Randomized trials of sodium reduction: An overview. *Am J Clin Nutr.* 1997;65: S643–S651.
23. Appel LJ, Moore TJ, Obarzanek E, et al. for the DASH Collaborative Research Group. A clinical trial of the effects of dietary patterns on blood pressure. *NEJM.* 1997;336(16): 1117–1124.
24. Stevens VJ, Obarzanek E, Cook NR, et al. Long-term weight loss and changes in blood pressure: Results of the Trials of Hypertension Prevention, phase II. *Ann Intern Med.* 2001;134: 1–11.
25. Haynes R. Is weight loss an effective treatment for hypertension? *Can J Physiol Pharmacol.* 1985;64: 825–830.
26. Neter JE, Stam BE, Kok FJ, Grobbee DE, Gelseijnse JM. Influence of weight reduction on blood pressure: A meta-analysis of randomized controlled trials. *Hypertension.* 2003;42: 878–884.
27. Ebrahim S, Smith GD. Lowering blood pressure: A systematic review of sustained effects of non-pharmacological interventions. *J Pub Health Med.* 1998;20(4): 441–448.
28. TOHP-1. The effects of nonpharmacologic interventions on blood pressure of persons with high normal levels. Results of the trials of hypertension prevention, phase 1. *JAMA.* 1992;267: 1213–1220.
29. Rocchini AP. Obesity and Blood Pressure Regulation. In *Handbook of Obesity,* Bray GA, Bouchard C, James WPT (eds.). New York: Marcel Dekker, 1998: 677–696.
30. Ferranini E, Buzzigoli G, Bonadonna R. Insulin resistance in essential hypertension. *NEJM.* 1987;317: 350–357.
31. Rocchini AP, Katch V, Kveselis D, Moorehead C, Martin M, Lampman R, Gregory M. Insulin and renal retention in the obese. *Hypertension.* 1989;14: 367–374.
32. Rocchini AP, Moorehead C, DeRemer S, Goodfriend TL, Ball DL. Hyperinsulinemia and the aldosterone and pressor responses to angiotensin II. *Hypertension.* 1990;15: 861–866.
33. Anderson EA, Hoffman RP, Balon TW, Sinkey CA, Mark AL. Hyperinsulinemia produces both sympathetic neural activation and vasodilation in normal humans. *J Clin Invest.* 1991;87: 2246–2252.
34. Tedde R, Sechi LA, Marigliano A, Scano L, Pala A. In vitro action of insulin on erythrocyte sodium transport mechanisms: Its possible role the pathogenesis of arterial hypertension. *Clin Exp Hypertension.* 1988;10: 545–559.
35. Walston J, Silven K, Bogardus C, et al. Time of onset of noninsulin dependent diabetes mellitus and genetic variation in β3-adrenergic receptor gene. *NEJM.* 1995;333: 343–347.
36. Dahl LK, Silver L, Christie RW. The role of salt in the fall of blood pressure accompanying reduction in obesity. *NEJM.* 1958;258: 1186–1192.

37. Fagerberg B, Andersson OK, Isaksson B, Björntorp P. Blood pressure control during weight reduction in obese hypertensive men: Separate effects of sodium and energy restriction. *Br Med J*. 1984;288: 11–14.

38. Reisen E, Abel R, Modan M, Silverberg DS, Eliahou HE, Modan B. Effect of weight loss without salt restriction on the reduction of blood pressure in overweight hypertensive patients. *NEJM*. 1978;298: 1–6.

39. Tuck MI, Sowers J, Dornfield L, Kledzik G, Maxwell M. The effect of weight reduction on blood pressure plasma renin activity and plasma aldosterone level in obese patients. *NEJM*. 1981;304: 930–933.

40. Maxwell MH, Kushiro T, Dornfeld LP, Tuck ML, Waks AU. BP changes in obese hypertensive subjects during rapid weight loss. Comparison of restricted v unchanged salt intake. *Arch Intern Med*. 1984;144: 1581–1584.

41. Elmer PJ, Obarzanek E, Vollmer WM, et al. for the PREMIER Collaborative Research Group. Effects of comprehensive lifestyle modification on diet, weight, physical fitness, and blood pressure control: 18-Month results of a randomized trial. *Ann Intern Med*. 2006;144: 485–495.

42. He J, Whelton PK, Appel LJ, Charleston J, Klag MJ. Long-term effects of weight loss and dietary sodium reduction on incidence of hypertension. *Hypertension*. 2000;35; 544–549.

43. Hypertension Prevention Trial Research Group. The hypertension prevention trial: Three-year effects of dietary changes on blood pressure. *Arch Intern Med*. 1990;150: 153–162.

44. Svetkey LP, Stevens VJ, Brantley PJ, et al. for the Weight Loss Maintenance Collaborative Research Group. Comparison of strategies for sustaining weight loss, the Weight Loss Maintenance randomized controlled trial. *JAMA*. 2008;299(10): 1139–1148.

45. Dornfield TP, Maxwell MH, Waks AU, Schroth P, Tuck MI. Obesity and hypertension: Long-term effects of weight reduction on blood pressure. *Int J Obes*. 1985;9: 381–389.

46. Reisen E, Frohlich ED. Effects of weight reduction on arterial pressure. *J Chron Dis*. 1982;33: 887–891.

47. Davis BR, Blaufox D, Oberman A, et al. Reduction in long-term antihypertensive medication requirements: effects of weight reduction by dietary intervention in overweight persons with mild hypertension. *Arch Intern Med*. 1993;153: 1773–1782.

48. Buchwald H, Avidor Y, Braunwald E, et al. Bariatric surgery: A systematic review and meta-analysis. *JAMA*. 2004; 292(14): 1724–1737.

49. Sjostrom CD, Peltonen M, Wedel H, Sjostrom L. Differential long-term effects of intentional weight loss on diabetes and hypertension. *Hypertension*. 2000;36: 20–25.

50. Sjöström CD, Peltonen M, Siöström L. Blood pressure and pulse pressure during long-term weight loss in the obese: The Swedish Obese Subjects (SOS) Intervention Study. *Obes Res*. 2001;9(3): 188–195.

51. Sjostrom CD, Lystig T, Lindroos AK. Impact of weight change, secular trends, and ageing on cardiovascular risk factors: 10-year experiences from the SOS study. *Int J Obes (Lond)*. November, 2011;35(11): 1413–1420. Doi: 10.1038/ijo.2010.282.

52. Simpson CC, LJ Appel, GJ Jerome, et al. *Relationship between Weight Regain and Blood Pressure in Phase 3 of the Weight Loss Maintenance Trial. Abstracts from the Joint Conference: Nutrition, Physical Activity and Metabolism and Cardiovascular, Epidemiology, and Prevention 2011 Scientific Sessions*; American Heart Association; 2011 Mar 22–25; Atlanta, GA. Abstract MP21, p. 126.

53. National Institutes of Health Technology Assessment Conference Panel. Methods for voluntary weight loss and control. *Ann Intern Med*. 1993;119: 764–770.

54. Institute of Medicine. Weighing the options: Criteria for evaluating weight management programs. 1995; Washington, DC: Govt. Pr Off.

55. Jeffery RW, Drewnowski A, Epstein LH, et al. Long-term maintenance of weight loss: Current status. *Health Psychol.* 2000 Jan; 19(1 Suppl): 5–16.
56. Kassirer J, Angell M. Losing weight—an ill-fated new year's resolution. *NEJM.* 1998;338: 52–54.
57. Wing RR, Phelan S. Long-term weight loss maintenance. *Am J Clin Nutr.* 2005;82(Suppl): S222–225S.
58. Bray GA. Nutrition, Diet, and Treatment of Overweight. Contemporary Diagnosis and Management of Obesity and the Metabolic Syndrome (3rd edn.). Newtown, PA: Handbooks in Health Care. 2003, Chapter 8: 202–239.
59. Svetkey LP, Ard JD, Stevens VJ, et al. For the Weight Loss Maintenance Collaborative Research Group. Predictors of long-term weight loss in adults with modest initial weight loss, by sex and race. *Obesity.* 2011 April 28. Epub ahead of print. PMID: 21527896
60. Goldstein DJ. Beneficial health effects of modest weight loss. *Int J Obes Relat Metab Disord.* 1992;16: 397–415.
61. Diabetes Prevention Program Research Group. Reduction in the incidence of type 2 diabetes with lifestyle intervention or metformin. *N Engl J Med.* 2002;346: 393–403.
62. Cutler JA. Randomized clinical trials of weight reduction in nonhypertensive persons. *Ann Epidemiol.* 1991;1: 363–370.
63. Svetkey LP. Management of pre-hypertension. *Hypertension.* 2005;45: 1056–1061.

5 Physical Activity and Blood Pressure Control

Deborah Rohm Young
University of Maryland School of Public Health

CONTENTS

Regular physical activity confers a number of health benefits. Physically active individuals have lower incidence of coronary heart disease, stroke, type 2 diabetes, some types of cancers, and obesity. Physical activity is known to reduce the incidence and prevalence of hypertension and to lower systolic blood pressure (SBP) and diastolic blood pressure (DBP). Given that only less than half of the U.S. population meets the federal guidelines for physical activity [1], it is no surprise that approximately 30% of the U.S. population has high BP [2]. This chapter reviews the evidence linking regular physical activity and lowering of BP, provides an overview of potential mechanisms for the association, clarifies recommendations on physical activity for controlling BP, and identifies interventions and policies to increase physical activity. The American College of Sports Medicine (ACSM) Position Stand "Exercise and Hypertension" is an excellent review document on this topic [3].

5.1   DEFINITIONS OF PHYSICAL ACTIVITY

Precisely, physical activity is any muscular contraction that results in bodily movement. Thus, typing this sentence is technically a physical activity. In more useful terms, we define physical activity as movement of large skeletal muscles (legs, arms), which requires energy expenditure substantially greater than that required during the resting state. Energy expended during physical activity can be conceptualized as multiples of resting metabolic rate, in which the resting metabolic rate is equal to 1 metabolic equivalent (MET). Physical activities are commonly categorized as light (1.5–2.9 METs), moderate (3.0–5.9 METs), and vigorous (≥6 METs) [4]. For example, brisk walking at 4 mph is defined as a 5-MET activity or an activity in which the energy expended is five times the energy expended at rest [5]. The term "exercise" is a subset of physical activity that is planned, structured, and goal-oriented to increase or maintain one or more types of physical fitness (aerobic fitness, muscular strength, muscular endurance, flexibility, body composition, etc.) [6].

Physical activity can also be defined as aerobic or nonaerobic. Aerobic physical activity uses the large muscle groups, uses oxygen as its primary source of energy, and can be carried out for relatively long periods. Walking, bicycling, kayaking, and raking leaves exemplify aerobic physical activity. In contrast, nonaerobic physical activity comprises short, high-intensity bursts of movement that cannot be sustained over time. During nonaerobic activities, the energy that is stored in muscles is rapidly depleted. Examples are heavy lifting and sprint running. Most of the health benefits associated with regular physical activity are from aerobic types of physical activity; they can occur from leisure, transportation, household, and work sources.

Individuals can be categorized in a variety of ways depending on how they engage in physical activities. Individuals who do not engage in moderate to vigorous physical activities are often defined as sedentary. Those who meet current federal guidelines are defined as physically active. However, federal guidelines have been in place since 2008 only, and physical activity assessment tools do not always result in data that can classify individuals as meeting guidelines. Further, it is often unclear how to define individuals who are neither sedentary nor active enough to meet the guidelines. They are sometimes termed inactive, insufficiently active, or moderately active. Because physical activity can be assessed by many ways (self-report instruments, interviews, objective measures), epidemiological studies often cannot be directly compared regarding the amounts and types of physical activity that are associated with health outcomes.

Physical activities can also be acute or chronic; health benefits confer from both. For example, the feeling of relaxation after completing a jogging session is the result of an acute bout of physical activity. In contrast, reduced risk of stroke results from numerous weekly sessions of physical activity carried out over months or years.

The above definitions can be summarized by the acronym FITT, which stands for frequency, intensity, time, and type. Frequency is the number of times per week or month that physical activity occurs (e.g., three times per week). Intensity is the amount of energy expended during a bout of physical activity (e.g., moderate to vigorous activity or a 5-MET activity). Time is the length of a particular bout of physical activity (e.g., 30 min of walking). Type is the kind of physical activity. This can include aerobic and nonaerobic activities or a particular type of these categories (e.g., walking, jogging).

5.2 CURRENT PHYSICAL ACTIVITY GUIDELINES AND RECOMMENDATIONS

5.2.1 NATIONAL GUIDELINES FOR AMERICANS

In October 2008, the U.S. Department of Health and Human Services published national guidelines for physical activity for all Americans. Those specific to adults are displayed in Table 5.1. More information and guidelines for youth, older adults, and adults needing special consideration (e.g., pregnancy, disabilities) can be found at http://www.health.gov/paguidelines/default.aspx. The guidelines are applicable for BP control; no specific alterations in recommendations are noted. While the U.S. Surgeon General published evidence-based recommendations for physical activity in 1996 to improve and maintain health of Americans [4], the 2008 national guidelines represent a major breakthrough that allows federal, state, and local policies and programs to support the guidelines. Of note, recommendations for physical activity and health have remained mostly consistent over this period, giving health professionals

---

TABLE 5.1

National (U.S.) Physical Activity Guidelines for Adults

	Recommendation
General	All adults should avoid inactivity. Some physical activity is better than none, and adults who participate in any amount of physical activity gain some health benefits.
Aerobic activity	For substantial health benefits, adults should do at least 150 min (2 h and 30 min) a week of moderate-intensity aerobic physical activity, or 75 min (1 h and 15 min) a week of vigorous-intensity aerobic physical activity, or an equivalent combination of moderate- and vigorous-intensity aerobic activity. Aerobic activity should be performed in episodes of at least 10 min, and preferably, it should be spread throughout the week.
Resistance activity	Adults should also do muscle-strengthening activities that are moderate or high intensity and involve all major muscle groups on 2 or more days a week, as these activities provide additional health benefits.

Source: Department of Health and Human Services, *Physical Activity Guidelines for Americans,* U.S. Department of Health and Human Services, Washington, DC, 2008. http://www.health.gov/paguidelines (accessed December 12, 2010).

and the public the confidence that the guidelines are stable and based on the best scientific evidence available.

5.2.2 Physical Activity and BP Control

Based on an evidence-based review of the literature on physical activity and BP, the 2004 position statement of the ACSM concludes that the optimal frequency, intensity, time, and type of physical activity for BP reduction are unclear [3]. Nevertheless, there are overwhelming data from randomized controlled trials for the position statement to conclude that aerobic physical activity reduces resting BP in persons with normal BP and in those with hypertension and that the response is greater in hypertensive persons. The position statement recommends that individuals with high BP follow the recommendations for the general population, which at that time was to accumulate at least 30 min of moderate-intensity physical activity on most, if not all, days of the week [7]. Although the benefits of strength exercise for BP control are thought to be modest, resistance or weight-lifting exercises (to enhance muscular strength and endurance) 2–3 days per week are also recommended as supplemental exercise to ensure a well-rounded physical activity program [8].

5.3 HIGHLIGHTS OF EVIDENCE SUPPORTING GUIDELINES OR RECOMMENDATIONS

5.3.1 Epidemiological Evidence

Large, prospective cohort studies provide evidence of associations between physical activity and prevention of hypertension. One of the first studies to report this association was conducted by Paffenbarger et al. Results from the Harvard Alumni Study indicated that men who reported vigorous physical activity had lower incidence of physician-diagnosed hypertension than men who reported no vigorous physical activity, after 6–10 years of follow-up [9]. Because of the nature of the cohort, the men were mostly whites and well educated. Pereira et al. used the Atherosclerosis Risk in Communities Study data set ($n = 7459$) to determine if the study results could be extended to women and blacks [10]. Over 6 years of follow-up, white men in the highest quartile of leisure-time physical activity had 34% reduced odds (95% CI: 0.47, 0.94) of incident hypertension compared with white men in the lowest quartile. The odds ratios for hypertension associated with a sport-activity index and a work-activity index (subscales of the study's physical activity instrument) for white men and all physical activity indices for white women, black men, and black women were not statistically significant. In the Coronary Artery Risk Development in Young Adults study on 3993 blacks and whites initially between 18 and 30 years of age, there were 634 cases of incidence of hypertension over 15 years of follow-up [11]. In the combined cohort analysis, the hazard rate ratio of physical activity was 0.83 (95% CI: 0.73, 0.93). When analyses were stratified by sex and race, the magnitude of the results was similar for all groups except for white women, although statistical significance was not attained. The lack of statistical significance for the subgroups is likely due to insufficient cases of incidence of hypertension, especially for the white women. These are merely some examples of the many published epidemiological studies examining physical activity and hypertension. Although the epidemiological evidence is less strong for the various population subgroups, there is no scientific reason to presume that the benefits of physical activity for reducing the risk of hypertension would not confer to all adults.

5.3.2 Randomized Controlled Trials

5.3.2.1 Aerobic Physical Activity

Published meta-analyses review the evidence supporting the role of physical activity interventions for reducing BP. Cornelissen and Fagard conducted the most recent meta-analysis of randomized controlled trials of aerobic exercise on resting BP among normotensive and hypertensive adults [12]. Fifteen trials included only nonhypertensive adults, 33 trials included participants with prehypertension, and 28 trials included participants with hypertension. The exercise interventions lasted between 4 and 52 weeks (median 16 weeks), with frequency ranging from 1 to 7 days per week (median 16 weeks), intensity ranging from moderate to vigorous intensity, and duration ranging from 15 to 63 min per session (median 40 min). As seen in Table 5.2, the meta-analysis demonstrates that physical activity significantly lowers SBP in those with and without hypertension and DBP in all but normotensive individuals. The effect is greatest in those with hypertension: mean reduction in SBP of 6.9 (95% CI: 9.1–4.6) and DBP of 4.9 (95% CI: 6.5–3.3) mmHg. However, the response is variable: across the individual trials, net mean change (control minus intervention) ranged from −20.0 to 9.0 mmHg in SBP and from −11.0 to 11.3 mmHg in DBP. Nonetheless, the results from the meta-analysis suggest that small effects on BP result from aerobic exercise training.

Although combining studies through meta-analytic techniques demonstrates the beneficial effects of physical activity for reducing BP, not all trials exhibit positive results. Investigators tend to discount unexpected or nonsignificant findings as a result of poor design or implementation. This is not always the case however, and

TABLE 5.2
Meta-analysis Results of the Effects of Aerobic Exercise on BP, Stratified by Baseline BP Status

	Systolic BP Change		Diastolic BP Change	
	Mean (mmHg)	95% CI	Mean (mmHg)	95% CI
Normal BP	−2.4	−4.2, −0.6	−1.6	−2.4, 0.7
Prehypertension	−1.7	−3.1, −0.3	−1.7	−2.6, −0.8
Hypertension	−6.9	−9.1, −4.6	−4.9	−6.5, −3.3

Source: Cornelissen, V.A. and Fagard, R.H., *J. Hypertens.*, 46, 667–75, 2005.

occasionally, well-designed trials do not yield BP-lowering benefits. For instance, Church et al. randomized postmenopausal women with prehypertension or stage 1 hypertension to four conditions: 50%, 100%, or 150% of recommended physical activity or control condition [13]. Supervised exercise training was conducted for 6 months at a similar frequency (3–4 times per week) and intensity (approximately three METs), but varying in duration from a mean of 72, 136, and 192 min per week for the 50%, 100%, and 150% groups, respectively. At follow-up, there were no differences in mean SBP or DBP change for any of the physical activity doses, compared with the control group. BP of the control group did decline, however, and regression to the mean that can occur without obtaining a stable measure of BP over a number of weeks both at baseline and follow-up may have contributed to the nonsignificant results.

5.3.2.2 Resistance Training

In addition to aerobic physical activity, a number of studies have investigated the effects of resistance training on BP control. The ACSM Position Stand in 2004 concluded that resistance training consistent with current physical activity recommendations reduces BP in normotensive and hypertensive individuals [3]. A meta-analysis report, published in 2005, was conducted on nine randomized controlled trials that included 12 study groups (three studies included hypertensive participants and nine included nonhypertensive participants; total $N = 341$) [14]. The exercise regimens varied: average frequency was 3 times per week, intensity was a mean of 61% of one repetition maximum (i.e., the heaviest weight that can be lifted one time) with a range 30%–90%, the number of exercises (e.g., bench press, lat pull) ranged from 1 to 14 (mean 9.9), and the number of sets ranged from 1 to 4 (mean 1.8), with the number of repetitions per set from 1 to 25. In 10 of the study groups, exercises included exercises for arms, trunk, and legs. The net response of resistance training was a pooled mean change of −3.2 (95% CI: −7.1 to 0.7) mmHg for SBP and −3.5 (95% CI: −6.1 to −0.9) mmHg for DBP. The meta-analysis found smaller reductions in BP in the hypertensive individuals than in nonhypertensive individuals, although there were only three trials with hypertensive individuals. Clearly, more well-designed trials are needed to determine the effects of resistance training on BP in individuals with hypertension.

The recommendation to include resistance training in regular physical activity routines for BP control is important, especially for older adults—the population subgroup that is most likely to have hypertension. Prior to the research on resistance training and BP, it was thought that resistance training would result in left ventricular hypertrophy and hypertension. It is well known that there is a transient but substantial increase in BP during resistance training, and there was concern that this would result in chronic elevated resting BP. Results from studies indicate that this concern was unfounded, and the limited evidence available suggests that there is little effect on BP after an acute resistance exercise bout [3]. Given that aging results in muscle atrophy, which can lead to loss of physical function and disability, and resistance training can maintain muscular strength, the added benefit of resistance training, that is, modest decline in BP can doubly benefit older adults [15].

5.4   POTENTIAL MECHANISMS EXPLAINING HOW AEROBIC EXERCISE REDUCES BP

The mechanisms by which regular aerobic exercise reduces BP are not definitive, but studies point to alterations in the sympathetic nervous system, the renin–angiotensin system, changes in vascular responsiveness, and structural adaptations [16,17]. These potential mechanisms may work independently or in concert. Animal and human studies together provide the body of evidence linking physiological and/or structural changes to lowering of BP after a period of physical activity training.

Two well-known physiological changes resulting from regular moderate to vigorous physical activity are reduction in vasomotor tone and decrease in activity of the sympathetic nervous system [16,17]. Given that activation of the sympathetic nervous system results in norepinephrine output and subsequent vasoconstriction and increased vascular resistance, which results in increased BP, most of the scientific evidence indicates that the chronic effects of physical activity modulate this response. Most studies demonstrate that exercise training reduces activity of the sympathetic nervous system and norepinephrine release in individuals with hypertension [16]. The effect of exercise on sympathetic tone may be mediated through insulin's effects on the sympathetic nervous system. Regular physical activity enhances uptake of glucose in muscles and improves insulin sensitivity [18], which may reduce activity of the sympathetic nervous system and thus reduce BP.

Endothelial dysfunction can also result in higher vascular resistance and increased BP [19]. Regular physical activity improves endothelial-dependent vasodilation through enhancement of nitric oxide release [20] and a number of other mechanisms [16,17]. This enhanced endothelial function may contribute to lower vascular resistance and reduce BP. Though the evidence is not consistent, it is also possible that effects on the renin–angiotensin system following exercise training will contribute to reduction in BP by affecting blood volume and vasomotor tone [16].

5.5   EFFECTS OF ACUTE PHYSICAL ACTIVITY ON BP

In addition to BP being influenced by regular physical activity, BP is also influenced by a single bout, or a session, of physical activity. After aerobic exercise, there is a reduction in resting BP. This phenomenon, first identified in the 1960s, is called *postexercise hypotension*, which occurs in nonhypertensive and hypertensive individuals [3]. This phenomenon appears to result from aerobic [21], but not resistance exercise [22]; at least for older adults with hypertension, it may persist for almost 24 h after a bout of physical activity [21]. The reduction in SBP is about 5 mmHg, as measured from ambulatory BP monitoring. While the actual FITT equation needed to produce this response is not known, the scientific evidence is sufficient for the ACSM Position Stand to state that there is a known BP-reducing benefit resulting from acute aerobic physical activity, especially for those with hypertension [3].

5.6 INCREASING PHYSICAL ACTIVITY: THE NATIONAL PHYSICAL ACTIVITY PLAN

In response to the 2008 physical activity guidelines for all Americans [23], the U.S. Government launched the National Physical Activity Plan in 2010. Based on the current evidence, if more Americans were physically active, the prevalence of high BP would be reduced. From Dr. Geoffrey Rose's population strategy for prevention, which states that a small reduction in risk in the entire population has greater societal benefits on morbidity and mortality compared with treating only a small number of individuals with a particular risk factor [24], it is clear that implementing a national physical activity plan can be of enormous benefit. The National Physical Activity plan can be found in its entirety at http://www.physicalactivityplan.org.

The plan is designed to be implemented across eight societal sectors: business and industry; education; health care; mass media; parks, recreation, fitness, and sports; public health; transportation, land use, and community design; and volunteer and nonprofit sectors. There are also five overarching strategies: (1) launch a grassroots advocacy effort to mobilize public support for the plan, (2) create a national physical activity education program, (3) disseminate best practice models of physical activity programs and policies, (4) create a national resource center to disseminate effective tools and strategies, and (5) establish a center for physical activity policy development and research that can be accessed across all the eight societal sectors.

The health care industry is identified as an important sector for implementing the plan. Using the "prevention" strategy, rather than the "high-risk" strategy, all patients should be assessed and counseled by health care providers to increase their physical activity, regardless of their individual risk status. Additional strategies for the health care sector include classifying physical inactivity as a treatable and preventable condition that is diagnosable, and hence can be covered as a fee-for-service condition, and providing medical coverage for physical activity programs for individuals. There are unique strategies identified for each of the societal sectors that can contribute to the plan.

There is no doubt that implementing a national physical activity plan that can change societal norms toward physical activity can have an impact on BP. One of the plan's societal sectors, transportation/land use/community design, is associated with physical activity and obesity [25,26], which may also influence BP. A recent study conducted in Portland, OR, found that individuals living in highly walkable neighborhoods had a decline in BP over a 1-year period, whereas those in low walkabiltity neighborhoods had BP increases [27]. After controlling for potential confounders, results indicated that high neighborhood walkability and residents' use of fast-food restaurants was associated with increased BP in low but not highly walkable neighborhoods. Evaluating the effects of community design and land-use patterns on the health status and health behaviors of residents is a complex undertaking, but data suggesting that the health status is improved when residents have access to walkable environments are beginning to emerge.

5.7   HEALTH CARE PROFESSIONALS AND
PHYSICAL ACTIVITY COUNSELING

Prevention and early intervention counseling by health care professionals is recognized as an effective strategy to increase physical activity among patients at high risk for developing hypertension and among the general population (http://www. physicalactivityplan.org). A 12-month, group-randomized trial involving counseling on physical activity given by the general practitioners of New Zealand to their patients resulted in increased physical activity among the patients compared with the patients who received usual health care advice [28]. There also was a reduction in SBP and DBP among those in the intervention group (SBP: −2.58, 95% CI: −4.02 to −1.13; DBP: −2.62, 95% CI: −3.62 to −1.61). However, there was a modest decline in BP among the control group, and thus, data were insufficient to detect between-group differences. Nonetheless, the results are encouraging and confirm the power of the messages health care providers can deliver to their patients. The intervention consisted of brief, individualized counseling by either the patient's primary care physician or a practice nurse using motivational interviewing techniques followed by telephone and mail support from individuals working at regional sports foundations. When health care providers are equipped with counseling techniques and facilitated with additional supports, physical activity can be increased, leading to potential BP-lowering benefits.

Physician advice/counseling is considered such an important recommendation that it is being monitored as part of the U.S. health surveillance system through both the National Health and Nutrition Examination (NHANES) and the Behavioral Risk Factor Surveillance System (BRFSS). Lopez et al., using NHANES data from 1999 to 2004, examined prevalence of counseling on lifestyle modification reported by almost 3500 hypertensive adults [29]. They reported that 79% of the participants received advice to exercise more and that 59% of the participants reported adhering to that advice. These results are remarkably similar to that reported by the BRFSS in which 76% of hypertensive individuals reported ever receiving advice from a health care professional to exercise to improve BP [30]. The data from the BRFSS suggested that those who were overweight or obese were more likely to receive advice than those who were of normal weight. These estimates of prevalence are encouraging and are higher than what has been reported for patients without chronic conditions [31,32]. As primary prevention guidelines are disseminated and implemented by primary care physicians, advice and counseling by health care professionals can extend beyond adults with hypertension to reach all of the population.

5.8   THE RISKS OF PHYSICAL ACTIVITY

The risk of musculoskeletal injuries from physical activity varies depending on the type and dose of the activity performed, personal characteristics of the individual, and environmental conditions. Noncontact activities (e.g., walking, swimming, playing tennis) have the lowest rates of injuries. A Finnish study reported that dancing, swimming, playing golf, and walking or cycling for transportation had the lowest report of injuries per 1000 hours of participation (<1 injury per 1000 hours) [33]. In contrast, contact sports such as karate, soccer, and basketball had higher rates of injuries (6.7, 7.8, and 9.1 per 1000 hours of participation, respectively). The same study found that 3.6 injuries were reported per 1000 hours of running. As running mileage increases, so does the risk of injury: Those who ran 40 miles per week were more than twice as likely to become injured compared with those who ran less than 10 miles per week [34]. It must be noted, however, that greater dose of physical activity is associated with greater health benefits.

The risk of developing injuries is increased from environmental factors. Proper-fitting protective gear such as bicycle helmets, knee pads, and elbow pads are essential to reduce injuries. Wearing bicycle helmets may reduce the risk of death from a crash by almost 75% [35]. Risks of heat and cold injuries from extreme inclement weather are rare and are reduced by wearing proper clothing and getting adequate hydration.

Of greatest clinical concern, there is an increased risk of adverse cardiovascular events during a bout of acute physical activity. This risk is most pronounced in high-intensity activity in which the cardiovascular system is taxed. Compared with sedentary activity, during vigorous activity, the relative risk is 2.4 (95% CI: 1.4–4.2) for experiencing a subarachnoid hemorrhage [36] and 2.1 (95% CI: 1.1–3.6) for myocardial infarction [37]. One study found that for a person who is usually sedentary, the relative risk of having an acute cardiac event while engaging in vigorous activity is 107 (95% CI: 67–171), whereas a peer who is regularly vigorously active had a relative risk of 2.4 for an acute event while being physically active (95% CI: 1.5–3.7) [38]. It is clear that the relative risks of having a cardiac event while exercising are dramatically lowered for persons with regular physical activity. The national recommendation for those with chronic conditions, and for all apparently healthy men of age 40 and above and women of age 50 and above, is to consult with a physician before starting a vigorous exercise program. Similarly, individuals with severe or uncontrolled hypertension should not start any physical activity program before being evaluated by a physician [3]. When resting BP is greater than 200 mmHg systolic or 115 mmHg diastolic, physical activity should be avoided [39].

Despite these precautions, the benefits of being regularly active outweigh the risks (http://www.physicalactivityplan.org). Those who are regularly active and/or highly fit have lower risks of both musculoskeletal [40] and cardiac injury [37,38,41]. In addition, regular physical activity is recommended for individuals with uncontrolled hypertension [42,43]. For persons starting a physical activity program, most musculoskeletal injuries can be minimized by slowly progressing the frequency, duration, and intensity of the activity until weekly volume goals are reached. Table 5.3 displays a progression plan for a walking program that minimizes the risk of injury. The program provides a plan for reaching the U.S. guidelines of aerobic activity, that is, 2.5 h a week.

TABLE 5.3
Example Walking Plan to Minimize Musculoskeletal Injuries

Week	Frequency (per week)	Intensity	Time (in minutes)
1	2	Comfortable pace (3 mph)	20
2	3	Comfortable pace (3 mph)	20
3	3	Comfortable pace (3 mph)	30
4	4	Brisk pace (3.5–4 mph)	20
5	4	Brisk pace (3.5–4 mph)	30
6	5	Brisk pace (3.5–4 mph)	30

Note: Generally, for a healthy 60-year-old woman who is currently sedentary with no walking for transportation or leisure, the goal is to meet the physical activity recommendations of walking 150 min/week.

5.9 INTERNATIONAL ISSUES REGARDING BP AND PHYSICAL ACTIVITY

The dual public health problem of elevated BP and physical inactivity is not unique to the United States. The World Health Organization estimated that 60% of all deaths in 2005 were due to chronic diseases, of which 80% occurred in low- and middle-income countries [44]. A Disease Control Priorities Project report states that high BP is the reason behind 9.3% of all deaths in high-income countries and 5.6% of deaths in low- and middle-income countries [45]. A surveillance program of chronic-disease risk factors in five Asian countries (nine survey sites in Bangladesh, India, Indonesia, Thailand, and Vietnam) reported the prevalence of elevated BP ranging from 9.3% in Bangladesh to 27.7% in Thailand [46]. Prevalence of low physical activity was approximately 50% in four of the nine sites. Worldwide, physical inactivity is estimated to account for 1.9 million deaths per year [47]. The World Health Organization recommendations include interventions to reduce the prevalence of physical inactivity as one of its major objectives in its 2008–2013 Action Plan for the Global Strategy for the Prevention and Control of Non-communicable Diseases [48]. The action plan includes a recommendation for all countries to establish a national physical activity plan, as the plan that has already been accomplished in Australia, France, Kuwait, Switzerland, Sweden, and the United States. Many other countries have physical activity policies and action plans that are not yet at the national level of implementation.

5.10 CONCLUSION

Key messages from this chapter are illustrated in Table 5.4. The benefits of regular physical activity are numerous and include reduction in the risk for developing hypertension, as well as modest lowering of both SBP and DBP. Moderate-intensity aerobic exercise, such as brisk walking for 30 min per day, on most days of the week is a physical activity that is sufficient to lower BP. Compelling data exist to suggest

TABLE 5.4

Summary: Take-Home Messages

Key Evidences	Recommendation for Health Care Practitioners
• Meta-analysis results demonstrate that regular physical activity (aerobic physical activity and resistance training) reduces BP for individuals with hypertension and normal BP • National physical activity guidelines call for Americans to participate in regular physical activity. The amount of physical activity recommended by the guidelines is sufficient to reduce BP • The benefits of physical activity greatly outweigh the risks	• Ask all patients about their current physical activity level • Inform all patients about physical activity guidelines and encourage adherence • If possible, help patients identify barriers and solutions • Encourage patients to start slowly and gradually increase the duration, frequency, and intensity of physical activity to meet national guidelines • Follow up and provide support and encouragement after initial counseling

that resistance training also may contribute to lowering of BP; therefore, resistance training also should be included in a well-rounded physical activity program. In today's society that is highly mechanized and replete with an abundance of attractive and entertaining sedentary leisure options, the challenge is to provide environments, policies, and programs that encourage greater physical activity. The National Physical Activity Plan provides a framework for comprehensive physical activity policies that integrate across all the U.S. societal sectors. Physicians and other health care professionals can play an important role in implementing the plan, which can help millions of Americans prevent or control hypertension.

REFERENCES

1. Carlson SA, Fulton JE, Schoenborn CA, Loustalo, F. Trend and prevalence estimates based on the 2008 physical activity guidelines for Americans. *Am J Prev Med.* 2010; 39:305–13.
2. Yoon S, Ostchega Y, Louis T. *Trend in Hypertension Awareness, Treatment, and Control—U.S. Adults, 1999–2008.* NCHS Data Brief, no. x. Hyattsville, MD: National Center for Health Statistics, 2007.
3. American College of Sports Medicine. Position Stand. Exercise and hypertension. *Med Sci Sports Exerc.* 2004; 36:533–53.
4. Ainsworth BA, Haskell WL, Whitt MC. Compendium of physical activities. An update of activity codes and MET intensities. *Med Sci Sports Exerc.* 2000; 32S:498–504.
5. Caspersen CJ, Powell KE, Christenson GM. Physical activity, exercise, and physical fitness. *Public Health Rep.* 1985; 100:125–31.
6. U. S. Department of Health and Human Services. *Physical Activity and Health: A Report of the Surgeon General.* 1996. Atlanta, GA: U. S. Department of Health and Human Services, Centers for Disease Control and Prevention, National Center for Chronic Disease Prevention and Health Promotion.
7. Pate RR, Pratt M, Blair SN, et al. Physical activity and public health: A recommendation from the Centers for Disease Control and Prevention and the American College of Sports Medicine. *JAMA.* 1995; 273: 402–7.

8. Williams MA, Haskell WL, Ades PA, et al. Resistance exercise in individuals with and without cardiovascular disease: 2007 update. A scientific statement from the American Heart Association Council on Clinical Cardiology and Council on Nutrition, Physical Activity, and Metabolism. *Circulation.* 2007; 116:572–84.

9. Paffenbarger RS Jr, Wing AL, Hyde R T, Jung, DL. Physical activity and incidence of hypertension in college alumni. *Am J Epidemiol.* 1983; 117:245–57.

10. Pereira MA, Folsom AR, McGovern PG, et al. Physical activity and incident hypertension in black and white adults: The Atherosclerosis Risk in Communities Study. *Prev Med.* 1999; 28:301–12.

11. Parker ED, Schmitz KH, Jacobs DR Jr, Dengel DR, Schreiner PJ. Physical activity in young adults and incident hypertension over 15 years of follow-up: the CARDIA study. *Am J Public Health.* 2007; 97:703–9.

12. Cornelissen VA, Fagard RH. Effects of endurance training on blood pressure, blood pressure-regulating mechanisms, and cardiovascular risk factors. *J Hypertens.* 2005; 46:667–75.

13. Church TS, Earnest CP, Skinner JS, Blair SN. Effects of different doses of physical activity on cardiorespiratory fitness among sedentary, overweight or obese postmenopausal women with elevated blood pressure. A randomized controlled trial. *JAMA.* 2007; 297:2081–91.

14. Cornelissen VA, Fagard RH. Effect of resistance training on resting blood pressure: a meta-analysis of randomized controlled trials. *J Hypertens.* 2005; 23:251–9.

15. Williams MA, Stewart KJ. Impact of strength and resistance training on cardiovascular disease risk factors and outcomes in older adults. *Clin Geriatr Med.* 2009; 25:703–14.

16. Fagard RH. Effects of exercise, diet, and their combination on blood pressure. *J Human Hypertens.* 2005; 19:S20–4.

17. Joyner MJ, Green DJ. Exercise protects the cardiovascular system: Effects beyond traditional risk factors. *J Physiol.* 2009; 587:5551–8.

18. McArdle WD, Katch FI, Katch VL. Exercise physiology. Energy, nutrition, and human performance. Baltimore, MD: Lippincott Williams & Wilkins, 1996.

19. Meadows JL, Vaughan DE. Endothelial biology in the post-menopausal obese woman. *Maturitas.* 2011;120–5. Epub 2011 May 6.

20. Kingwell BA, Sherrard D, Jennings GM, Dart AM. Four weeks of cycle training increases basal production of nitric oxide from the forearm. *Am J Physiol.* 1997; 272:H1070–7.

21. Ronda MUPB, Alves MJNN, Braga AMFW, et al. 2002. Postexercise blood pressure reduction in elderly hypertensive patients. *J Am Coll Cardiol.* 2002; 39: 676–82.

22. Roltsch MH, Mendez T, Wilund KR, Hagberg JM. Acute resistive exercise does not affect ambulatory blood pressure in young men and women. *Med Sci Sports Exerc.* 2001; 33:881–6.

23. Department of Health and Human Services. *2008 Physical Activity Guidelines for Americans.* Washington, DC: U.S. Department of Health and Human Services. 2008. Available at http://www.health.gov/paguidelines (accessed December 12, 2010).

24. Rose G. *The Strategy of Preventive Medicine.* Oxford, UK: Oxford University Press, 1992.

25. Lopez R. Urban sprawl and risk for being overweight or obese. *Am J Public Health.* 2004; 94:1574–9.

26. Saelens BE, Sallis JF, Frank LD. Environmental correlates of walking and cycling: Findings from the transportation, urban design, and planning literature. *Ann Beh Med.* 2003; 25:80–91.

27. Li F, Harmer P, Cardinal BJ, Vongjaturapat N. Built environment and changes in blood pressure in middle aged and older adults. *Prev Med.* 2009; 48:237–241.

28. Elley CR, Kerse N, Arroll B, Robinson E. Effectiveness of counseling patients on physical activity in general practice: Cluster randomized controlled trial. *BMJ.* 2003; 326:1–6.

29. Lopez L, Cook EF, Horng MS, Hicks LS. Lifestyle modification counseling for hypertensive patients: Results from the National Health and Nutrition Examination Survey 1999–2004. *Am J Hypertens.* 2009; 22:325–31.

30. Carlson SA, Maynard LM, Fulton JE, Hootman JM, Yoom PW. Physical activity advice to manage chronic conditions for adults with arthritis or hypertension, 2007. *Prev Med.* 2009; 49:209–12.

31. Kreuter MW, Scharff DP, Brennan LK, Lukwago SN. Physician recommendations for diet and physical activity: Which patients get advised to change? *Prev Med.* 1997; 26:825–33.

32. Wee CC, McCarthy EP, Davis RB, Phillips RS. Physician counseling about exercise. *JAMA.* 1999; 282:1583–8.

33. Parkkari J, Kannus P, Natri A, et al. Active living and injury risk. *Int J Sports Med.* 2004; 25:209–16.

35. Attewell RG, Glase K, McFadden M. Bicycle helmet efficacy: A meta-analysis. *Accid Anal Prev.* 2001; 33:345–52.

36. Vlak MHM, Rinkel GJE, Greebe P, van der Bom JG, Algra A. Trigger factors and their attributable risk for rupture of intracranial aneurysms. A case-control study. *Stroke.* 2011; 42:1878–82.

37. Willich SN, Lewis M, Lowel H, et al. Physical exercise as a trigger of acute myocardial infarction. *New Engl J Med.* 1993:329:1684–90.

38. Mittleman MA, Maclure M, Tofler GH, et al. Triggering of acute myocardial infarction by heavy physical exertion. *New Engl J Med.* 1993; 329:1677–83.

39. American College of Sports Medicine. ACSM's guidelines for exercise testing and prescription. Sixth edition. Philadelphia, PA: Lippincott Williams & Wilkins, 2000.

40. Hootman JM, Macera CA, Ainsworth BE, Martin M, Addy CL, Blair SN. Association among physical activity levels, cardiorespiratory fitness, and risk of musculoskeletal injury. *Am J Epidemiol.* 2001; 154:251–8.

41. Giri S, Thompson PD, Kiernan FJ, et al. Clinical and angiographic characteristics of exertion-related acute myocardial infarction. *JAMA.* 1999; 282:1731–1736.

42. Ham OK, Yang SJ. Lifestyle factors associated with blood pressure control among those taking antihypertensive medication. *Asia Pac J Public Health.* Epub ahead of print Oct 12, 2009.

43. Ahmed MI, Pisoni R, Calhoun DA. Current options for the treatment of resistant hypertension. *Expert Rev Cardiovasc Ther.* 2009; 7:1385–93.

44. World Health Organization. *a Guide for Population-Based Approaches to Increasing Levels of Physical Activity. Implementation of the Who Global Strategy on Diet, Physical Activity, and Health.* Geneva, Switzerland: World Health Organization, 2007.

45. Lopez AD, Mathers CD, Ezzati M, Jamison DT, Murray CJL. Global and regional burden of disease and risk factors, 2001: Systematic analysis of population health data. *Lancet.* 2006; 367:1747–57.

46. Ng N, Minh HV, Juvekar S, et al. Using the INDEPTH HDSS to build capacity for chronic non-communicable disease risk factor surveillance in low and middle-income countries. 2009. *Global Health Action Supplement.* 2009; 1:7–17.

47. World Health Organization. *The World Health Report. Reducing Risks, Promoting Healthy Life.* Geneva, Switzerland: World Health Organization, 2002.

48. World Health Organization. *2008–2013 Action Plan for the Global Strategy for the Prevention and Control of Noncommunicable Diseases.* Geneva, Switzerland: World Health Organization, 2008.

Section II

Implementation of Lifestyle Intervention for Blood Pressure Control

OVERVIEW

Laura P. Svetkey

In order for efficacious nutritional or lifestyle interventions to improve BP control, these behaviors must be adopted in the real world. In this book, we deliberately refer to "lifestyle change" rather than "going on a diet" or "starting an exercise program" to indicate that we are promoting sustained change in how one lives. It is difficult to change behavior, particularly when there are pressures against change. In the United States, and increasingly in the global society, the pressures against healthy dietary pattern, weight control, and physical activity are formidable. Nonetheless, there is ample evidence that sustained behavior change is achievable. Successful behavior change can be promoted by interventions that are grounded in behavioral theory, that use established behavior-change strategies, and that are provided at both the individual and the system levels.

Behavioral theory suggests that people change when they are ready and when they have the appropriate tools. Tools that promote behavior change go beyond information. For example, many people understand that overweight is unhealthy and that reducing energy balance leads to weight loss. However, that knowledge is generally insufficient for achieving successful weight control. Behavioral tools include concrete strategies for making change, such as goal setting, action planning, and relapse prevention. Motivation is the key, and it can be strengthened through techniques of motivational interviewing. Chapter 6 introduces behavioral theory and practices and explains how motivational interviewing techniques apply this theory to successful lifestyle change.

Behavioral interventions make use of behavioral theory and behavior-change tools in various ways, but most involve strategies to increase awareness and understanding, helping people adopt behavior-change tools and enhancing motivation, social support, monitoring of progress, and feedback. These strategies can be applied to improve lifestyles for BP control at the individual level (i.e., behavioral intervention directed at hypertensive or prehypertensive patients) or at the system level (i.e., behavioral intervention directed at a health system or a health care team that is providing treatment for hypertension). Chapter 7 reviews evidence concerning strategies for implementing behavior change for BP control at the individual level, and Chapter 8 provides evidence concerning implementation at the provider level.

Thus, in this section, we review the evidence and make recommendations related to promoting successful lifestyle change to improve BP control using behavioral theory and practice, applied at both the individual and the health-provider levels.

6 Motivational Interviewing in Hypertension Management

Denise Ernst
Denise Ernst Training and Consultation

Marlyn Allicock
University of North Carolina at Chapel Hill

Marci K. Campbell
University of North Carolina at Chapel Hill

CONTENTS

6.1   INTRODUCTION

Lifestyle changes are keys to managing chronic health conditions such as hypertension. These changes often include modifying dietary intake, increasing physical activity, controlling or losing weight, and adhering to prescribed medications. All of these changes require daily motivation and self-monitoring to be successful. In the absence of symptoms, many patients with conditions such as hypertension drift back to old habits, and nonadherence is a major factor inhibiting optimal disease management [1]. As health professionals, we may find nonadherence to be extremely frustrating as we may feel that our expert health advice is having little or no effect on patients' behavior.

Motivating people to adopt healthier patterns requires an understanding of human behavior and how people actually change. Effective health communication can facilitate behavior change, particularly by providing powerful, positive messages that speak to the interests, desires, and concerns of community members. Programs and messages that are based on an understanding of health behavior and that use effective communication strategies have a much greater traction in producing positive change. However, ultimately, it is the patient's choice as to whether he or she will initiate or maintain recommended changes. Free choice and self-motivation are key elements of human behavior. Strategies that encourage patients to realize and express their own motivations and commitments to change will be more effective than those that persuade or scare people into changing.

One promising strategy that can address patient motivation and treatment efficacy is motivational interviewing (MI). Originally developed for treating substance abuse [2], MI's success in changing seemingly intractable behaviors in this arena fostered its expansion to many other health-related fields, including health behavior, therapeutic adherence, and mental health [3–5]. The evidence for the efficacy of MI in these fields continues to build from many clinical trials, other research efforts, and practice-based studies [3–4].

This chapter reviews the evidence on the application of MI to the management of chronic diseases such as hypertension and diabetes, which require adherence to medication and behavior regimens. The chapter also discusses the theoretical underpinnings of MI techniques in influencing behaviors, provides concrete steps for practitioners to incorporate MI skills in their encounters with patients, and outlines specific recommendations for using MI with hypertensive patients.

6.2 WHAT IS MI?

MI is a collaborative, person-centered form of guiding to elicit and strengthen motivation for change [6]. It was developed in the early 1980s; its brief and effective method can be learned and used by a wide variety of health professionals to help patients tackle complex health issues and concerns [2]. The traditional approach to behavior change, often practiced in health care settings, involves providers delivering brief advice and giving explicit recommendations to patients [7]. MI, on the other hand, operates from the viewpoint that the patient has a central role in determining his or her own behavior change and has freedom of choice in his or her treatment. The clinician collaborates with the patient to determine which behavior change approach would be most suitable. Thus, orientation of MI is interpersonal, egalitarian, and empathic. It is a client-centered "way of being" that manifests through specific techniques and strategies, such as reflective listening and agenda setting. MI helps individuals to work through their ambivalence about behavior change, surmount their own barriers, and explore potential untapped sources of motivation [2]. In MI, the patient is expected to do much of the psychological work, although the counselor facilitates and guides the process. Counselors establish a safe, nonconfrontational, and supportive climate, where clients feel comfortable expressing both positive and negative aspects of their current behavior, as well as the pros and cons for change. To achieve these ends, MI counselors rely heavily on reflective listening and positive affirmations rather than on persuasion or advice giving.

Two major components of MI are (1) the underlying spirit and style of the interaction between the provider and the patient and (2) technical focus on strategically influencing the patient's talk in the direction of change. Miller and Rose [8] hypothesize that both these elements—the relational (MI spirit) and the technical (influencing change talk)—determine MI's efficacy. Evidence indicates that both the components contribute to the method's effectiveness and that they operate synergistically [8].

The spirit of MI has clearly evolved from the client-centered approach of Carl Rogers [9]. It draws heavily on the role of empathy and acceptance. In addition, MI focuses on actively collaborating with the patient on the agenda, goals, plans, and actions to be taken. MI attempts to elicit or evoke from the patient his or her ideas, values, strengths, knowledge, suggestions, concerns, reasons for change, and commitment. Lastly, the deep valuing of the patient's autonomy, decision-making capacity, and responsibility for his or her choices is central to MI's spirit. Miller and Rose [8] state that the MI spirit as exhibited by the counselor has a direct relationship to patient outcomes. Findings from several studies support the hypothesis that the therapeutic conditions created by the counselor promote positive change [10–14].

The second component of MI that contributes to its efficacy is its technical focus, which, Miller and Rose [8] state, serves to increase the patient's change talk during the counseling session and decrease talk in favor of continuing the negative behavior/resistance against change. This improved change talk predicts patient behavior. The strategic focus on patient speech involves how the conversation is structured, what the provider asks for and responds to, the strategies that are employed, and how the provider guides the patient in the direction of change. Several studies [15–17] have shown that the counselor's use of MI's consistent style elicits change talk and reduces resistance. Further evidence suggests that change talk predicts behavior change [18–22]. Using MI techniques, the provider elicits patients' statements about their desire, ability, reasons, and need for change. As commitment language is drawn out, behavior change is more likely. Both relational and technical components are important to the provider's delivery of effective MI and the subsequent changes in patient behavior.

6.3   MI AS A STRATEGY FOR AIDING IN BEHAVIOR CHANGE

Consolidated evidence supports the effectiveness of MI for addressing many health behaviors including diet [5,23], physical activity [24,25], weight loss [26], and conditions requiring adherence [27–30], such as hypertension and diabetes.

Unhealthy dietary intake and a sedentary lifestyle are risky behaviors that often lead to diseases or health conditions such as diabetes, high blood pressure, obesity, heart disease, and some cancers. When addressing diet and physical activity behaviors, the intent is generally to modify, rather than eliminate, and to reshape, rather than abstain, untoward behaviors [31]. The goal is often tangible, such as eating the recommended daily servings of fruits and vegetables, reducing fat intake, and engaging in physical activity for a specified number of days/minutes per week. Changes to improve physical activity and dietary behaviors may be viewed as problematic for individuals in two realms. First, engaging in physical activity and having a healthy diet for chronic disease prevention often require long-term changes that may be viewed as burdensome and thus increase individuals' ambivalence about making healthy changes [5]. Second, modifying one's diet or physical activity may require giving up or reducing favorite foods or sedentary behaviors, which may be perceived as an unpleasant sacrifice.

MI can serve as a way to help individuals work through their ambivalence by reframing the need for change in positive terms (what is to be gained vs. what is to be lost), coming to terms about the chronic nature of changes required, and identifying ways to reduce perceptions of change as burdensome [5].

Several reviews and meta-analyses examine the evidence for using MI to change diet and physical activity behaviors. Dunn et al. [32] reviewed 29 studies that delivered MI face-to-face and involved MI monitoring, random assignment, inclusion of a control group, and measurement of behavioral and health outcomes in the areas of substance abuse, smoking, HIV risk behaviors, and diet and exercise. They reported that diet and physical activity interventions demonstrated the most significant effects, whereas the most modest effects were found for smoking.

VanWormer et al. [33] conducted a meta-analysis (four studies) on the effectiveness of MI in diet modification. Significant effects were found in three of the four studies. The review pointed out that MI can be effective even in small doses. It also encouraged more frequent contacts between providers and patients as a way to enhance behavior change.

Rubak et al. [34] conducted a meta-analysis to examine the effectiveness of MI across 72 randomized controlled trials. In 74% of the 72 studies reviewed, there was demonstrated effectiveness for using MI. The analysis included 13 studies targeting physiological problems such as weight loss, decreasing blood lipids, increasing physical activity, and managing diabetes and asthma. In 77% of these studies, an effect was reported. In addition, MI outperforms some of the traditional approaches such as giving advice, is effective in brief doses, and may be conducted by a variety of practitioners.

Martins and McNeil [4] discuss 24 published studies that used MI intervention to modify diet and/or physical activity. Overall, the studies showed support for MI's effectiveness in diet and physical activity behaviors both as a single strategy and in combination with other interventions. Patients receiving the MI intervention reported increased self-efficacy related to diet and exercise, reduced caloric intake, and increased consumption of fruits and vegetables. Additionally, patients who received MI showed decreases in BMI.

In a recent review and meta-analysis of the effectiveness of MI in weight-loss interventions, Armstrong et al. [26] identified 12 studies that met the strict inclusion criteria. Compared with controls, the MI group was associated with a greater loss of weight and reduction in BMI. The authors report that increased effect size was found if weight loss was the primary goal, when the MI was an adjunct to a behavioral weight-loss program, if the duration of treatment was longer than 6 months and if a good treatment fidelity measure was used to ensure quality.

Patients who have chronic diseases such as diabetes and hypertension are expected to manage such conditions by adhering to particular diets, incorporating exercise into their routines, taking medications as prescribed, and undertaking other self-care regimens. A departure from any of the prescribed regimens may lead to poor patient-health outcomes. For example, poor medication adherence can be a costly and troublesome issue for health providers and a serious health risk for patients. Forgetfulness is often cited as a major reason for poor adherence. Remedies to counteract forgetfulness (e.g., pillboxes, timers, beepers, and similar strategies) may still fail when there are underlying reasons that relate to side effects of the medication, ambivalence about the disease or treatment, and fear of or harm from the treatment. On the one hand, individuals may recognize the benefits of taking medication, but on the other hand, they may want to avoid side effects and associated inconveniences or to deny their illness. MI may be effective for those whose adherence is related to ambivalence about the value or utility of taking their medications or for those who have not come to terms with the implications of their condition.

Evidence suggests that MI-based treatment is indeed promising for diabetes and hypertension control. Woollard et al. [35] reported significant decreases in both weight and blood pressure of hypertensive patients receiving the high (6 in-person appointments) intervention treatment compared with those in the low (1 in-person appointment and 5 telephone appointments) intervention and control arms. Similarly, others have shown that MI counseling have led to maintenance of medication adherence [28,36], lowering of blood pressure [28], improved glycemic control [37], improved knowledge of diabetes, beliefs about treatment, motivation for behavior change [38], and short-term weight loss [39,40].

6.4   THEORY AND BEHAVIOR CHANGE

A number of social psychological theories address key constructs in promoting effective behavior change. MI is a counseling technique that draws from multiple theoretical and practical sources in order to create a patient-centered, empathic style of communication. MI encourages individuals to voice their concerns and motivations; to consider issues such as values, barriers, and competing demands; and to ultimately come up with their own reasons and commitments for changing behavior. This type of communication style has proven effective for promoting behavioral adherence [5,23–25] in several areas such as substance abuse, obesity prevention and treatment, dietary change, and chronic disease management.

What is a theory anyway? A *theory* is a set of interrelated concepts, definitions, and propositions that presents a systemic view of events or situations in order to explain and predict future events or situations. Behavioral theories attempt to explain behavior and suggest ways to achieve desired changes. In other words, theories should help us to understand why people behave the way they do now, and by knowing this, we should be able to predict whether they are likely to change. It is particularly important that theories are generalizable; that is, they are broadly applicable across populations and certain kinds of health behaviors. Some theories can help explain the dynamics of the behavior, the internal processes people often use to facilitate changing the behavior, and the effects of external influences on the behavior, such as social and environmental determinants.

As noted above, Miller and Rose [8] hypothesize the underlying processes of MI that are said to influence and predict behavior change. However, other theories are also relevant to MI. The following section provides an overview of some of the theories and constructs that underpin key elements of MI as it may apply to behavioral adherence to lifestyle change.

Health Belief model [41]: What makes people decide to engage in a healthy behavior change? Knowledge is necessary, but not sufficient, for helping people to follow guidelines for medication adherence. People must have the motivation to change. If they believe that they are at increased risk for a particular health problem, that lifestyle change will decrease their risk, and that the benefits of changing outweigh the costs or barriers, then this theory posits that people are more likely to change. The Health Belief model examines many of these issues and provides some important concepts for conveying health information effectively [41]. Through specific techniques and strategies, MI allows health care providers to engage in conversations in which information regarding knowledge, individual perception of risk, and benefits and barriers to engaging in a particular behavior can be elicited and discussed.

Perceived *susceptibility* to a health problem and perceived *severity* or seriousness of the condition and its consequences combine to form the perception of *threat*. Effective health communications should assess the patient's current perceptions about these factors and present feedback or information to help the patient compare their perception with actual risk along with a strategy to reduce the sense of threat by taking the recommended action. Too high a level of perceived threat, induced by fear messages or "over the top" kinds of communications, can actually backfire and result in inaction and fatalism [42]. In addition to considering risk and severity, individuals weigh the perceived *benefits* of the advised action (what will I gain?) against the *barriers* and costs of change (what makes it hard and/or what will I lose?) before deciding to act. Barriers can be very important inhibitors of behavior change. Examples of barriers to healthy eating behavior include the perceived financial cost of purchasing healthier foods, taste preferences for high-sodium or high-fat choices, and lack of support from family members or friends to eat healthy foods. It is important to try to elicit the relevant barriers and the importance of those barriers for each individual, rather than to make assumptions or try to advise people about how to remove them. Often, people express barriers but can also come up with their own solutions to overcoming those barriers. MI provides some ways to help facilitate this process based on the realization that when people come up with their own solutions, they are more likely to follow through with the change compared with that when a professional tries to solve the problems for them. People often (rightly) feel that professionals cannot know what it is like to walk in their shoes and that their lives are so different that a professional's advice may be discounted or even resented. Unwanted or personally irrelevant advice typically leads to greater resistance to change, which is not the desired outcome of counseling.

Self-efficacy (confidence) regarding one's ability to perform the behavior is sometimes considered part of the Health Belief model. Self-efficacy is defined as an individual's degree of confidence in his or her ability to perform a specific behavior. Self-efficacy is not the same thing as self-confidence, which is more of a global sense of efficacy, whereas behavioral self-efficacy is specific to the behavior of interest. So, for example, one might be very confident in one's ability to take medication daily but not very confident about one's ability to be physically active five or more days per week for 30 min at a time. Self-efficacy includes degree of confidence, strength of persistence in the face of obstacles, and commitment to continuing the behavior in different situations and over time.

Behavioral and cognitive strategies to increase self-efficacy include setting small goals at first and gradually increasing the challenge, modeling behavior changes, offering opportunities to practice the behavior, giving constructive feedback, and encouraging positive "self-talk." In individual-level interventions, self-help and computer-interactive strategies can be designed to increase self-efficacy by allowing individuals to select goals, obtain feedback on their progress, and learn concrete skills that are needed to succeed with the behavior change. MI practitioners use importance and confidence rulers as tools to gauge a client's level of confidence for making a behavior change. However, taking the first steps toward a change in behavior depends on a combination of both importance and confidence. Thus, practitioners ask clients to rate both importance of making the change and their confidence that they could follow through with particular plans for achieving their goals. Importance means not only how important it is to a person to make a particular change but also the personal benefits they see to making this change. Often, people understand the benefits of making a particular change, but they may have other pressing needs or priorities in their lives. Confidence means how confident or sure a person is about his or her ability to do something different in life. Confidence is a key factor in making changes. A person may understand that a change is important but may not have the confidence to proceed. People sometimes feel less confident because they had tried to make a similar change before and had been less than successful or there were barriers, such as not knowing what to do first or how to fit this change into their already overloaded life.

MI practitioners first ask clients to rate the importance of the change, and then using the same scale, they ask about confidence. For example, *"How confident are you that you could monitor your blood pressure daily if you decided to? On a scale of 0 to 10, with 0 being not confident at all, and 10 being very confident, where would you place yourself?"* Then the practitioner asks, *"Why did you choose ___, and not a lower number like 1 or 2?"* Clients' answers to this question tell what helps them to feel confident. Finally, the practitioners ask, *"What would it take to move your number a little higher?"* The answers tell you what would increase their confidence.

Stages of change [43]: Changing lifestyle behaviors to control conditions such as hypertension is more or less difficult depending on where the person is in the decision process to attempt a specific change at a given time. For example, even though someone may be aware that eating high-sodium foods can contribute to elevated blood pressure levels, he or she may not be ready or willing to switch to low-sodium alternatives. This may be true for many reasons. It may be that because of competing demands and the need to set priorities, the person has decided (perhaps reasonably) that other health actions, such as quitting smoking, are more important. The person may have ingrained habits, possibly since childhood or culturally based, that he or she does not believe are changeable, such as traditions of eating salted or cured meats on certain occasions or having a "taste" for salty snacks. Perhaps, the individual is ready to change but lacks knowledge or skills to behave differently.

The Stages-of-Change transtheoretical model was developed by Prochaska and DiClemente in the context of smoking cessation behavior; it has its roots in earlier stage models of health behavior [43]. The model's central assumption is that behavior change is a dynamic process involving several cognitively distinct stages. According to the stages-of-change approach, people can be categorized according to their readiness to change. The stages constitute a cycle rather than a linear progression, and people can enter or exit at any point. For example, individuals may progress to action but then relapse and go through some of the stages several times before succeeding in maintenance. The stages include precontemplation (unaware, not interested in change), contemplation (thinking about changing, usually within 6 months), preparation (ready to change soon, e.g., in the next 30 days), action (currently trying to change), and maintenance (maintaining the new, healthier habits for at least 6 months). Some model iterations include the stages of relapse (returning to the old behavior) and termination (new behavior is so established that relapse is not an issue).

MI as a client-centered, directive approach used as a means for enhancing a patient's intrinsic motivation to change is a natural complement with the transtheoretical model. MI seeks to explore motivation required to move a patient through the different stages of change. MI is a useful application at any time regardless of the stages. However, MI is thought to be especially applicable to individuals who are in the precontemplation and contemplation stages [44]. Individuals in the precontemplation stage may not want specific action techniques when they are not ready or thinking about change. Similarly, those who are contemplating change but have not yet decided to change are more resistant to traditional approaches that force change when they are not ready. The guiding principles of MI encourage counselors to express empathy and to accept (i.e., "roll with") resistance to allow the patient to determine the best course of action.

The literature on health education indicates that "one-size-fits-all" programs may fail to motivate large segments of the population who are at different stages of readiness [45]. By applying this idea to the issue of hypertension management, interventions can be tailored to the needs and concerns of individuals at each stage of the change process. MI uses the stages as one element of assessing clients' motivational readiness, realizing that people must feel ready, as well as willing and able, if they are going to seriously address the health issue and modify behavioral choices.

Self-determination theory [46]: Another theory that merits discussion in the context of MI is self-determination theory (SDT) [46]. SDT focuses on human motivation and as such is informative particularly for interventions where enhancing motivation is the key. SDT bases its assumptions on three main human values that underlie behavior: desire for autonomy, competence, and relatedness. SDT interventions often assess the roles of two kinds of motivation in determining behavior change: *intrinsic* or motivation coming from within the individual to perform a behavior "for its own sake" and *extrinsic* or motivation applied from external sources to perform the behavior "for the sake of others." Examples of intrinsic motivation include desire for more control over one's health, wanting to feel better about oneself, and wanting to be a good role model. Examples of extrinsic motivation include exhortations from family members to change behavior, feeling guilty or ashamed about what others think, and feeling pressured by the health provider to change. In general, extrinsic motivation may change behavior in the short term, but this change tends to be less lasting compared with the behavior change coming from intrinsic motivation. Therefore, interventions tend to focus on building intrinsic motivation through actions such as self-assessment, reflection, exercising volitional control over change, and helping people commit to changes they want to make for themselves. These types of strategies are core elements of MI counseling.

6.5 PRACTICAL APPLICATION

Our premise in promoting provider–patient interactions grounded in MI is that any amount of time that is available for the conversation can be used to strengthen the patient's motivation to change. In current medical practice, prolonged counseling by the primary provider is generally not feasible, and trained counseling staff are often not available. In this section, we provide guidelines for MI counseling under optimal circumstances, recognizing that these techniques can be useful to whatever extent it is feasible to provide them [34].

In *Motivational Interviewing in Health Care: Helping Patients Change Behavior*, Rollnick and colleagues [7] identify three core skills used in these conversations: asking, listening, and informing. MI involves specific and strategic use of these skills to guide the conversation toward the negotiated behavioral goal (e.g., increasing exercise, taking medication regularly, and adopting the DASH diet) and to shape the conversation in a way that the patient "talks himself or herself into change." Table 6.1 provides detail and examples of these skills. In general, the provider should move away from reliance on closed-ended questions ("How many pounds do you want to lose?") to the use of open-ended questions ("What concerns have you had about your weight?") that prompt the patient to talk more. The provider then uses listening skills such as reflecting and then summarizing what the patient has said in order to reinforce the patient's reasons to change and to convey empathy and understanding. Lastly, the act of informing the patient, a routine act in any medical care encounter, is done in a way that promotes the patient's sense of choice and autonomy, minimizes the chance of resistance, and encourages the patient to actively engage the information.

The strategic use of the skills discussed in Table 6.1 can increase the likelihood of change even if delivered in small, short doses. Miller and Rose [8] hypothesize that the behavior change is mediated through "change talk" or the patient's voicing the arguments and reasons for change. The technical components of MI are used to facilitate an increase in "change talk." In the dialogue below (Table 6.2), you will see that the providers do this by choosing carefully what questions they ask and what they respond to. Both theory and research suggest that the patient arguing against change or expressing "resistance" to change is associated with a decreased likelihood of behavior change [47]. So the MI provider also uses the skills to avoid arguing with the patient, to roll with the resistance rather than confront it, and to minimally respond to (not completely ignore) the patient's reasons to keep the *status quo*. This guides the conversation toward the behavior change in a collaborative and patient-centered manner, drawing on the patient's motivation.

TABLE 6.1

Core Motivational Interviewing Skills, Examples, and Goals of the Encounter

Key Provider Skills	Example MI Responses	Goals of Encounters: What You Want the Patient to Do in the Conversation
Ask **open-ended questions** that encourage the patient to • Think broadly and deeply about their situation • Tell their story • Elaborate on their own hopes, goals, desires, and motivation • Stay focused in the current effort to change, not simply reporting the past • Develop their own plan for change and process for monitoring • State their intention to change explicitly	• What are your reasons for wanting to keep your blood pressure in the normal range? • What concerns do you have about your health? • Where would you like to be with your health in the next year? • What are some of the specific benefits you are experiencing (or hope to experience) from exercising more or following a healthy eating pattern? • To be successful, how would you go about making this change? • What is your first step? • What are you going to do?	• Elaborate on their own personal reasons to get or stay healthy/change their lifestyle/develop positive habits • Connect the current change to their overall goals and hopes • Articulate their strengths and confidence • Develop a plan that will be their own and is likely to succeed • State their intention to change
Listen to the patient and reflect: • Respond in an empathic, nonjudgmental, and supportive manner • Reflect back to the patient what you hear and understand • Reflective responses can (1) validate their struggle, emotions, and concerns; (2) affirm their strengths, hope, and goals; and (3) reinforce their reasons, plans, and intentions for change	• You have been having a hard time juggling a lot of personal responsibilities and having to deal with managing your high blood pressure makes your life seem more complicated • On the one hand, taking care of your health feels overwhelming at times, and on the other hand, it is important to you to find a way to manage your blood pressure • You have already made changes to your diet and you feel ready to think about other ways to help you manage your weight • It is important to you to get your blood pressure under control so that you can (reflect the patient's reason) and you plan to (reflect the patient's plan)	• Experience being heard and understood by the provider • Utilize the created safe environment to explore the change • See themselves from another perspective • Tap into their inner motivation for health

TABLE 6.1 (continued)
Core Motivational Interviewing Skills, Examples, and Goals of the Encounter

Key Provider Skills	Example MI Responses	Goals of Encounters: What You Want the Patient to Do in the Conversation
Provide information/ suggestions/ advice to the patient: • Ask permission to share your opinion • Offer information in a neutral tone; avoid using words like "you should" or "you must" • Prioritize the information and give only the most important • Avoid telling the patient what they already know • Ask the patient about their thoughts on the information/suggestion/ advice • Affirm the patient's choice to act or not to act on that information	• Would you mind if I share my thoughts about some things that might be appropriate in this case? • Can I tell you what some other patients have found helpful to them? • As your provider, I think the most important thing in terms of managing your blood pressure is to find a way for you to take the medication regularly. What do think about that? • What do you already know about how to keep your blood pressure in the normal range? • It seems like you have a pretty good handle on knowing when and how to check your blood pressure but you are unsure of the side effect of the medications. Would you like some information about that? • We have discussed three different options to help you manage your weight. What do you think might work for you? • It is really up to you what you choose to start with. You are the only one who can know what will work in your life.	• Not respond with resistance that is normal when being told what to do • Willingly hear the information • Actively process or "chew" on the information • Ask for more details, specifics, follow-up • Determine the relevance of the information to their own life • Begin the process of choosing to act on the information

Working with motivation requires a shift in thinking and focus from just providing information or advice to actively eliciting the patient's knowledge, ability, strengths, and internal motivation. This shift changes the overall dynamics in the conversation such that it is more collaborative, bidirectional, and engaging. This may be a very different way of interacting with patients than the provider was trained to do, and the ability to shift takes effort and practice. With practice, the shift can be incorporated into routine visits, preventive care, educational visits, or even urgent care.

The dialogue in Tables 6.2 and 6.3 provides a glimpse into the use of MI skills and strategies in a provider–patient conversation about blood pressure. The intention

TABLE 6.2

A Dialogue about Blood Pressure: Motivational Interviewing in Action

	MI Techniques and Theoretical Constructs Addressed
Provider: We briefly discussed the fact that your blood pressure seems to be going up a little each time you come back for a check up. You seem concerned about that. **What concerns you**?	Ask an open-ended question to encourage the patient to express change talk (their concerns about their condition, risk factors, health in general).
Patient: Well, both my grandmas died of a stroke. It was awful. I know they struggled with high blood pressure. It scares me.	This is an example of patient change talk and also perceived susceptibility, one good reason to keep blood pressure in control.
Provider: *You saw what they went through and you would like to avoid having a stroke if possible.* **What else concerns you?**	Reflect the change talk and acknowledge the patient's concerns by reflecting the underlying meaning. Ask for more information and seek elaboration.
Patient: I really don't want to have to take medication. Do you think I will have to?	This is change talk and another reason to control blood pressure. It is also an indication of the patient's ambivalence about medication, a possible barrier to treatment.
Provider: *You'd like to keep your blood pressure in the normal range without medication.* There are a lot of other strategies that can be explored. Many people are able to keep their blood pressure at normal levels without medication. **What have you heard about what you can do to keep it down?**	Reflect the change talk. You do not have to immediately answer the question; you can reflect the meaning of the question. Avoid resistance; provide information in a neutral manner without telling them what they should do. Ask the patient what they already know about changing the condition or risk factor.
Patient: I know that salt was banned from the house when my grandma had her first stroke. Everyone pitched a fit. I've also heard that losing weight can help. I've been working on that for years and as you can see, I haven't had much success in the long run.	The patient has first-hand knowledge about blood pressure. Voicing that knowledge serves to enhance self-efficacy and be a cue to action.
Provider: *It is important to you to do what you can to stay healthy.* And you are right, both the reduction (not necessarily banning altogether) of salt and weight loss are common strategies that can be effective at keeping the blood pressure in a good range. In addition, certain other dietary changes such as increasing fruits and vegetables or low-fat dairy products can be helpful. And, of course, adding in more physical activity on a regular basis helps not only to lower your blood pressure but also to lower other risk factors of heart disease. **What do you think about those things?**	Reflect the underlying value in a positive way. You do not have to respond immediately to the sense of failure. Validate the patient's knowledge. Provide information that adds to their knowledge and avoid educating them about what they already know. Ask for their thoughts about these and encourage them to actively process the new information.

TABLE 6.2 (continued)
A Dialogue about Blood Pressure: Motivational Interviewing in Action

	MI Techniques and Theoretical Constructs Addressed
Patient: It is funny. I just joined an exercise class with a friend. I love it. I never minded exercising but always found it difficult to fit in to my life with everything else I had to do. This class is something new for me and I love doing it with my friend. I think we can keep it up. Maybe it will help with my blood pressure too.	This is patient change talk about physical activity and blood pressure. She is expressing the benefits of exercise. The statement also provides evidence of the patient's deeper values and self-efficacy for exercise.
Provider: *That is great. For you, the class ties into at least two things you really value; your health and your friendship.* Doing that regularly should help with the blood pressure. I also wanted to say that your decision several years ago to quit smoking was very significant. You might well be on medication already if you hadn't done that. *I know it was tough but you did it. You stuck with it.* You might be able to use some of what you learned in that effort to help you make any changes now that you would like to make. **How do you think your success with quitting smoking might help you now?**	Reflect and affirm the patient's efforts, both past and present, highlighting strengths such as perseverance, personal decisions to change, and the possibilities to learn from those efforts. Ask about the patient's successful efforts in the past and link them with the current change effort. This builds confidence and self-efficacy.
Patient: I'd almost forgotten about that! It was hard but I kept thinking about my kids. I could see the disappointment in their faces every time I lit up. I couldn't stand it. I had to show myself that I could be in charge and not let the nicotine be in charge. I do feel a little bit like that with the exercise. My kids are grown now and they are active and healthy. I want to keep up. I want to be a hip grandma when the time comes. My poor grandma never really got to enjoy having grandchildren. It was sad. I really want to stay healthy.	The patient reflects on the past effort and her motivation at the time. She then brings it into the current effort to keep exercising. She gives four more reasons to change. She also takes what sounds like extrinsic motivation and internalizes it.
Provider: *You want to be in charge of your life because your family is important to you. You want to be an active part of their lives for a long time.*	Reflect the important personal values that underlie the desire to stay healthy.
Patient: Yep, nothing is more important to me than my family. Hey, I have a friend whose doctor told her to drink a glass of red wine everyday with dinner for her heart. What do you think about that?	

(continued)

TABLE 6.2 (continued)
A Dialogue about Blood Pressure: Motivational Interviewing in Action

	MI Techniques and Theoretical Constructs Addressed
Provider: I'm glad that you brought up the alcohol. There is a lot of conflicting information out there about how alcohol affects your heart and your blood pressure. For people who don't have other problems with alcohol, drinking a glass a day can be beneficial for one's health. It is important to remember that a glass of wine is 5 ounces. If a person increases the amount, the benefits begin to go away and the risks increase. Higher levels of drinking are associated with elevated blood pressure. So, a little is good for your heart, but more is not. **How do you see your alcohol use fitting in with this?**	Affirm the patient's engagement and questions. Provide information in a way that the patient can easily understand and respond to.
Patient: Well, I have never been a big drinker. Except maybe in college. But I have started to enjoy a glass of good wine once in a while. I don't let myself have too much because of the calories. I'd rather have the dessert than the second glass of wine. I have always been concerned about calories. Lot of good it did me.	The patient once again brings up the issue of unsuccessful weight loss efforts.
Provider: *On the one hand, it sounds like you feel a bit hopeless about the weight and on the other hand, you are determined to keep trying to find a way to stay healthy.*	Reflect on the patient's feelings about their situation.
Patient: Well I do keep trying, that's for sure. I have spent so much money, so much time, and so much energy on trying to lose these 30 pounds. I have lost it a few times and then back it comes. I've tried lots of diets; they all work for a while, then life takes over.	These are all reasons to maintain the status quo or not to change (sustain talk). It provides evidence for a lack of self-efficacy to lose weight and potential barriers to success.
Provider: I do have a little different perspective on the weight issue. Would it be OK if I share it?	The provider chooses not to focus on the sense of failure directly but to offer an alternative perspective. Ask permission to share your opinion, thoughts, and suggestions.
Patient: Sure	
Provider: Well, achieving and maintaining a healthy weight is a good goal. However, the things we have been talking about such as increasing physical activity and eating a healthy diet can have a positive impact on your health even if there isn't weight loss. Really, a person can be healthier, more fit, and feel better even	Avoid giving suggestions as a directive or as the only way a patient can proceed. Ask the patient to reflect on the opinion/advice/ suggestion.

TABLE 6.2 (continued)

A Dialogue about Blood Pressure: Motivational Interviewing in Action

	MI Techniques and Theoretical Constructs Addressed

with that extra 30 pounds. For some people, focusing less on the weight and more on getting healthy leads to more success. **What do you think?**

Patient: I do think that is probably true for me. When I joined this exercise class, I wasn't really thinking about the weight. I was just thinking about being active and having fun with my friend. It is just so easy to get down on yourself about packing around the extra weight. It seems like it should be easy to control and people are always telling you that.

Provider: *For you, the exercise has a lot of benefits even without weight loss.* I would encourage you to think about all of your successes and all of the positive things that you are doing for your health. And we can work together to develop a plan for keeping your blood pressure in the normal range. How's that?

Encourage the patient to remember their success. Offer to collaborate and work together to support the patient's goals.

Patient: Sounds good to me. Where should I start?

Provider: We should start with what you feel is most likely to be successful. We have talked about a lot of things. *You are most interested in keeping the blood pressure under control so that you can possibly avoid taking medication and suffering the consequences of hypertension. You have already accomplished some significant gains by quitting smoking. You have some knowledge about the dietary issues involved and in the past have focused on weight loss. You have recently started an exercise class that you are very excited about and feel may be a good fit for your lifestyle at this time. You are already on your way.* **What other things would you like to consider at this time?**

Emphasize that the patient is in the driver's seat for any change; they can chose where to start. Summarize the patient's story with an emphasis on their strength, success, desire to change, and reasons for moving forward. Ask for the patient's plans and goals.

Patient: Definitely keep up the exercise class. I have also been thinking about seeing if my daughter would be interested in walking with me on the weekends. I don't get to see her much and it could be fun. I'm a little hesitant to focus too much on the diet stuff but I would like some information about what kind of diet helps with blood pressure. That way I can start thinking about.

(continued)

TABLE 6.2 (continued)

A Dialogue about Blood Pressure: Motivational Interviewing in Action

	MI Techniques and Theoretical Constructs Addressed
Provider: *Sounds like a good plan.* I have some information to give you. We can talk about it at your next visit if you want. I have a question for you. *You sound confident that you can continue the exercise class and possibly add the walking.* **What gives you confidence?**	Affirm the patient's plans. Offer support and information. Ask the patient about their confidence.
Patient: Because I have paid for it! We had to pay for 10 classes in advance. No way I cannot go. Plus, I always loved to dance and this class has a lot of dance. I enjoy it. I get excited thinking about it. And my friend and I made a pact. Gotta do what you make a pact about, right?	
Provider: *You are committed and determined. You follow through with what you say you are going to do.* I also have confidence that you will be able to find a way to keep that physical activity in your life. I'll look forward to the update when you come back next time.	Affirm the patient's strengths and qualities that will help them accomplish their goals. Express confidence and hope in the patient. Offer to follow-up with the patient.

is not to suggest that a provider would use all of these in one visit but to illustrate the method. The dialogue is set in the context of an ongoing provider–patient relationship. From an MI standpoint, the relationship is a critical component and the skills can be used to build that relationship and maintain it. The skills identified in Table 6.1 are also highlighted (**open-ended questions in bold**, *reflections and summaries in italic*, and <u>informing responses in underlined</u>) in the dialogue, and commentary is included to the right. In addition, the patient's comments, in particular, change talk, that are relevant to the change effort are also highlighted in gray. In MI, the strategic use of the skills to elicit very specific types of patient comments is thought to build motivation for change.

6.6 SUMMARY

Health care providers understand the critical role that patients play when it comes to managing and optimizing their health. Patients' choices about their level of physical activity, dietary habits, adherence to treatments, and behavioral habits are strong determinants of their overall health, well-being, and ability to manage chronic conditions. Providers are often frustrated by the fact that many patients do not follow through with the recommendations they make about these choices. Many factors, supported by multiple theoretical models (i.e., Health Belief model, Transtheoretical model or Stages of Change, and SDT), are involved in patient decisions, and the research indicates that providers can exert influence on those decisions and on the subsequent behavioral choices (Table 6.4).

TABLE 6.3

Sample Dialogue with an "Unsuccessful" Patient

Dialogue	MI Techniques and Commentary
Provider: OK Jim, here is your prescription for the antibiotic. That should take care of you within a couple of days. If it is all right with you, I'd like to check in with you about your blood pressure and the goals you set the last time you were here. OK?	Provide transition from the clinical conversation to the focus on goals and lifestyle change Ask permission to talk about the new topic. The patient most likely did not come in to talk about his lifestyle
Patient: I guess, I don't remember what I was going to do but I'm pretty sure that I haven't done anything. There has just been too much going on	The patient is expressing his sense of failure that is seen as a reason not to change
Provider: My notes say that you were going to try to figure out how to eat better when you travel. You were travelling a lot for work at that time	Remind the patient about his goals in a neutral, nonjudgmental, and objective way. This should be delivered as a statement (reflection) as opposed to a question
Patient: Oh right. I still am travelling almost every week for a couple of days. So it is hotel food, lots of business meetings, and fast food at the airport. Hasn't changed	The patient is giving more reasons to keep the status quo
Provider: *So the plan for making changes when travelling hasn't worked so well.* We can get back to that but first **tell me what has been going well for you in terms of your health**	Acknowledge that the plan as opposed to the person has not worked Give an opportunity to come up with something that has worked
Patient: Well, I did take that information on the blood pressure diet home and talk about it with my wife. Come to think of it, we have made some changes at home. We switched to low-fat milk. That was really hard at first but I'm getting used to it. And we started experimenting with different fruits and vegetables. That has been kind of fun. I've tried a lot of funny looking things!	This whole passage is the reporting of past success. While technically not "change talk," it gives the provider great information to draw from later in the conversation
Provider: *You have been successful in making some small but important changes in your diet*	Acknowledge the change efforts stressing the value of the effort and naming it as a success
Patient: Yeah but is my blood pressure any better? No. And I have put on a couple of pounds. Probably the cheese sauce on those vegetables. I don't think change is possible with my job the way it is	The patient persists at focusing on the lack of progress and failure
Provider: *You kinda feel like nothing can change right now*	Acknowledge the patient's frustrations about change
Patient: Well, there has to be a way. I can't just give up. I know where that leads	The patient responds by turning and moving toward change

(continued)

TABLE 6.3 (continued)
Sample Dialogue with an "Unsuccessful" Patient

Dialogue	MI Techniques and Commentary
Provider: *You are determined to find a way to keep that blood pressure in control.* Let me ask you this. On a scale from 0 to 10 with 0 being not at all important and 10 being the most important thing, how important is it to you right now to get your blood pressure under better control?	Reflect the personal strengths that are evident. This builds on his motivation to make another attempt. The MI strategy using the ruler is a useful tool for eliciting change talk and getting a deeper understanding of the dilemma that the patient faces
Patient: Well, it should be a 10 but I'd say it is a 6. There are just too many other things	Patient is still expressing failure
Provider: **So what makes it a 6 and not a 0?**	This is a direct request for change talk; the question asks for reasons that it are important
Patient: When I am home and my wife is reminding me, it seems to be important. She is always talking to me about this and that thing to stay healthy. But when I am on the road, it is out of sight, out of mind and I just don't like to think about it	Patient talks mostly about the importance of extrinsic motivation, in this case, his wife to making an effort
Provider: *Your wife's concern makes it important for you.* **Why is it so important to her?**	Reflection reframes the wife's talking as concern and asks for elaboration
Patient: She is making big plans to travel when we retire in a couple of years. She is really healthy, exercises all the time. She wants me to be able to keep up with her. Sometimes she threatens to go without me if I can't. That would be a bummer!	Patient continues to talk about his wife but at this point, he turns it around and indicates that he wants to be able to keep up, to go with her. It becomes internalized
Provider: *Sounds like you'd like to enjoy your retirement with your wife and to keep up!* **What else makes it important?**	Reflection reinforces the internalization
Patient: Well, I just know that my friends who take the medication have problems that I don't want to have if you know what I mean	Patient gives another reason to deal with the blood pressure
Provider: I do. And I would like to work with you to find a way to do this without the medication. Let me ask you this, **what do you think would have to change or be different for this to become an 8 or 9 in importance?**	Provider offers collaboration This question asks the patient to think forward and to look at the possibility of this becoming more important
Patient: I hate to say it, but if something scares me, I usually respond. I mean I don't want to have a stroke or anything but that would probably do it. That sounds pretty bad doesn't it?	Patient expresses distress with his own response to the question. It doesn't sit well with him
Provider: *You're concerned that something really bad would have to happen for you to make big changes*	Provider reflects that discomfort
Patient: Ouch! I know I'm not a wimp. I should do something now	Patient expresses strength and a need to take action

TABLE 6.3 (continued)

Sample Dialogue with an "Unsuccessful" Patient

Dialogue	MI Techniques and Commentary
Provider: *It might be the time to start.* So, another question. On that same scale of 0–10, with 0 being no confidence and 10 being totally confident, how confident are you that you could make changes to control your blood pressure if you did decide that now was the right time?	Provider reflects that action with a slightly tentative "might" to avoid pushing the patient The ruler is being used here to actively assess and build confidence
Patient: Well, an 8 at home and probably a 4 or 5 on the road	Patient continues to express ambivalence about the change and his confidence
Provider: **What makes up that confidence? Why are you as high as you are?**	Provider asks directly for the patient's statement of confidence, ignoring the discrepancy for now
Patient: When I am at home, my wife really helps me with that. She supports me and works with me. She makes it easy to eat differently and even to get some exercise. We have already done a lot as I said before	Patient indicates that his wife's support is a primary contributor to his confidence
Provider: Well what about that 4 or 5 on the road. **What gives you confidence then?**	Provider asks for more about the confidence, particularly when his wife isn't there to provide support
Patient: Well, I have been able to take some control over the travel time. Last week, I checked out the hotel ahead of time for the dining options and exercise facilities. Didn't use it but I know what's there for next time	This change talk is called "taking steps," actions that have occurred in the last week to support the change effort. The patient sees this as a confidence booster
Provider: *So you know that you do have some control over your travel time.* **What would help you to be more confident on the road?**	Provider reflects the meaning of the change talk and asks for the patient to think ahead to what it takes for him to build confidence
Patient: Probably just trying one thing	Change talk, a possible solution
Provider: *You have made some good first steps with the changes at home and working closely with your wife.* **How can you build on that success?**	Provider reinforces earlier success and asks the patient to build on it
Patient: I tell you what. I'll talk with her again, go over the information, and see what more we can do at home. But I spend so much time on the road and she isn't there to be the food police!	This change talk is commitment language, a statement about what the patient is actually going to do. Change talk is frequently surrounded by reasons not to change, as is the case here
Provider: *What is important for you is to find something that you have control over, that you are willing to do, and you feel confident about doing? Probably something small to start with.* **What do you think would work for you?**	Provider gives a brief summary of what the patient has said will work The question asks for the patient to begin problem solving and generating solutions
Patient: Well I wonder if I could get her to help me take food with me when I travel. I always end up grabbing something fast and full of fat at the airport. With some planning I could see having my own food. I really don't even like most of the fast foods that much	Patient is actively voicing the solutions, what it will take to do them, and how to go about it

(continued)

TABLE 6.3 (continued)
Sample Dialogue with an "Unsuccessful" Patient

Dialogue	MI Techniques and Commentary
Provider: *Sounds like a good thing to work on.* **What seems reasonable to you to start with?**	Provider affirms the patient's plan and asks for next/ first steps
Patient: I travel this week. I have a long flight out. I will try taking something for that. I don't know what but I'm sure we can come up with something	This is commitment language again, a statement of what the patient will do, even if it is "trying"
Provider: *Good plan. Let me see if I got it all. You came in feeling like you hadn't accomplished any of your goals related to managing your blood pressure. This is mostly due to your very busy travel schedule at work and the difficulties of trying to control that. You have made some significant changes at home with the help of your wife and she is an important part of your success and confidence. You are hoping for a long, healthy retirement with her with some pleasure travel. You also want to avoid the medication if possible. You see yourself as capable of making changes and taking control even in difficult situations and you'd like to do that before anything bad happens. And you are planning to enlist the help of your wife with even more changes at home and starting to explore carrying food with you when you travel.* Did I get it all?	Provider affirms the plan again. Then he summarizes the conversation, being sure to include the change talk that the patient has given along the way. The provider does not ignore the patient's failure to reach his goals or his reasons for that. However, the emphasis in on the reasons to change and the plans made
Patient: Yes and you know what else? My son has been asking me to hike the Pacific Trail with him. I want to do that too!	Patient adds to the change talk with another reason to manage his blood pressure, something that is important to him
Provider: *Lots of good reasons to get that blood pressure in line.* Since I probably won't see you for a while, I'd like to encourage you to continue building on your successes. It is easy to get all over ourselves for what we see as failure. That is where you started today. Yes, our plans don't always work out the way we want, we don't always make all the changes we think we should. And, there are almost always seeds of hope and success in there too. Pay attention to those and keep them growing. **What do you think about that?**	Provider reinforces the patient's desire to change Provider offers encouragement, support, and confidence to the patient. He asks the patient to consider changing what he pays attention to. He then asks what the patient thinks about that
Patient: It's true. It is easy to overlook or even forget what I do right. I'll work on that. Thanks Doc	Patient agrees with commitment language and appreciation

TABLE 6.4
Summary: Take-Home Messages

Key Evidences	Recommendation for Health Care Providers

• Motivational interviewing is a collaborative, person-centered form of guiding to elicit and strengthen motivation for change
• MI is founded on behavioral theories including the Health Belief theory, Stages of Change, and self-determination model
• Research has shown the efficacy of applying MI in changing lifestyle behaviors
• Research indicates that practicing MI does not require a specific professional background [34]. It requires a desire to learn it, a willingness to practice, and a commitment to make the effort
	• All providers are encouraged to consider taking steps to learn and apply MI. It will benefit patients' health by improving lifestyle behaviors and is a very useful tool in all health providers' toolbox. The following steps are suggested for providers to learn more about MI and to practice this method:
	• Read *MI in Health Care* [7]. Practice the skills and strategies detailed in this book
	• Pursue training, feedback, and coaching in MI. A list of MI trainers (organized by country and state) can be found on the Web site www.motivationalinterviewing. org. This combination of learning strategies can produce long-term changes in provider behaviors [12]
	• If formal training is not available and you are interested in taking small steps to improve your practice, you can utilize the strategies and skills demonstrated in the sample dialogue in this chapter. We suggest the following:
	  a. Develop a list of good open-ended questions (those designed to encourage the patient to give you change talk) that can be used in your conversations with patients
	  b. Try out the strategies such as the importance and confidence rulers with patients
	  c. Practice your listening skills and develop your capacity to convey empathy to your patients
	  d. Practice the Ask–Provide–Ask strategy
	    i. What do you already know about … ?
	    ii. Ask permission to provide information or give advice
	    iii. Provide tailored information in a neutral, nonjudgmental manner
	    iv. What do you make of that?

MI is a method of communication that effectively facilitates behavior change with a wide variety of behaviors, in many different settings, and is used by all types of providers. MI draws on an underlying spirit of collaboration, empathy, and support for patient autonomy. MI is effective in small doses and is easily adapted to most health care settings. The basic skills are straightforward and simple: asking, listening, and informing. These skills are used strategically and deliberately to help the patient explore their own reasons, motivation, confidence, plans, and commitment to change. The MI provider guides the conversation toward behavior change. Although learning MI and integrating it into practice is not easy, it is doable and worthwhile.

REFERENCES

1. Haynes RB, Ackloo E, Sahota N, McDonald HP, Yao X. Interventions for enhancing medication adherence (Review). *The Cochrane Collaboration.* 2008. New York: Wiley & Sons.
2. Miller W, Rollnick S. *Motivational Interviewing: Preparing People for Change.* 2002. New York: Guilford Press.
3. Apodaca TR, Longabaugh R. Mechanisms of change in motivational interviewing: a review and preliminary evaluation of the evidence. *Addiction.* 2009;104(5):705–715.
4. Martins RK, McNeil DW. Review of motivational interviewing in promoting health behaviors. *Clin Psychol Rev.* 2009;29(4):283–293.
5. Resnicow K, Dilorio C, Soet JE. Motivational interviewing in medical and public health settings. In: Miller WR, Rollnick S, Eds., *Motivational Interviewing: Preparing People for Change*, (pp. 251–269). 2002, 2nd ed. New York: Guilford Press.
6. Miller WR, Rollnick S. Ten things that motivational interviewing is not. *Behav Cogn Psychother.* 2009;37:129–140.
7. Rollnick S, Miller WR, Butler CC. *Motivational Interviewing in Health Care: Helping Patients Change Behavior.* 2007. New York: Guilford Press.
8. Miller WR, Rose GS. Toward a theory of motivational interviewing. *American Psychologist.* 2009;64(6):527–537.
9. Rogers CR. A theory of therapy, personality, and interpersonal relationships as developed in the client-centered framework. In: Koch S, Ed. *Psychology: The Study of a Science. Vol 3. Formulations of the Person and the Social Contexts*, (pp. 184–256). 1959, New York: McGraw-Hill.
10. Gaume J, Gmel G, Daeppen, J-B. Brief alcohol interventions: Do counselors' and patients' communication characteristics predict change? *Alcohol Alcohol.* 2008;43:62–69.
11. Moyers T, Miller W, Hendricksen S. How does motivational interviewing work? Therapist interpersonal skill predicts client involvement within motivational interviewing sessions. *J Consult Clin Psychol.* 2005;73:590–598.
12. Miller WR, Yahne CE, Moyers TB, Martinez J, Pirritano M. A randomized trial of methods to help clinicians learn motivational interviewing. *J Consult Clin Psychol.* 2004;72(6):1050–1063.
13. Boardman T, Catley D, Grobe J, Little T, Ahluwalia J. Using motivational interviewing with smokers: Do therapist behaviors relate to engagement and therapeutic alliance? *J Subst Abuse Treat.* 2006;31:329–339.
14. Catley D, Harris KJ, Mayo MS, Hall S, Okuyemi KS, Boardman T, Ahluwalia J. Adherence to principles of motivational interviewing and client within-session behavior. *Behav Cogn Psychother.* 2006;34:43–56.
15. Miller WR, Benefield RG, Tonigan JS. Enhancing motivation for change in problem drinking: A controlled comparison of two therapist styles. *J Consult Clin Psychol.* 1993;61:455–461.
16. Amrhein PC, Miller WR, Yahne C, Knupsky A, Hochstein, D. Strength of client commitment language improves with therapist training in motivational interviewing. *Alcohol Clin Exp Res.* 2004;28(5):74A.
17. Houck JM, Moyers TB. *What you do matters: Therapist influence on client behavior during motivational interviewing sessions.* Presented at the International Addiction Summit; 2008. Melbourne, Australia.
18. Amrhein PC. The comprehension of quasi-performance verbs in verbal commitments: New evidence for componential theories of lexical meaning. *J Mem Lang.* 1992;31:756–784.
19. Amrhein PC, Miller WR, Yahne CE, Palmer M, Fulcher L. Client commitment language during motivational interviewing predicts drug use outcomes. *J Consult Clin Psychol.* 2003;71:862–878.

20. Aharaonovich E, Amrhein PC, Bisaga A, Nunes EV, Hasin DS. Cognition, commitment language, and behavioral change among cocaine-dependent patients. *Psychol Addict Behav*. 2008;22:557–562.

21. Gollwitzer PM. Implementation intentions: Simple effects of simple plans. *Am Psychol*. 1999;54:493–503.

22. Strang J, McCambridge J. Can the practitioner correctly predict outcome in motivational interviewing? *J Subst Abuse Treat*. 2004;27(1):83.

23. Peterson KE, Sorenson G, Pearson M, et al. Design of an intervention addressing multiple levels of influence on dietary and activity patterns of low-income, postpartum women. *Health Educ Res*. 2002;17:531–540.

24. Bennett JA, Lyons KS, Winters-Stone K, Nail LM, Scherer J. Motivational interviewing to increase physical activity in long-term cancer survivors: A randomized controlled trial. *Nurs Res*. 2007;56(1):18–27.

25. van Keulen HM, Mesters I, Ausems M, van Breukelen G, Campbell M, Resnicow K, Brug J, de Vries, H. Tailored print communication and telephone motivational interviewing are equally successful in improving multiple lifestyle behaviors in a randomized controlled trial. *Ann Behav Med*. 2011;41(1):104–118.

26. Armstrong MJ, Mottershead TA, Ronksley PE, Sigal RJ, Campbell TS, and Hemmelgarn BR. Motivational interviewing to improve weight loss in overweight and/or obese patients: A systematic review and meta-analysis of randomized controlled trials. *Obes Res*. 2011: 1–15.

27. Knight KM, McGowan L, Dickens C, Bundy C. A systematic review of motivational interviewing in physical health care settings. *Br J Health Psychol*. 2006;11:319–332.

28. Ogcdcgbc G, Chaplin W, Schocnthalcr A, Statman D, Berger D, Richardson T, Phillips E, Spencer J, Allegrante JP. A practice-based trial of motivational interviewing and adherence in hypertensive African Americans. *Am J Hypertens*. 2008;21(10): 1137–1143.

29. Scala D, D'Avino M, Cozzolino S, Mancini A, Andria B, Caruso G, Tajana G, Caruso D. Promotion of behavioural change in people with hypertension: An intervention study. *Pharm World Sci*. 2008;30(6):834–839.

30. Spahn JM, Reeves RS, Keim KS, Laquatra I, Kellogg M, Jortberg B, Clark NA. State of the evidence regarding behavior change theories and strategies innutrition counseling to facilitate health and food behavior change. *J Am Diet Assoc*. 2010;110(6):879–891.

31. Resnicow K, Jackson A, Braithwaite R, et al. Healthy body/healthy spirit: A church-based nutrition and physical activity intervention. *Health Educ Res*. 2002;17: 562–573.

32. Dunn C, Deroo L, Rivara FP. The use of brief interventions adapted from motivational interviewing across behavioral domains: A systematic review. *Addiction*. 2001;96(12):1725–1742.

33. VanWormer JJ, Boucher JL, Pronk NP, Thoennes, JJ. Lifestyle behavior change and coronary artery disease: Effectiveness of a telephone-based counseling program. *J Nutr Educ Behav*. 2004;36(6):333–334.

34. Rubak S, Sandbaek A, Lauritzen T, Christensen B. Motivational interviewing: A systematic review and meta-analysis. *Br J Gen Pract*. 2005;55(513):305–312.

35. Woollard J, Beilin L, Lord T, Puddey I, MacAdam D, Rouse I. A controlled trial of nurse counseling on lifestyle change for hypertensives treated in general practice: Preliminary results. *Clin Exp Pharmacol Physiol*. 1995;22(6–7):466–468.

36. Lawrence DB, Allison W, Chen JC, Demand M. Improving medication adherence with a targeted, technology-driven disease management intervention. *Dis Manag*. 2008;11(3):141–144.

37. Hawkins SY. Improving glycemic control in older adults using a videophone motivational diabetes self-management intervention. *Res Theory Nurs Pract*. 2010;24(4):217–232.

38. Rubak, S., Sandbaek, A., Lauritzen, T., Borch-Johnsen, K., Christensen, B. General practitioners trained in motivational interviewing can positively affect the attitude to behaviour change in people with type 2 diabetes. One year follow-up of an RCT, Addition Denmark. *Scand J Prim Health Care.* 2009,27(3):172–179.
39. Greaves CJ, Middlebrooke A, O'Loughlin L, Holland S, Piper J, Steele A, Gale T, Hammerton F, Daly M. Motivational interviewing for modifying diabetes risk: A randomised controlled trial. *Br J Gen Pract.* 2008;58(553):535–540.
40. West DS, DiLillo V, Bursac Z, Gore SA, Greene PG. Motivational interviewing improves weight loss in women with type 2 diabetes. *Diabetes Care.* 2007;30(5):1081–1087.
41. Rosenstock, I. Historical origins of the Health Belief Model. *Health Educ Monogr.* 1974;2(4):328–335.
42. Talbert PA. The relationship of fear and fatalism with breast cancer screening among a selected target population of african american middle class women. *J Social Behav Health Sci.* 2008;2:96–110.
43. Prochaska JO, DiClemente CC. Stages and processes of self-change of smoking: Toward an integrative model of change. *J Consult Clin Psychol*, 1983;51:390–395.
44. DiClemente CC, Velasquez MM. Motivational interviewing and the stages of change. In: Miller WR and Rollnick S, Eds., *Motivational Interviewing*, 2nd ed., (pp. 201–216). 2002. New York: The Guilford Press.
45. Kreuter MW, Strecher VJ, Glassman B. One size does not fit all: The case for tailoring print materials. *Ann Behav Med.* 1999;21(4):276–83.
46. Deci E, Ryan R. (Eds.). *Handbook of Self-Determination Research.* 2002. Rochester, NY: University of Rochester Press.
47. Moyers, TM, Martin, T, Christopher PJ, Houck JM, Tonigan JS, Amrhein PC. Client language as a mediator of motivational interviewing efficacy: Where is the evidence? *Alcohol Clin Exp Res.* 2007;31(s3):40s–47s.

7 Self-Management and Hypertension

Hayden B. Bosworth
Veterans Affairs Medical Center and
Duke University

CONTENTS

7.1   INTRODUCTION

Chronic diseases such as hypertension have become the leading cause of death and disability in most countries of the world [1]. Hypertension is the major modifiable risk factor for cardiovascular disease, stroke, chronic heart failure, and renal diseases [2–4]. The prevalence of hypertension is increasing, which will likely lead to an even greater burden of these secondary diseases [5]. Unhealthy behaviors, including those that lead to hypertension (poor dietary pattern and sedentary lifestyle), account for as much as 40% of premature deaths in the United States, whereas deficiencies in health care delivery account for only 10% [6]. Thus, the anticipated increase in health care expenses due to rising rates of hypertension has called for a burning platform for prevention of hypertension. Hence, clinical and public health interventions must aim at reducing the burden of hypertension, at least in part, through self-management by those affected or at risk.

Managing a chronic illness, such as hypertension, is a time-consuming and complex process. Yet, often chronically ill patients themselves are called on to manage the broad array of factors that contribute to their health. Programs that provide patient support for chronic diseases—so-called self-management support—have been developed in recognition that treating chronic illnesses requires a unique model of care. In 2003, the Institute of Medicine defined self-management support as "the systematic provision of education and supportive interventions by health care staff to increase patients' skills and confidence in managing their health problems, including regular assessment of progress and problems, goal setting, and problem-solving support." Engaging patients in their own care (patient activation) is a widely agreed-upon self-management goal for chronic diseases. Enhancing patient activation can lead to positive self-management behavior changes in patients with chronic conditions [7].

Addressing the increased incidence of chronic diseases is one of the most important challenges for health systems. In contrast to the traditional management of acute conditions, often characterized by a short period of patient adherence to following the doctor's orders, management of a chronic disease requires that patients take a more active role in the day-to-day decisions about the management of their illness [8]. This disease paradigm requires that there be a working patient–provider "partnership" that involves effective treatment within an integrated system of collaborative care, which includes self-management education and follow-up [9]. Thus, both patient and provider have important roles in the treatment of chronic conditions. Patients are expected to do what is needed to manage the condition on a daily basis; health care providers act as consultants, interpreters of symptoms, and resource persons, and they offer treatment suggestions [10,11].

The Chronic Care model developed by Wagner et al. [12] (Table 7.1) and the *Innovative Care for Chronic Conditions* [13], edited by the World Health Organization, propose that ideal care for chronic conditions is achieved when health

---

TABLE 7.1

Components of the Chronic Care Model

- The Chronic Care model identifies the elements of a health care system that encourage high-quality chronic disease care.
- *Community*—Mobilize community resources to meet needs of patients.
- Example: A health system forms a partnership with a local senior center that provides exercise classes as an option for older patients.
- *Health System*—Create a culture, organization, and mechanisms that promote safe, high-quality care.
- Example: Healthcare Effectiveness Data and Information Set measures (HEDIS) and other quality measures.
- *Self-management Support*—Empower and prepare patients to manage their health and health care.
- Using a collaborative approach, providers and patients work together to define problems, set priorities, establish goals, create treatment plans, and solve problems along the way.
- *Delivery System Design*—Assure the delivery of effective, efficient clinical care and self-management support.
- The delivery of effective, efficient clinical care through appropriate use of all team members, planned patient interactions, regular follow-up, and case management are all important parts of delivery system design (e.g., primary medical center home) [12].
- *Decision Support*—Promote clinical care that is consistent with scientific evidence and patient preferences.
- *Clinical Information Systems*—Organize patient and population data to facilitate efficient and effective care.

care providers interact with informed patients. An essential ingredient of effective treatment for chronic conditions is the partnership between patients and health professionals because it offers the opportunity to empower patients to become more active in managing their health. When patients are more informed, involved, and empowered, they interact more effectively with health care providers and strive to take actions that will promote healthier outcomes [9,14]. In addition, the partnership between the patient and the health professional allows for the care plan to be individualized and to address the specific knowledge patients must have and the behaviors they must change to manage the condition effectively. Patients are supported in self-management education that is focused on providing them with the skills to live as active and meaningful a life as possible with their chronic conditions. The patient is central to defining the "disease-related problems" and the self-management program assists them with problem solving and in gaining the self-efficacy and confidence to deal with these problems [11]. Evidence suggests that when self-management programs support the patient's assessment of their condition, there is greater patient satisfaction with care, better patient adherence with treatment, and higher likelihood that health care relationships will be continuously maintained [15].

Self-management education programs are distinct from simple patient education or skills training in that they are designed to allow people with chronic conditions to take an active part in the management of their own condition. Quality improvement interventions that have attempted to improve outcomes of chronic care without a component that supports patient self-management have not been found to affect patient outcomes [16]. The inclusion of recommendations for self-management support in a number of guidelines solidifies self-management support as a key dimension of the quality of care for chronic conditions. Self-management programs are expected to reduce costly health crises and improve outcomes for chronically ill patients, including those with hypertension.

7.2 REVIEW OF SELF-MANAGEMENT PROGRAMS IN HYPERTENSION AND RELATED CONDITIONS

It is predicted that by 2025, more than 1.5 billion individuals worldwide will have hypertension, accounting for up to 50% of the risk for heart diseases and 75% of the risk for stroke [17]. For several decades, it has been well known that lowering blood pressure (BP) with lifestyle modification, medications, or both can substantially reduce a patient's subsequent risk for diseases [18]. For each 10-mmHg decrease in systolic blood pressure (SBP), the average risk of mortality due to heart diseases and stroke decreases by 30% and 40%, respectively [19]. Meta-analyses have shown that weight loss [20], following the Dietary Approaches to Stop Hypertension (DASH) diet (a diet that is low in saturated fat and total fat and rich in low-fat dairy products, fruits, vegetables, calcium, potassium, and fiber [21]), reduced sodium intake [22], and aerobic exercise [23] significantly lower BP [21,24,25]. Despite the clear benefits of treatment, only half of those with hypertension have adequate BP control [26–28].

During the past several decades, patient self-management programs have been developed to foster self-care among patients with chronic diseases [9,29,30]. In general, however, self-management interventions have achieved modest successes in trials with control groups. In the most recent Cochrane review of interventions used to improve control of BP in patients with hypertension [31], 72 randomized clinical trials were identified representing the following 6 intervention types: (1) self-monitoring, (2) educational interventions directed to the patient, (3) educational interventions directed to the health professional, (4) health professional–led care (from nurse or pharmacist), (5) organizational interventions that aimed to improve the delivery of care, and (6) appointment reminder systems. In this review of the evidence, self-monitoring was associated with modest, but statistically significant, net reduction in SBP [weighted mean difference (WMD): −2.5 mmHg; 95% CI: −3.7 to −1.3 mmHg] and diastolic blood pressure (DBP) (WMD: −1.8 mmHg; 95% CI: −2.4 to −1.2 mmHg). Trials of educational interventions directed at patients or health professionals appeared unlikely to be associated with large net reductions in BP by themselves [31]. Nurse- or pharmacist-led care may be a promising way forward, with the majority of randomized controlled trials being associated with improved BP control and reduction in mean SBP and DBP [31,32]. Results of studies examining appointment reminder systems were heterogeneous and hence were not clear, but the majority of trials increased the proportion of individuals who attended follow-up visits, and in two small trials, this also led to improved BP control [31]. Fahey et al. conclude that an organized system of registration, recall, and regular review allied to a vigorous stepped care approach to antihypertensive drug treatment appears the most likely way to improve the control of high BP [33].

Health professional–led care appears to be a promising way of delivering care but requires further evaluation. A recent meta-analysis identified 298 clinical trials in the United States that evaluated pharmacist-provided direct patient care for hypertension and various other chronic conditions and that showed significant improvements in BP, as well as in hemoglobin A1c and LDL-cholesterol levels, adverse drug events, medication adherence, quality of life, and patient knowledge [34]. This meta-analysis found a mean reduction in SBP of 9.3 mmHg when pharmacists managed therapy or recommended medications to the physicians compared with a reduction of 4.8 mmHg when nurses conducted the interventions [34].

Lay-led self-management education programs may lead to small, short-term improvements in participants' self-efficacy, self-rated health, cognitive symptom management, and frequency of aerobic exercise within the context of hypertension. In a Cochrane review of lay-led self-management programs for people with chronic conditions, seven studies showed a small, statistically significant increase in self-reported aerobic exercise. Results are based on 17 studies that involved over 7442 people with chronic conditions, including hypertension [35]. There were no statistically significant differences between groups in physicians' or general practitioners' encounters (9 studies). There were also no statistically significant differences between groups for hospital visits (6 studies). There was a small statistically significant improvement in self-efficacy (e.g., confidence to manage the condition) (10 studies). Thus, there is currently no evidence to suggest that such programs improve psychological health and symptoms of health-related quality of life or that they significantly alter health care use. In general, at this time, we lack conclusive data to suggest that lay-led interventions significantly and clinically result in improved BP.

7.3 DEVELOPING OR IMPLEMENTING A SELF-MANAGEMENT PROGRAM

An initial step in choosing or building a self-management program is to decide where in the health care system the program will be positioned. Variation exists in terms of the program components, location of the program within the health care system, and staff involvement [36]. A key question is, "Will it be managed and administered within the patient's primary care setting or external to it?" The answer to this question often has important ramifications for the degree to which self-management support is integrated with other aspects of the patient's chronic care and thus who the players are, the quantity and kind of data available to support it, and the nature of the administrative oversight and support.

Patients play a fundamental role in public health as they ultimately make decisions regarding how to lead their own lives; the important choices they make have an impact on their health, the effectiveness of prescribed treatments, and their use of medical resources. Health care providers also play a critical role in patients' decision-making; most patients with chronic diseases such as hypertension receive the majority of the information about their disease and all of their treatment in primary care office settings. Therefore, in order to improve the health of patients, the role of health care professionals will likely need to be extended beyond practicing evidence-based medicine in a typical clinical setting. This extension will require providing patients with easy-to-understand assessment of their hypertension risk and means to modify their risks in a more convenient environment, such as one's home, that potentially improves access to care.

Other reasons why the office setting may not be ideal for managing hypertension and promoting self-management may be due to competing issues that arise during routine office visits or due to lack of accessibility to primary care. Limitations include clinical inertia in part because of excessive workloads on the part of physicians [37–40]; unmet information needs and poor adherence to hypertension treatment [41]; and differing thresholds at which health professionals and patients would choose to start or intensify treatment [42]. Moreover, the primary care office visit is often devoted to multiple tasks, including guideline-directed screening (e.g., for cancer), medication refill, adult vaccination, and payment issues, making it even more difficult to concentrate on any given disease. In addition, solely focusing on patients receiving treatment in health care settings may lead to underrepresentation of patients with chronic diseases, who are disenfranchised from the health care system. To improve hypertension control through the primary care setting, testing novel approaches to treatment interventions for enhancing self-management, with assessment of effects on quality indicators and costs, needs to be considered.

Alternative methods of service delivery are needed to improve outcomes for patients with chronic disease such as hypertension [43]. The use of nonphysicians to implement interventions may enhance our ability to achieve high-quality, guideline-concordant care. In general, while pharmacists, particularly community pharmacists, have been found to be the most effective in improving BP [44], both pharmacists and nurses, for example, are effective at bringing hypertensive individuals in concordance with national guideline goals [45–50] and can improve patient adherence to BP medications and improve BP control [51–54]. Case management by nurse-led teams has been shown to be an efficacious strategy to improve management of cardiovascular risk factors, including management of hypertension, in many studies [55,56]. Nurses, for example, have demonstrated successful strategies for improving BP [56–60] by serving as a bridge to physician care and by adhering more strictly to management algorithms, including many counseling features that may not necessarily be feasible within the time frame of a busy physician in practice [61].

In general, there is growing evidence that intensive programs improve hypertension control, yet earlier lifestyle-intervention trials have generally relied on initial intensive intervention for all individuals and have gradually decreased in intensity over time irrespective of improvements [62,63], raising concerns about the potential for widespread dissemination and sustainability of intensive intervention effects. More contacts and longer intervention duration are usually better than fewer contacts and shorter intervention duration; however, these average effects obscure the widely varying experiences of individuals. Some individuals respond quickly and require little additional support, while others benefit from more intensive and/or more prolonged intervention. Hypertension management strategies that involve progressively more intense intervention have several potential advantages, including the fact that a larger number of patients can be targeted than if a "one-size-fits-all" paradigm is used. That is, a low-intensity first step can be widely delivered as a first-line offering at scale with very low fixed costs. Only those individuals with inadequate BP control would progress to more intensive intervention components. Second, the progressive intensity approach is potentially cost-effective as technology and human capital are utilized optimally. Thus, given the increasing prevalence of hypertension and limited resources, it is becoming more important to provide the right level of hypertension care at the right place if we are to improve the quality of hypertension control. However, the use of a step-care approach that involves increasing treatment intensity has not been effectively evaluated and would require further examination before implementation could be recommended.

7.4 COMPONENTS OF A SELF-MANAGEMENT PROGRAM TO CONSIDER

Factors to consider in implementing a self-management program include staffing, content of the program, patient population served, supporting material, protocols for how staff members are to provide support, staff training, communication with patients, communication between health care providers, and self-management support (Table 7.2). For a program that seeks to change patient behavior, such as nutrition or exercise, a key underlying consideration is the need to include both supportive coaching interventions and educational interventions as part of the program content. Although patient education is necessary, it alone is not sufficient. Rather than being prescriptive or hierarchical, self-management programs should be patient-centered and tailored to the needs and concerns defined by patients and their situations. An enhanced level of physician trust has been documented as a

TABLE 7.2

Factors to Consider in Hypertension Self-Management Programs

- Staffing
- Content of the program
- Patient population served
- Supporting material
- Protocols for how staff members are to provide support
- Emphasis and training staff to interact with patients (e.g., MI)
- Facilitate communication between self-management staff and health care providers (e.g., closing the clinical loop—ensuring all parties are up to date with ongoing treatments)

contributing factor to pharmacological and nonpharmacological adherence, making the strengthening of patient–provider relationships a priority [64,65].

Basic components of self-management programs that rely on nonclinical providers consist of closely monitoring symptoms; knowing what symptoms may require action and when to respond with appropriate actions (e.g., adjust medications, initiate call to a health care provider); promoting major lifestyle changes (e.g., modify diet, lose weight, increase exercise, stop smoking, and consume alcohol moderately); promoting adherence to medication regimens, some of which may be inconvenient or produce side effects; and facilitating and encouraging regular office visits for lab tests and clinician consultations.

Another goal of self-management support programs is to reduce health care costs and workplace costs related to the reduced productivity of chronically ill workers. Offering patients better support is hypothesized to help them stay healthier, prevent expensive exacerbations and complications, and decrease utilization of health care services, thereby reducing costs for providers, insurers, employers, and other large purchasers of health care services, as well as for the patients themselves.

Empowerment strategies for patients address the complex interaction of motivations, cues, perceptions, consequences, expectations, and environmental and cultural influences inherent in patients to effectively motivate them to change their behaviors. One such patient empowerment intervention, motivational interviewing (MI), has been demonstrated to be an effective tool for improving patient self-management and lifestyle modification [66]. MI, discussed in more detail in Chapter 6, is a client-centered, goal-oriented method for enhancing intrinsic motivation to change by exploring and resolving ambivalence [66]. This method avoids well-intentioned advice or scare tactics, and it allows patients to play a central role in their treatment [66]. Furthermore, MI is not based on the information model but is rather shaped by an understanding of what triggers change. In the primary care setting, interventions should be brief and emphasize the three underlying assumptions of MI: collaboration, evocation, and autonomy. Collaboration refers to the creation of a partnership that creates the space for change to occur by honoring the client's expertise and perspective. Evocation means that the collaborative process allows the resources for change that reside within the client to emerge; thus, the interventionist's task is to focus on eliciting the client's rationale for seeking behavioral change. Autonomy means that the responsibility for behavior change lies with the individual.

Although these techniques differ in style and application in the clinical setting, they are all based on the premise of enhancing intrinsic motivation to behavior change by exploring and resolving ambivalence.

Integrated communications channels involve multiprovider-level communication with patients regarding the importance of self-management. Health care providers charged with communicating these adherence-enhancing messages to patients include physicians, pharmacists, nurses, and case managers, among others. Health care providers should negotiate a plan with the patient and anticipate and address problems as they arise.

A majority of work to date has focused on how people initiate change in health behaviors. However, the treatment of chronic diseases such as hypertension requires long-term sustained changes in relevant health-risk behaviors. Yet, people generally have challenges when undertaking long-term change in health behaviors. In a recent meta-analysis of self-management programs in diabetes, sharp declines in benefits were found only a few months after the interventions ended, thus illustrating poor levels of maintenance of learned behaviors [67]. Among the demographic and intervention characteristics examined in the meta-analysis, only the duration of the intervention predicted a program's success. This finding mirrors well-established patterns of relapse after interventions promoting weight loss [68] and smoking cessation [69,70]. Further work is needed to address maintenance of behavior change.

Among one of the few successful studies to demonstrate long-term maintenance was the Weight Loss Maintenance study [71], which involved 1685 overweight/obese adults with hypertension and/or dyslipidemia, who were initially provided a weight loss intervention consisting of 20 weekly group sessions. The phase I intervention emphasized BP-related lifestyle goals. Those who succeeded in losing at least 4 kg were eligible for randomization to one of three 30-month maintenance conditions ($n = 1032$): a Personal Contact intervention with monthly phone (9 per year) or face-to-face (3 per year) contact with an interventionist, an Interactive Technology intervention with unlimited access to an interactive Web site designed to promote weight loss maintenance, or a Self-Directed control condition. The majority of individuals who successfully completed an initial 6-month behavioral weight loss program maintained weight below their entry level after 30 additional months. Monthly brief personal-contact sessions provided modest benefit in sustaining weight loss, whereas an Internet-based intervention provided early but transient benefit. Thus, further work is needed to determine the level of intensity of self-management programs that is needed to maintain effects, with a potential consideration of *booster shots*.

A limitation of extant work is that it typically has focused on change in a single specific health-related behavior. In the case of hypertension, current national guidelines for the prevention and treatment of high BP include five nonpharmacologic interventions [72], each of which has been proven in clinical trials to significantly lower BP, and most have been shown to prevent the development of hypertension. These five treatments include the DASH dietary pattern [73–76], weight loss in overweight patients [20,77], reduced sodium intake [77,78], regular moderate-intensity physical activity [23,79], and moderation of alcohol intake [80]. Despite the focus on a specific behavior such as weight loss or exercise, increasing work is demonstrating potential benefits of focusing on multiple hypertension-related behaviors simultaneously. For example, a hypertension lifestyle intervention study (PREMIER, $n = 810$), demonstrated that, after 6 months, change in multiple behaviors improved SBP. The improvement was linked specifically to weight loss, increased physical activity, DASH dietary changes, and reduced sodium intake [81]. Because changes in the various lifestyle factors were generally not associated with each other (e.g., few dietary changes were linked to increased exercise), it appears that some patients may have successfully controlled hypertension through exercise, others through weight loss or dietary pattern, and still others through reduction of sodium intake. However, the intervention approach addressed all of these factors.

Similarly, in the Take Control of Your Blood Pressure study, the combination of BP monitoring at home and a tailored brief behavioral intervention focusing on the five nonpharmacological interventions, as well as medication adherence, resulted in a statistically significant improvement in BP control and decreases in SBP and DBP at 24 months, with minimal costs [59]. These recent studies further support the idea that patient self-management interventions that focus on multiple behaviors and long-term maintenance may be valuable tools for improving BP control rates.

7.5 SOCIAL SUPPORT AND SELF-MANAGEMENT

A wealth of literature has shown that higher social support is associated with better adherence to health behaviors (e.g., diet, exercise) and emotional well-being, improved clinical outcomes, and lower mortality [82,83]. Among patients with hypertension, social support could be marshaled to enhance self-management and, ultimately, patient outcomes [82,84,85]. To this end, spouses/life partners represent a potentially important source of social support [86].

One rationale for including spouses/partners in health interventions is that they are the most common source of influence on people's health behaviors [87,88]. Lifestyle changes may be difficult to initiate and maintain if there are inconsistencies within one's contextual environment [89]. For example, it may be difficult to make dietary changes when the individual attempting dietary changes is not involved in cooking meals or shopping for groceries [90]. Decades of research has confirmed that social context influences morbidity and mortality [91–94], in part, because social support enhances adherence [94–101]. Spouse/partner support includes emotional support (i.e., the provision of empathy, feedback, trust, and love) and instrumental support (i.e., physical care, transportation, finances, and help with errands). Spouses/partners may positively influence patients' health by providing instrumental assistance (e.g., preparing healthier foods) or emotional support (e.g., empathy, positive reinforcement). Another rationale for couple-based interventions is that they may improve the physical or psychological health of spouses/partners (partner effect) [102]; spouses/partners with the same condition as patients may accrue direct health benefits, whereas spouses/partners without the same condition as patients may benefit from lifestyle changes (e.g., diet, exercise) or derive psychological benefits (e.g., less worry or stress) by helping their partner achieve improved health status and outcomes [103–105]. In general, studies have suggested that adherence to health behaviors may be enhanced by social support [94–101].

7.6   TELEMEDICINE AND SELF-MANAGEMENT

There is an increasing mismatch between a rising demand for services (particularly with regard to management of chronic illness) and the supply of service providers [106], together with increasing cultural expectations for just-in-time services. With the preponderance of care shifting to the management of chronic conditions and the importance of both prevention and disease management, many of these health care interactions can take place *virtually.*

For example, BP monitoring at home is a self-management strategy that has been examined as a method to improve BP control by engaging patients in monitoring their own health parameters [59]. Individual BP monitoring is believed to improve the recognition of BP control, which may lead to improved medication adherence, adherence to lifestyle recommendations, and ultimately better BP control [107–109]. A meta-analysis of 18 randomized controlled trials that compared BP monitoring at home to usual care found that BP monitoring at home independent of other interventions resulted in small improvements in BP control [110]. A joint call to action by the American Heart Association, American Society of Hypertension, and Preventive Cardiovascular Nurses Association recommends that BP monitoring at home should become a routine component of BP measurement in the majority of patients with known or suspected hypertension; it is particularly of value in patients with diabetes, in whom tight BP control is of paramount importance. This call-to-action paper concludes that BP monitoring at home has the potential to improve the quality of care while reducing costs and therefore should be reimbursed by third-party payers [110].

Another example of virtual BP management is *telemedicine* or remote monitoring in patients' homes, which has been offered as a plausible solution to improving ambulatory medical care. To date, most telemedicine efforts showing improved outcomes have utilized telephone-based interventions [111]. However, a number of Internet- and Web-based tools have emerged to further enable communication between patients and providers and among providers. One study, for example, demonstrated that Web-based communication with pharmacist care management improved BP control in hypertensive patients [112]. Web-based monitoring may be more acceptable and effective compared with clinic-based monitoring and management; in addition, it is more scalable and cost effective compared with traditional disease management or telephone-based programs. The degree to which Web-based communication coupled with a Web-based, tailored disease management and education program can improve BP control beyond traditional telemedicine disease management provided by health care personnel is unknown, but research in this area is ongoing [113].

7.7   CONCLUSION

Patient self-management is defined as the implementation of strategies that enhance the patient's ability to monitor and manage daily health and symptoms, solve problems, overcome barriers encountered, modify lifestyle risk factors, and communicate with clinical providers as active collaborators in defining and achieving health and therapeutic goals. With an expected shortage of primary care providers in the United States health care system, an increase in the number of individuals entering

TABLE 7.3

Summary: Take-Home Messages

Key Evidences	Recommendation for Practitioners
• Patient self-management involves strategies that enable the patient to monitor and manage daily health and symptoms, solve problems, overcome barriers encountered, modify lifestyle risk factors, and communicate with clinical providers as active collaborators in defining and adhering to health and therapeutic goals. • Components of self-management programs consist of closely monitoring symptoms and when to respond with appropriate actions (adjust medications, initiate call to a health care provider, reduce salt intake). • Social support could be marshaled to enhance self-management and, ultimately, patient outcomes. • Health information technology, including electronic records and e-prescription, can help provide the necessary data infrastructure.	• Continuity of care and follow-up are essential not only at initiating a behavior but also for maintaining behavioral changes. • Be patient-centered, addressing the patient's preferences, concerns, lifestyle, culture, and beliefs. • Focus on empowering patients to become more active in managing their disease by providing the skills to treat their hypertension. • Interventions should be holistic, encompassing an understanding of the patient's overall medical condition. • Interventions should include multiple components, using a variety of tools and incentives tailored to the individual patient's characteristics and needs. • Use technology support when possible and feasible.

the health care system as a result of health care reform, and the rising prevalence of hypertension among Americans, which is expected to surpass 70 million in coming years, the need to implement and evaluate innovative ways to improve patient self-management will grow. Self-management programs will need to be patient-centered, that is, addressing the patient's preferences, concerns, lifestyle, culture, and beliefs. Interventions should be holistic, encompassing an understanding of the patient's overall medical condition, and should include reconciliation of all self-management recommendations. Interventions should include multiple components and the use of a variety of tools and incentives tailored to the individual patient's characteristics and needs. Services delivered outside the physician practice (e.g., counseling by pharmacists) should engage directly with the prescribing physician, with appropriate privacy safeguards. Health information technology, including electronic platforms for delivery of lifestyle self-management interventions, provides opportunities for widespread dissemination (Table 7.3) [114].

ACKNOWLEDGMENT

This research is supported by Established Investigator Award from the American Heart Association and a career Scientist Award from Health Services Research and Development, Veterans Affairs Medical Center (08-027). The views expressed in this manuscript are those of the authors and do not necessarily represent the views of the Department of Veterans Affairs.

REFERENCES

1. American Heart Association. *Heart Disease and Stroke Statistics—2009 Update*. Dallas, TX: American Heart Association; 2010.
2. Stamler J, Stamler R, Neaton J. Blood pressure, systolic and diastolic, and cardiovascular risks: U.S. population data. *Arch Intern Med*. 1993;153:598–615.
3. Perry H, Roccella EJ. Conference report on stroke mortality in the southeastern United States. *Hypertension*. 1998;31:1206–1215.
4. Kannel W. Blood pressure as a cardiovascular risk factor. Prevention and treatment. *JAMA*. 1996;275:1571–1576.
5. Fields LE, Burt VL, Cutler JA, Hughes J, Roccella EJ, Sorlie P. The burden of adult hypertension in the United States 1999 to 2000. A rising tide. *Hypertension*. 2004;44:398–404.
6. Schroeder SA. Shattuck Lecture. We can do better—Improving the health of the American people. *N Engl J Med*. 2007;357(12):1221–1228.
7. Hibbard JH, Mahoney ER, Stock R, Tusler M. Do increases in patient activation result in improved self-management behaviors? *Health Serv Res*. 2007;42(4):1443–1463.
8. Anderson RM, Funnell MM. Patient empowerment: Myths and misconceptions. *Patient Educ Couns*. 2010;79(3):277–282.
9. Bodenheimer T, Lorig K, Holman H, Grumbach K. Patient self-management of chronic disease in primary care. *JAMA*. 2002;288(19):2469–2475.
10. Azarmina P, Prestwich G, Rosenquist J, Singh D. Transferring disease management and health promotion programs to other countries: Critical success factors. *Health Promot Int*. 2008;23(4):372–379.
11. Lorig K. Self-management education: More than a nice extra. *Med Care*. 2003;41(6):699–701.
12. Wagner EH, Austin BT, Von Korff M. Improving outcomes in chronic illness. *Manag Care Q*. Spring 1996;4(2):12–25.
13. WHO. *Innovative Care for Chronic Conditions: Building Blocks for Action*. World Health Organization, Geneva, Switzerland; 2002.
14. Coleman K, Austin BT, Brach C, Wagner EH. Evidence on the Chronic Care Model in the new millennium. *Health Aff (Millwood)*. 2009;28(1):75–85.
15. Fischer D, Stewart AL, Bloch DA, Lorig K, Laurent D, Holman H. Capturing the patient's view of change as a clinical outcome measure. *JAMA*. 1999;282(12):1157–1162.
16. Renders CM, Valk GD, Griffin S, Wagner EH, Eijk JT, Assendelft WJ. Interventions to improve the management of diabetes mellitus in primary care, outpatient and community settings. *Cochrane Database Syst Rev*. 2001(1):CD001481.
17. Kearney PM, Whelton M, Reynolds K, Muntner P, Whelton PK, He J. Global burden of hypertension: Analysis of worldwide data. *Lancet*. 2005;365(9455):217–223.
18. Chobanian AV, Bakris GL, Black HR, et al. Seventh report of the Joint National Committee on Prevention, Detection, Evaluation, and Treatment of High Blood Pressure. *Hypertension*. 2003;42(6):1206–1252.
19. Lewington S, Clarke R, Qizilbash N, Peto R, Collins R. Age-specific relevance of usual blood pressure to vascular mortality: A meta-analysis of individual data for one million adults in 61 prospective studies. *Lancet*. 2002;360(9349):1903–1913.
20. Neter JE, Stam BE, Kok FJ, Grobbee DE, Geleijnse JM. Influence of weight reduction on blood pressure: A meta-analysis of randomized controlled trials. *Hypertension*. 2003;42(5):878–884.
21. Appel L, Moore TJ, Obarzanek E, Vollmer WM, Svetkey LP, Sacks FM, Bray GA, Vogt TM, Cutler JA, Windhauser MM, Lin P-H, Karanja N, for the DASH Collaborative Research Group. A clinical trial of the effects of dietary patterns on blood pressure. *N Engl J Med*. 1997;336:1117–1124.

22. Jurgens G, Graudal NA. Effects of low sodium diet versus high sodium diet on blood pressure, renin, aldosterone, catecholamines, cholesterols, and triglyceride. *Cochrane Database Syst Rev.* 2004(1):CD004022.

23. Whelton SP, Chin A, Xin X, He J. Effect of aerobic exercise on blood pressure: A meta-analysis of randomized, controlled trials. *Ann Intern Med.* 2002;136(7):493–503.

24. Sacks FM, Svetkey LP, Vollmer WM, et al. Effects on blood pressure of reduced dietary sodium and the Dietary Approaches to Stop Hypertension (DASH) diet. DASH-Sodium Collaborative Research Group. *N Engl J Med.* 2001;344(1):3–10.

25. Elmer PJ, Obarzanek E, Vollmer WM, et al. Effects of comprehensive lifestyle modification on diet, weight, physical fitness, and blood pressure control: 18-month results of a randomized trial. *Ann Intern Med.* 2006;144(7):485–495.

26. Joint National Committee on Detection Evaluation, and Treatment of High Blood Pressure. *The sixth report of the Joint National Committee on Detection, Evaluation, and Treatment of High Blood Pressure (JNC VI).* Bethesda, MD: U.S. Department of Health and Human Services, National Institutes of Health; 1997.

27. Burt V, Whelton P, Roccella EJ, et al. Prevalence of hypertension in the US adult population: Results from the third National Health and Nutrition Examination Survey. 1988–1991. *Hypertension.* 1995;25:305–313.

28. Psaty BM, Manolio TA, Smith NL, et al. Time trends in high blood pressure control and the use of antihypertensive medications in older adults: The cardiovascular health study. *Arch Intern Med.* 2002;162(20):2325–2332.

29. Lorig KR, Sobel DS, Ritter PL, Laurent D, Hobbs M. Effect of a self-management program on patients with chronic disease. *Eff Clin Pract.* 2001;4(6):256–262.

30. Bodenheimer T, Wagner EH, Grumbach K. Improving primary care for patients with chronic illness: The chronic care model, Part 2. *JAMA.* 2002;288(15):1909–1914.

31. Glynn LG, Murphy AW, Smith SM, Schroeder K, Fahey T. Interventions used to improve control of blood pressure in patients with hypertension. *Cochrane Database Syst Rev.* 2010;17(3):CD005182.

32. Carter BL, Foppe van Mil JW. Comparative effectiveness research: Evaluating pharmacist interventions and strategies to improve medication adherence. *Am J Hypertens.* 2010;23(9):949–955.

33. Fahey T, Schroeder K, Ebrahim S. Interventions used to improve control of blood pressure in patients with hypertension. *Cochrane Database Syst Rev.* 2006(4):CD005182.

34. Chisholm-Burns MA, Lee JK, Spivey CA, et al. US Pharmacists' Effect as Team Members on Patient Care: Systematic Review and Meta-Analyses. *Med Care.* 2010;48(10):923–933.

35. Pearson M, Mattke S, Shaw R, Ridgely MS, Wiseman SH. *Patient Self-Management Support Programs: An Evaluation.* Final Contract (Prepared by RAND Health under contract No. 282-00-0005). AHRQ publication *No. 08-0011.* Rockville, MD: Agency for Healthcare Research and Quality; 2007.

36. Bosworth HB, Powers BJ, Oddone EZ. Patient self-management support: Novel strategies in hypertension and heart disease. *Cardiol Clin.* 2010;28(4):655–663.

37. Black HR. Management of older hypertensive patients: Is there a difference in approach? *J Clin Hypertens (Greenwich).* 2003;5(6 Suppl 4):11–16.

38. Ghosh AK. Care of the elderly: The problem of clinical inertia. *Minn Med.* 2002;85(11):6.

39. O'Connor PJ. Overcome clinical inertia to control systolic blood pressure. *Arch Intern Med.* 2003;163(22):2677–2678.

40. Phillips LS, Branch WT, Cook CB, et al. Clinical inertia. *Ann Intern Med.* 2001;135(9):825–834.

41. Jones J, Gorkin L, Lian JF, Staffa JA, Fletcher AP. Discontinuation of and changes in treatment after start of new courses of antihypertensive drugs: A study of the United Kingdom population. *BMJ.* 1995;311:293–295.

42. Steel N. Thresholds for taking antihypertensive drugs in different professional and lay groups: Questionnaire survey. *BMJ.* 27 2000;320(7247):1446–1447.

43. Ostbye T, Yarnall KS, Krause KM, Pollak KI, Gradison M, Michener JL. Is there time for management of patients with chronic diseases in primary care? *Ann Fam Med.* 2005;3(3):209–214.

44. Carter BL, Rogers M, Daly J, Zheng S, James PA. The potency of team-based care interventions for hypertension: A meta-analysis. *Arch Intern Med.* 26 2009;169(19):1748–1755.

45. Borenstein JE, Graber G, Saltiel E, et al. Physician-pharmacist comanagement of hypertension: A randomized, comparative trial. *Pharmacotherapy.* 2003;23(2):209–216.

46. Denver EA, Barnard M, Woolfson RG, Earle KA. Management of uncontrolled hypertension in a nurse-led clinic compared with conventional care for patients with type 2 diabetes. *Diabetes Care.* 2003;26(8):2256–2260.

47. New JP, Mason JM, Freemantle N, et al. Specialist nurse-led intervention to treat and control hypertension and hyperlipidemia in diabetes (SPLINT): A randomized controlled trial. *Diabetes Care.* 2003;26(8):2250–2255.

48. Vivian EM. Improving blood pressure control in a pharmacist-managed hypertension clinic. *Pharmacotherapy.* 2002;22(12):1533–1540.

49. Mehos BM, Saseen JJ, MacLaughlin EJ. Effect of pharmacist intervention and initiation of home blood pressure monitoring in patients with uncontrolled hypertension. *Pharmacotherapy.* 2000;20(11):1384–1389.

50. Boulware LE, Daumit GL, Frick KD, Minkovitz CS, Lawrence RS, Powe NR. An evidence-based review of patient-centered behavioral interventions for hypertension. *Am J Prev Med.* 2001;21(3):221–232.

51. Bosworth HB, Olsen MK, Gentry P, et al. Nurse administered telephone intervention for blood pressure control: A patient-tailored multifactorial intervention. *Patient Educ Couns.* 2005;57(1):5–14.

52. Bosworth HB, Olsen MK, Oddone EZ. Improving blood pressure control by tailored feedback to patients and clinicians. *Am Heart J.* 2005;149(5):795–803.

53. Bosworth HB, Olsen MK, Goldstein MK, et al. The veterans' study to improve the control of hypertension (V-STITCH): Design and methodology. *Contemp Clin Trials.* 2005;26(2):155–168.

54. Krass I, Taylor SJ, Smith C, Armour CL. Impact on medication use and adherence of Australian pharmacists' diabetes care services. *J Am Pharm Assoc.* 2005;45(1):33–40.

55. Allen JK, Dennison CR. Randomized trials of nursing interventions for secondary prevention in patients with coronary artery disease and heart failure: Systematic review. *J Cardiovasc Nurs.* 2010;25(3):207–220.

56. DeBusk RF, Miller NH, Superko HR, et al. A case-management system for coronary risk factor modification after acute myocardial infarction. *Ann Intern Med.* 1994;120(9):721–729.

57. Hill MN, Han HR, Dennison CR, et al. Hypertension care and control in underserved urban African American men: Behavioral and physiologic outcomes at 36 months. *Am J Hypertens.* 2003;16(11):906–913.

58. Bosworth HB, Olsen MK, Dudley T, et al. Patient education and provider decision support to control blood pressure in primary care: A cluster randomized trial. *Am Heart J.* 2009;157(3):450–456.

59. Bosworth HB, Olsen MK, Grubber JM, et al. Two Self-management Interventions to Improve Hypertension Control: A Randomized Trial. *Ann Intern Med.* 2009;151(10):687–695.

60. Bosworth H, Powers BJ, Olsen MK, McCant F, Grubber J, Smith V, Gentry P, Rose C, Van Houtven C, Wang V, Goldstein MK, Oddone EZ. Home blood pressure management and improved blood pressure control: Results from a randomized controlled trial. *Arch Intern Med.* 201;171(13):1173–1180.

61. Sikka R, Waters J, Moore W, Sutton DR, Herman WH, Aubert RE. Renal assessment practices and the effect of nurse case management of health maintenance organization patients with diabetes. *Diabetes Care.* 1999;22(1):1–6.
62. Writing Group of the PREMIER Collaborative Research Group (WGOTPCR). Effects of comprehensive lifestyle modification on blood pressure control: main results of the PREMIER clinical trial. *JAMA.* 2003;289(16):2083–2093.
63. Hollis JF, Gullion CM, Stevens VJ, et al. Weight loss during the intensive intervention phase of the weight-loss maintenance trial. *Am J Prev Med.* 2008;35(2):118–126.
64. Traylor AH, Schmittdiel JA, Uratsu CS, Mangione CM, Subramanian U. Adherence to cardiovascular disease medications: Does patient-provider race/ethnicity and language concordance matter? *J Gen Intern Med.* 2010;25(11):1172–1177.
65. Traylor AH, Schmittdiel JA, Uratsu CS, Mangione CM, Subramanian U. The predictors of patient-physician race and ethnic concordance: A medical facility fixed-effects approach. *HSR.* 2010;45(3):792–805.
66. Butterworth SW. Influencing patient adherence to treatment guidelines. *J Manag Care Pharm.* 2008;14(6 Suppl B):21–24.
67. Norris SL, Lau J, Smith SJ, Schmid CH, Engelgau MM. Self-management education for adults with type 2 diabetes: A meta-analysis of the effect on glycemic control. *Diabetes Care.* 2002;25(7):1159–1171.
68. Perri MG, Nezu AM, McKelvey WF, Shermer RL, Renjilian DA, Viegener BJ. Relapse prevention training and problem-solving therapy in the long-term management of obesity. *J Consult Clin Psychol.* 2001;69(4):722–726.
69. Lancaster T, Hajek P, Stead LF, West R, Jarvis MJ. Prevention of relapse after quitting smoking: A systematic review of trials. *Arch Intern Med.* 2006;166(8):828–835.
70. Fu SS, Partin MR, Snyder A, et al. Promoting repeat tobacco dependence treatment: Are relapsed smokers interested? *Am J Manag Care.* 2006;12(4):235–243.
71. Svetkey LP, Stevens VJ, Brantley PJ, et al. Comparison of strategies for sustaining weight loss: The weight loss maintenance randomized controlled trial. *JAMA.* Mar 12 2008;299(10):1139–1148.
72. Chobanian AV, Bakris GL, Black HR, et al. The seventh report of the joint national committee on prevention, detection, evaluation, and treatment of high blood pressure: The JNC 7 report. *JAMA.* 2003;289(19):2560–2571.
73. Karanja N, Obarzanek E, Lin PH, McCullough ML, Phillips KM, Swain JF, et al. Descriptive characteristics of the dietary patterns used in the Dietary Approaches to Stop Hypertension Trial. DASH Collaborative Research Group. *J Am Diet Assoc.* 1999;99:S19–S27.
74. Sacks FM, Appel LJ, Moore TJ, et al. A dietary approach to prevent hypertension: A review of the Dietary Approaches to Stop Hypertension (DASH) Study. *Clin Cardiol.* 1999;22(7 Suppl):III6-10.
75. Svetkey L, Sacks FM, Obarzanek E, et al., for the DASH-Sodium Collaborative Research Group. The DASH diet, sodium intake and blood pressure trial (DASH-sodium): Rationale and design. *J Am Diet Assoc.* 1999;99:S96–S104.
76. Svetkey L, Simons-Morton D, Vollmer WM, Appel LJ, Conlin PR, Ryan DH, Ard J, Kennedy BM, for the DASH research group. Effects of dietary patterns on blood pressure: Subgroup analysis of the Dietary Approaches to Stop Hypertension (DASH) randomized clinical trial. *Arch Intern Med.* 1999;159(3):285–293.
77. The effects of nonpharmacologic interventions on blood pressure of persons with high normal levels. Results of the Trials of Hypertension Prevention, Phase I. *JAMA.* 1992;267(9):1213–1220.
78. Cutler JA. Randomized clinical trials of weight reduction in nonhypertensive persons. *Ann Epidemiol.* 1991;1(4):363–370.

79. Kelley GA, Kelley KS. Progressive resistance exercise and resting blood pressure: A meta-analysis of randomized controlled trials. *Hypertension.* 2000;35(3):838–843.
80. Xin X, He J, Frontini MG, Ogden LG, Motsamai OI, Whelton PK. Effects of alcohol reduction on blood pressure: A meta-analysis of randomized controlled trials. *Hypertension.* 2001;38(5):1112–1117.
81. Obarzanek E, Vollmer WM, Lin PH, et al. Effects of individual components of multiple behavior changes: The PREMIER trial. *Am J Health Behav.* 2007;31(5):545–560.
82. Martire L, Lustig A, Schulz R, Miller G, Helgeson V. Is it beneficial to involve a family member? A meta-analysis of psychosocial interventions for chronic illness. *Health Psychol.* 2004;23(6):599–611.
83. Tower RB, Kasl SV, Darefsky AS. Types of marital closeness and mortality risk in older couples. *Psychosomatic Med.* 2002;64(4):644–659.
84. Berg CA, Upchurch R. A developmental-contextual model of couples coping with chronic illness across the adult life span. *Psychol Bull.* 2007;133(6):920–954.
85. Martire L, Schulz R. Involving family in psychosocial interventions for chronic illness. *Curr Direct Psychol Sci.* 2007;16(2):90–94.
86. Kiecolt-Glaser JK, Newton TL. Marriage and health: His and hers. *Psychol Bull.* 2001;127(4):472–503.
87. Rook KS, Thuras PD, Lewis MA. Social control, health risk taking, and psychological distress among the elderly. *Psychol Aging.* 1990;5(3):327–334.
88. Tucker JS, Mueller JS. Spouses' social control of health behaviors: Use and effectiveness of specific strategies. *Pers Soc Psychol Bull.* 2000;26(9):1120–1130.
89. Sherman AM, Bowen DJ, Vitolins M, et al. Dietary adherence: Characteristics and interventions. *Control Clin Trials.* 2000;21(5 Suppl):206s–211s.
90. Carmody T, Fey S, Pierce D, Connor W, Matarazzo J. Behavioral treatment of hyperlipidemia: Techniques, results, and future directions. *J Behav Med.* 1982;5(1):91–116.
91. Berkman LF. The role of social relations in health promotion. *Psychosomatic Med.* 1995;57(3):245–254.
92. Cohen S. Psychosocial models of the role of social support in the etiology of physical disease. *Health Psychol.* 1988;7(3):269–297.
93. Cohen S. Social relationships and health. *American Psychologist.* 2004;59(8):676–684.
94. DiMatteo MR. Social support and patient adherence to medical treatment: A meta-analysis. *Health Psychol.* 2004;23(2):207–218.
95. McCann BS, Retzlaff BM, Dowdy AA, Walden CE, Knopp RH. Promoting adherence to low-fat, low-cholesterol diets: Review and recommendations. *J Am Diet Assoc.* 1990;90(10):1408–1414.
96. Bovbjerg VE, McCann BS, Brief DJ, et al. Spouse support and long-term adherence to lipid-lowering diets. *Am J Epi.* 1995;141(5):451–460.
97. Catz SL, Kelly JA, Bogart LM, Benotsch EG, McAuliffe TL. Patterns, correlates, and barriers to medication adherence among persons prescribed new treatments for HIV disease. *Health Psychol.* 2000;19(2):124–133.
98. Sherbourne CD, Hays RD, Ordway L, DiMatteo MR, Kravitz RL. Antecedents of adherence to medical recommendations: Results from the Medical Outcomes Study. *J Behav Med.* 1992;15(5):447–468.
99. Ogedegbe G, Harrison M, Robbins L, Mancuso CA, Allegrante JP. Barriers and facilitators of medication adherence in hypertensive African Americans: A qualitative study. *Ethn Dis.* Winter 2004;14(1):3–12.
100. Molassiotis A, Nahas-Lopez V, Chung WY, Lam SW, Li CK, Lau TF. Factors associated with adherence to antiretroviral medication in HIV-infected patients. *Int J STD AIDS.* 2002;13(5):301–310.

101. Voils CI, Steffens DC, Flint EP, Bosworth HB. Social support and locus of control as predictors of adherence to antidepressant medication in an elderly population. *Am J Geriat Psych.* 2005;13(2):157–165.
102. Kenny D. Models of non-independence in dyadic research. *J Soc Pers Relat.* 1996;13:279–294.
103. Martire LM, Lustig AP, Schulz R, Miller GE, Helgeson VS. Is it beneficial to involve a family member? A meta-analysis of psychosocial interventions for chronic illness. *Health Psychol.* 2004;23(6):599–611.
104. Kiecolt-Glaser JK, Newton TL. Marriage and health: His and hers. *Psychol Bull.* 2001;127(4):472–503.
105. Martire LM, Schulz R, Helgeson VS, Small BJ, Saghafi EM. Review and meta-analysis of couple-oriented interventions for chronic illness. *Ann Behav Med.* 2010;40(3):325–342.
106. Shineski E. Secretary of Veterans Affairs Nominee Eric Shineski Confirmation Testimony before the Senate Committee on Veterans Affairs. US Senate Committee on Veterans Affairs, 14 January 2009.
107. Bosworth HB, Olsen MK, McCant F, et al. Hypertension Intervention Nurse Telemedicine Study (HINTS): Testing a multifactorial tailored behavioral/educational and a medication management intervention for blood pressure control. *Am Heart J.* 2007;153(6):918–924.
108. Rogers MAM, Small D, Buchan DA, et al. Home monitoring service improves mean arterial pressure in patients with essential hypertension. *Ann Intern Med.* 2001;134(11):1024–1032.
109. Reed S, Li Y, Oddone EZ, et al. Economic evaluation of home blood pressure monitoring with or without telephonic behavioral self-management in patients with hypertension. *Am J Hypertens.* 2010;23(2):142–148.
110. Pickering TG, Miller NH, Ogedegbe G, Krakoff LR, Artinian NT, Goff D. Call to action on use and reimbursement for home blood pressure monitoring: Executive summary: A joint scientific statement from the American Heart Association, American Society of Hypertension, and Preventive Cardiovascular Nurses Association. *Hypertension.* 2008;52(1):1–9.
111. Roth A, Malov N, Steinberg DM, et al. Telemedicine for post-myocardial infarction patients: An observational study. *Telemed J E Health.* 2009;15(1):24–30.
112. Green BB, Cook AJ, Ralston JD, et al. Effectiveness of home blood pressure monitoring, Web communication, and pharmacist care on hypertension control: A randomized controlled trial. *JAMA.* 2008 2008;299(24):2857–2867.
113. Shah BR, Adams M, Peterson ED, et al. Secondary prevention risk interventions via telemedicine and tailored patient education (SPRITE): A randomized trial to improve postmyocardial infarction management. *Circ Cardiovasc Qual Outcomes.* 2011;4(2):235–242.
114. Thinking outside the pillbox: A system-wide approach to improving patient medication adherence for chronic disease. Available at http://www.nehi.net/publications/44/thinking_outside_the_ pillbox_a_systemwide ed trial.

8 Implementing Behavioral Change for Blood Pressure Control at the Provider Level

Elena Salmoirago-Blotcher and Ira Ockene
University of Massachusetts Medical School

CONTENTS

8.1 INTRODUCTION

Hypertension affects about 65 million people in the United States, and its prevalence remains at 30%, which did not significantly change over the past 10 years (1999–2008) [1]. Based on data from the National Health and Nutrition Examination Survey (NHANES) (2003–2004), it was found that awareness about high blood pressure (BP) (i.e., a positive response to the question, "Have you ever been told by a doctor or health professional that you had hypertension, also called high blood pressure?") was 76% and that 65% of patients were receiving treatment. However, BP control (i.e., BP levels <140 mmHg systolic and <90 mmHg diastolic) [2] was achieved only in 37% of patients. According to more recent NHANES data [3], these figures have improved between 2007 and 2008, with 50.1% of individuals having a BP below 140/90. Interestingly, lifestyle changes are not a likely reason for the observed improvement in BP control since most patients with hypertension are still obese [4] and their dietary habits have deteriorated [5]. Despite this progress, it is evident that adequate BP control is not achieved in about half of patients with high BP, particularly in specific age groups (less than 40 and over 60 years old) and in Hispanic patients [3].

Hypertension is almost entirely managed in primary care settings. Based on the available evidence, several complex behavioral educational strategies and intensive counseling programs have been recommended both as first-line therapy and in addition to the pharmacological treatment of hypertension [6–13]. It is not clear, however, how best the primary care team can organize and deliver effective care, including behavioral strategies to improve BP control.

In this chapter, we summarize the current evidence for the efficacy of behavioral interventions in promoting better BP control, focusing primarily on behavioral interventions directly targeting BP levels and/or (predefined) BP control that are offered, delivered, or implemented at the provider level. The definition of "provider" in this chapter is rather wide, referring to nurse practitioners, primary care physicians or their offices, and pharmacists. Throughout this chapter, the reader should also keep in mind that studies of provider-level behavioral interventions often employ multiple strategies that do not fit in a single category and that there are differences in the populations examined across studies and in the criteria used to define BP control. Moreover, since strategies often overlap, it is difficult to draw definitive conclusions on the effect of individual components of complex interventions. Of particular relevance here, strategies that target lifestyle treatment often also target medication treatment, and differential effects cannot be determined. With that caveat, we start by reviewing interventions targeting providers' behavior and education, with a special focus on technical support; we then address patient-centered strategies, followed by a review of the evidence for the efficacy of interventions implemented at the system level. We then conclude with a series of practical recommendations for primary care providers.

8.2   PROVIDER-CENTERED INTERVENTIONS

Why do we need to educate providers? Providers seem reluctant to modify medications or reinforce lifestyle changes even when the patient has not reached optimal BP control. Phillips et al. [14] have defined this phenomenon, known as *clinical inertia*, as "the failure of health care providers to initiate or intensify therapy when indicated." According to a study conducted in the 1990s, approximately 40% of patients still had a BP equal to or higher than 160/90 mmHg despite having seen their providers for hypertension-related visits, on an average, more than six times per year [15].

There are multiple reasons for clinical inertia to occur. First, clinicians tend to overestimate their adherence to hypertension treatment guidelines [16]. Oliveria et al. [17] reported that physicians did not change or begin a new hypertension treatment usually when the systolic BP (SBP) recorded at a specific visit was at least

150 mmHg, as compared to when the diastolic BP (DBP) was at least 91 mmHg. This indicates that physicians consider diastolic readings more important than systolic readings and suggests that physicians may be familiar with hypertension treatment guidelines without necessarily transferring this knowledge into clinical practice. Other reasons for not following recommendations include the provider's belief that the recorded BP is not representative of the patient's typical BP, hypertension not being a clinical priority for a specific visit, patients' nonadherence to medications [18], or the clinicians' lack of concern for small elevations in BP above the recommended goals [19].

8.2.1 TECHNICAL SUPPORT

Educational strategies targeting provider's education have been implemented using electronic, automated, telephone-based, or paper-based (i.e., flowcharts) technical support. Broadly, they have included provider reminders, that is, feedback reminders alerting the clinician to conditions such as missing appointments, prescription refills, or anomalous blood-test results, and decision-support systems, that is, systems that prompt the provider to consider changes in the treatment when a certain goal has not been reached [11,20].

8.2.2 PROVIDER REMINDERS

A review of educational and organizational interventions to improve the treatment of hypertension in primary care [21] found that appointment reminder systems [22–26] resulted in improved follow-up of patients, except for one trial [27], without affecting BP control. A recent review concluded that reminders increased the proportion of patients attending follow-up (OR: 0.41; 95% CI: 0.32, 0.51) in the majority of trials and improved BP control in two small trials (OR: 0.54; 95% CI: 0.41, 0.73); these data, however, require further confirmation due to the heterogeneity of the studies [28].

8.2.3 DECISION-SUPPORT SYSTEMS

Decision-support systems and clinical reminders work by linking hypertension guidelines to a patient, prompting the provider to take the necessary measures to implement current recommendations in that specific patient. In the early 2000s, a review of studies on physician education interventions alone or in combination concluded that reminders improved the follow-up of hypertension and that they may be useful in improving compliance with guideline recommendations; however, they had no effect on BP levels [29]. A 2×2 factorial randomized controlled trial of computer-displayed suggestions to physicians and pharmacists (physician intervention only, pharmacist intervention only, intervention by physician and pharmacist, and control) in 712 patients with uncomplicated hypertension failed to show relevant differences among groups with regard to BP levels, health-related quality of life, symptoms and side-effect profiles, number of emergency department visits and hospitalizations, and drug therapy compliance [30].

The Assessment and Treatment of Hypertension, Evidence-Based Automation Decision-Support System (ATHENA-HTN) [31,32] is an automatic guideline-based decision-support system designed to assist primary care providers in adhering to hypertension guidelines. Its main characteristic is its integration with existing electronic health record systems, enabling providers to see displayed hypertension management guidelines while they are seeing patients. ATHENA-HTN is one of the strategies used in the Hypertension Intervention Nurse Telemedicine Study (HINTS) [33], a study designed to improve BP control by involving different interventions at the patient level (tailored behavioral intervention and medication management), health system level (nurses are involved in intervention delivery), and provider education level (the ATHENA decision-support system).

A group of researchers at the Veterans Administration in Palo Alto, CA, conducted a cluster randomized trial involving geographically diverse primary care clinics of a university-affiliated Department of Veterans Affairs health care system [34]. A general intervention designed to improve concordance with guidelines for drug therapy of hypertension and to increase awareness of the importance of adequacy of BP control was delivered to 36 attending physicians and nurse practitioners, with findings based on 4500 hypertensive patients. The comparison group received the general intervention and a printed individualized advisory sent to clinicians at each patient's visit, indicating whether the patient's antihypertensive regimen was in agreement with current guidelines. The study's primary outcome was "change in the proportion of clinicians' patients with guidelines-concordant drug treatment." The prevalence of patients undergoing guideline-concordant treatments was 10.9% in the individualized intervention versus 3.8% in the general intervention, $p = .008$; however, there were no-between-group differences in BP control.

The Veterans' Study to Improve the Control of Hypertension (V-STITCH) [35] was a cluster randomized trial involving 30 primary care providers in the Durham VAMC Primary Care Clinic. Providers were randomly assigned to an intervention consisting in an electronically generated decision-support system delivering guideline-based recommendations to the provider at each patient's visit or to a control group receiving a reminder displaying the patients' most recent BP levels and current therapy. A sample of the providers' hypertensive patients ($n = 588$) was then randomly assigned to receive a nurse-delivered telephone intervention involving tailored behavioral and education modules to promote medication adherence and improve specific health behaviors or usual care. The primary outcome was the proportion of patients who achieved BP values ≤ 140/90 mmHg at each outpatient clinic visit over 2 years. There were no significant differences in BP control across the three groups compared with the control group. In particular, the decision-support system did not affect BP control, while secondary analyses showed that rates of BP control improved (from 40.1% to 54.4%, $p = .03$) among patients receiving the nurse-delivered phone intervention as compared to those not receiving a nurse intervention at 24 months of follow-up.

Rinfret et al. [36] conducted a randomized controlled trial of an intervention combining BP self-monitoring and access to an information technology–supported adherence and monitoring system providing nurses, pharmacists, and physicians with monthly BP reports compared to usual care in 223 primary care hypertensive subjects with hypertension confirmed by ambulatory monitoring. Change in the mean 24-h ambulatory BP for both SBP (-11.9 vs. -7.1 mmHg; $p < .001$) and DBP (-6.6 vs. -4.5 mmHg; $p = .007$), as well as the proportion of subjects achieving BP control as defined by the Canadian U.S. guidelines (46.0% vs. 28.6%, $p = .006$), was greater in the intervention subjects. In this study, the specific contribution of the BP-reminder component of the intervention is difficult to determine because patients assigned to the intervention received a combination of self-monitoring, reminder, and counseling (i.e., in response to the alerts generated by the system, patients were contacted by the nurses and were provided further education on hypertension and adherence).

Better BP control can be achieved when interventions directed at providers are combined with patients' education or counseling. A cluster randomized controlled trial [37] conducted in two hospital-based and eight community-based clinics in the Veterans Affairs Tennessee Valley Healthcare System involving 1341 veterans with essential hypertension assigned 182 providers to one of three interventions: (1) provider education [providers received e-mails with a Web-based link to the Seventh Report of the Joint National Committee on the Prevention, Detection, Evaluation and Treatment of High Blood Pressure (JNC 7) guidelines]; (2) provider education and alert (a patient-specific hypertension computerized alert); or (3) provider education, hypertension alert, and patient education (drug adherence and lifestyle modifications). Six-month follow-up data (available for 73% of patients) showed that a multifactorial intervention including patient education improved BP control as compared with provider education alone. Patients assigned to the patient-education group had better BP control (138/75 mmHg) than those assigned to the provider-education-and-alert or provider education–alone groups (146/76 and 145/78 mmHg, respectively). In the patient-education group, more patients had a SBP of 140 mmHg or less as compared to those in the provider education–alone or provider-education-and-alert groups (adjusted relative risk of BP control for the patient-education group, as compared with the provider education–alone group, is 1.31; 95% CI: 1.06–1.62; $p = .012$).

The Hypertension Improvement Project [38] was a randomized controlled trial with a 2×2 factorial design of a physician education intervention (8 primary care practices, 32 physicians) versus control and/or patient ($n = 574$) behavioral lifestyle intervention versus control. The physician intervention included Internet-based training, self-monitoring, and quarterly feedback reports, while the patient intervention included 20 weekly group sessions followed by 12 monthly telephone counseling sessions on weight loss, Dietary Approaches to Stop Hypertension dietary pattern, exercise, and reduced sodium intake. The primary outcome was "change in systolic BP at 6 months." The physician intervention had no effect (0.3 mmHg; 95% CI: 1.5–2.2), while the patient intervention resulted in a change in SBP by 2.6 mmHg (95% CI: 4.4–0.7; $p = .01$) at 6 months, with a significant interaction between the two interventions, showing that physicians' education, although not effective when alone, did increase the effect of the patient counseling intervention. No effect on BP was detected in patient, physician, or combined interventions at 18-months follow-up; however, the effect on dietary habits and weight loss was maintained.

In summary, decision support/clinical reminders improve clinicians' adherence to treatment guidelines; however, when used alone, they result in modest changes in

BP [39]. Furthermore, as reported in a thorough review of the role of health information technology in the management of hypertension [40], clinical reminders are not accepted well by clinicians. In general, they appear to perform better when integrated in clinical work and when designed to avoid the need for double entry of information in separate systems. Those clinical trials showing a positive effect often used reminders as part of multidisciplinary interventions and usually included counseling and educational components.

8.2.4 COMMUNICATION AND CLINIC ORGANIZATION

Although technically not "interventions," communication skills and good clinic organization are essential components of a provider's care. Thus, we want to conclude this section commenting on these particular aspects of hypertension treatment at the provider level.

Independent of the efficacy of the prescribed medications or of how careful and up-to-date is the physician/provider, the patient's motivation to take that medication or adopt a specific lifestyle change is what will ultimately determine if the treatment is successful [41]. The patient's motivation and, consequently, the clinical outcomes will improve if a patient's relationship with his or her physician is based on trust and empathy [42–44]. A second important component is the clinic organization. According to Phillips et al., physicians are not trained to achieve therapeutic goals, and practices may not be appropriately organized to facilitate such intervention [14]. Patients will often base their overall opinion of their physician's care on the type of service they receive, including minimal waiting time, good bedside manners, and an easily accessible, comfortable office environment [11].

8.3 PATIENT-CENTERED INTERVENTIONS

Educational strategies directed to the patient have been recommended both as first-line therapy and in addition to the pharmacological treatment of hypertension [6–13]. However, despite the potential for decreasing treatment-associated costs and improving patients' compliance with pharmacological therapy, the implementation of counseling and patient's education in primary care settings has been difficult due to time constraints and uncertainties about reimbursement policies. Other barriers include patients' noncompliance, inadequacy of teaching materials, lack of counseling training, low confidence of the physician in the efficacy of counseling intervention, and patients' demographic, insurance, and perceived health characteristics [45–47]. Patient education, however, does not necessarily imply referring patients for specialized counseling or systematic group training; rather, patient education may begin in the office, with the physician providing advice regarding diet, exercise, and other lifestyle recommendations. However, only a minority of patients receive even simple advice/counseling from their primary care providers regarding behavioral changes that are important in the management of high BP [48,49]. A Center for Disease Control study [49] using data from the 2008 Health Styles survey to estimate the prevalence of self-reported hypertension advice received from health professionals showed that only 21%–24.4% of patients reported receiving advice regarding lifestyle changes relevant for hypertension management such as weight loss, exercise, and reduction of dietary sodium intake. Primary care providers do not seem to consider lifestyle modification counseling as a good investment of their time even though research has shown that advice from a health care provider seems to be predictive of subsequent attempts to modify lifestyle habits [50–52], suggesting that "routine" advice given by doctors and other health professionals may have some effectiveness.

Provider-implemented behavioral interventions aimed at patients' education overall include three basic strategies: printed materials, counseling, and structured training courses. Printed materials usually include booklets, leaflets, or brochures containing relevant hypertension-related information (e.g., importance of achieving BP control, reasons for treating high BP even when the patient is asymptomatic, cardiovascular risk factors, need for life-long treatment, available drugs to treat hypertension, and healthy lifestyle for the prevention or management of hypertension) that can be mailed to the patients or offered at the clinic. Counseling may have an individual format or a group format, and even when group-delivered, it is usually personalized with individuals or group members often sharing their personal experiences. Structured training courses usually have a classroom format with a prespecified curriculum and one or more instructors. Counseling and training courses may include multiple components, such as encouraging weight loss, healthy diet choices, exercise, and other lifestyle changes. Furthermore, both counseling and educational interventions are usually combined with other interventions, including traditional pharmacological treatment.

8.3.1 EDUCATIONAL INTERVENTIONS

Overall, educational interventions based on the delivery of information using leaflets, mailings, or printed materials to the patients have not been effective in reducing BP levels [53–56]. A recent randomized clinical trial assessing the effectiveness of educational materials mailed to patients with mildly uncontrolled hypertension ($n = 162$) versus that of usual care ($n = 150$) did not show a significant effect on mean BP; however, there was an improvement in patient's self-reported knowledge and patient's satisfaction with the care [57].

A recent meta-analysis [58] reports that educational interventions directed to the patient (16 clinical trials included) resulted in a trend toward improved BP control (OR: 0.83; 95% CI: 0.75, 0.91), while results were heterogeneous for mean differences in SBP and DBP. However, the definition of "BP control" differed across studies. Furthermore, definitions of patient-directed educational intervention were broad or not provided, and they included interventions ranging from mailings to training classes. Other limitations were the lack of treatment fidelity assessments, blinding issues, and that there were only usual-care controls—no attention control groups were included.

8.3.2 BEHAVIORAL INTERVENTIONS

Boulware et al. [59] conducted a systematic review and meta-analysis of the literature to assess the independent and additive effects of three behavioral interventions on BP control (counseling, self-monitoring, and structured training courses). The authors selected 15 articles focusing exclusively on the former techniques. Counseling resulted in significant DBP improvement in four studies [60–63] and in 11.1-mmHg improvement in SBP (95% CI: 4.1–18) [60,62], compared with usual care. Counseling was also superior to training courses in a study comparing counseling and usual care or training [63]. Finally, combined interventions [64–67] in which counseling was delivered together with either self-monitoring or training courses were not superior to counseling alone, except for one study showing a reduction in SBP [65]. However, as the authors point out in the discussion, due to the author's choice of eligibility criteria, this review resulted in the exclusion of studies examining counseling, training, and self-monitoring in combination with other interventions. Furthermore, these studies differed in duration, content, and the type of provider delivering the intervention [59]. In fact, a recent study [68] evaluating the combined effect of self-monitoring and counseling showed positive results for the combined intervention. This was a 2×2 factorial randomized clinical trial ($n = 636$) comparing usual care, a behavioral intervention (bimonthly tailored, nurse-administered telephone intervention targeting hypertension-related behaviors), BP monitoring at home (3 times weekly), and behavioral intervention plus BP monitoring at home. At 24 months (with 25% of patients lost to follow-up), the primary outcome (improvement in BP control relative to the usual-care group) was 4.3% (95% CI: −4.5%,12.9%) in the behavioral intervention group, 7.6% (95% CI: −1.9%, 17.0%) in the group monitoring BP at home, and 11.0% (95% CI: 1.9%, 19.8%) in the combined behavioral plus self-monitoring group, with only the combined home monitoring and tailored behavioral telephone intervention significantly improving BP control relative to usual care.

The most promising results have been observed in interventions that creatively combined different strategies targeting the patient's and the provider's education at the same time. Roumie et al. [37] showed that 59.5% of patients receiving a multicomponent intervention combining provider education and alerts and patient education and about 40% in the provider-education-alone group and in the combined provider education and alert group achieved the SBP goal of 140 mmHg or less. Likewise, the Hypertension Improvement Project has shown a significant interaction between interventions targeting physician education and counseling of patients, resulting in a significantly higher reduction in SBP at 6 months of follow-up compared with intervention alone [38]. Therefore, combining behavioral intervention strategies clearly can benefit BP control; the challenge is to design strategies that are practical, affordable, and easy for long-term implementation.

8.4 INTERVENTIONS IMPLEMENTED AT THE SYSTEM LEVEL

This section examines interventions aimed at improving the delivery of care at higher and more complex levels than at the provider level. The general organization of the health care system does not always facilitate the efficient delivery of effective treatments, and several attempts have been made to intervene at this level. Interventions at the system level may involve changes in management of hypertension strategies, introduction of new members to the clinical team or team change, or creating new roles for traditional providers such as nurses or pharmacists.

Counseling and training patients can be particularly effective when delivered as a team effort. Subgroup analyses have shown that pharmacist- or nurse-led counseling interventions result in greater reductions of BP [59]. A systematic review examining the effectiveness of quality improvement strategies in lowering BP has shown that despite differences across studies (such as the number of providers involved and BP measurement techniques), a team-change strategy in which a provider other than the patients' primary care physician shared some responsibility for the patient's BP management was the most effective strategy [39,69]. Glynn et al. reported that the majority of randomized trials of nurse- or pharmacist-led care were associated with improved BP control with a range of mean differences from −13 to 0 mmHg for mean SBP ($n = 10$ RCTs) and from −8 to 0 mmHg for DBP ($n = 12$ RCTs) [28]. In particular, involvement of pharmacists leads to a significant improvement in BP control [70–76], and continued interventions by pharmacists may be necessary to maintain high rates of BP control, especially in patients whose BP begins to increase [77]. A downside of team-change strategies is that they may result in a discontinuity in the relationship between the patient and the primary care provider, which may in turn lead patients to be less satisfied with the quality of care they receive [78].

A Cochrane-based systematic review and meta-analysis of interventions designed to improve BP control [28] presented the pooled results of several studies of organizational interventions targeting the delivery of care. The review documented heterogeneous results largely driven by the largest study, the Hypertension Detection and Follow-Up Program. This seminal trial recruited 11,237 hypertensive patients in 14 U.S. communities, stratified by entry DBP (90–104, 105–114, and 115+ mmHg), and randomly assigned them either to a systematic antihypertensive treatment program (stepped care) or to usual sources of care (referred care). The stepped-care approach consisted of a standardized program of stepwise-defined dose increments and/or addition of specified drugs until BP control was achieved [79]. Furthermore, several measures, such as pill counts to monitor drug adherence, providing the participants with free antihypertensive drugs, clinic visits, laboratory tests, and transportation to the clinic, were undertaken in the stepped-care arm to enhance compliance with antihypertensive treatment. Clinic organization was improved by minimizing waiting times and by holding clinics at convenient hours. After 1 year, 80.4% of the participants receiving stepped care remained in active therapy compared with 50.6% in the referred care group [79]. All-cause mortality at 5 years of follow-up in the stepped-care group was reduced compared with that in the referred-care group (6.4% vs. 7.7%, $p < .01$, 17% reduction), particularly in the group with DBP of 90–104 mmHg at study entry (5.9% vs. 7.4%, $p < 0.01$, a 20% reduction) [80]. This study finding indicates that systematic, effective management of hypertension has a great potential for reducing mortality for a large segment of the population with hypertension.

8.5 NEW DEVELOPMENTS

We conclude this chapter by reporting on the recent developments in this field. The recently published studies in this field all have in common the use of newer technologies to deliver educational interventions, namely, short message service (SMS) via mobile phone, Web services, and interactive DVD story telling.

The first study [81] tested the effect of an 8-week intervention using SMS (text messages) via cellular phone and Internet to improve BP control, weight control, and serum lipids of obese patients with hypertension. Patients in the intervention group were asked to record their BP and body weight weekly in a Web-based diary accessed via the Internet or cellular phone, and they received weekly recommendations by both cellular phone and Internet. The authors reported a significant postintervention decrease in SBP and DBP (9.1 and 7.2 mmHg, respectively; $p < .05$) in the intervention group, as well as decreases in body weight and waist circumference and an increase in high-density lipoprotein cholesterol. Despite the limitations (small sample size, quasi-experimental design, and very short duration of follow-up) warranting replication in a larger population, these results are interesting and appear to be particularly promising in older, low-income, less educated patients, and in minorities such as African Americans and Hispanics who frequently do not own or do not use a computer [82].

The effectiveness of Web-delivered hypertension care has been tested in a recent randomized controlled trial [75], the Electronic Communications and Home Blood Pressure Monitoring study, enrolling 778 participants aged 25–75 years with uncontrolled essential hypertension and Internet access who were randomly assigned to usual care, BP monitoring at home, and secure Website training or to both BP monitoring at home and Website training plus pharmacist care management delivered through Web communication. While the study failed to demonstrate the efficacy of BP monitoring at home and Web-delivered patient training in attaining better BP control compared with the usual care group, the addition of Web-based pharmacist care to BP monitoring at home and Web training significantly increased BP control. Although with some caveats, such as the exclusion of about 20% of patients (usually minorities, less educated patients, and older patients) because they did not have Internet access, this was the first randomized trial testing the efficacy of Web-delivered care for hypertension, showing that Web delivery can be a safe and useful tool to provide effective BP care.

Houston et al. [83] tested the effect of storytelling, a powerful tool for health promotion in vulnerable populations, on BP levels in 299 (71% women) hypertensive African Americans with baseline uncontrolled hypertension, who were recruited in an inner-city safety-net clinic in the southern United States. Participants were randomly assigned to receive three DVDs containing peer-delivered interactive hypertension-care storytelling or an attention control DVD. Despite its limitations (about 75% of patients retained and short duration of follow-up), this study showed a reduction of both SBP (11.21 mmHg; 95% CI: 2.51–19.9 mmHg; $p = .012$) and DBP (6.43 mmHg; CI: 1.49–11.45 mmHg; $p = .012$) at 3 months in the intervention group compared with the attention control group, with between-group differences maintained at 6 months.

8.6 CONCLUSION

The available evidence indicates that among the strategies implemented at the provider level, those involving health care team change, patient education, and facilitation of transfer of clinical information were the most effective in achieving better

TABLE 8.1

Practical Suggestions

Intervention	Level of Evidence	Recommendations
Communication skills	Unknown	Good bedside manners and communication
Clinic organization	Modest/unknown	Provide easy access to patients (including phone and e-mail contact)
		Contact patients to confirm appointments and follow up patients who missed appointments
		Make clinic comfortable, including convenient access hours
		Schedule next appointment before patient leaves office
Technical support	Moderate	Use appointment reminders, preferably computer-based
	Greater effect when used in association with counseling/ team change	Use a computer-based approach for BP monitoring and follow-up
		Periodically audit patients' files to assess compliance with guidelines, goals, and recommendations
Educational materials (booklets, brochures)	Modest	Printed materials containing instructions regarding lifestyle changes are useful
	May increase patients' knowledge	
Counseling	Good	Provide simple advice for lifestyle changes
	Greater effect when combined with provider education and self-monitoring of BP	Propose participation in formal, intensive counseling
Team change	Good	Collaborate with other health care professionals (nurses, physician assistants, pharmacists, dentists, registered dietitians, etc.) to deliver counseling/education about lifestyles changes and medication adherence

Source: Chobanian, A.V. et al., *Hypertension*, 42, 1206–1252, 2003.

BP control [69]. Among patient-focused interventions, provider-delivered counseling may improve BP levels and may be an important addition to traditional pharmacological treatment, particularly when delivered by pharmacists. Combined counseling and structured training courses may lead to further improvements, while training courses alone do not appear to be effective compared with counseling or usual care. The most effective strategies creatively employed multiple interventions targeting the patient, the provider, and the health care system at the same time [37,38,75] and often included technical support facilitating the transfer of information between the patient and the provider. Further development may come from the use of new technologies (text messaging, use of social networks,

Web-based interventions) to deliver counseling interventions, and promising results have been shown by the use of peer-delivered forms of counseling, such as storytelling. Future research should aim at achieving a better understanding of the specific role of single intervention components in BP control, include treatment fidelity assessments, and plan for longer durations of follow-up since the effects were not maintained over time in some studies. Finally, there is limited evidence that the observed improvement in BP control over time has been achieved through lifestyle changes, as most hypertensive patients are still obese and have unhealthy dietary habits [4,5,38]. This indicates that further improvement in BP control could probably be obtained by directly targeting dietary and exercise habits, and additional efforts should be invested in promoting healthy dietary and exercise behaviors (Table 8.1).

REFERENCES

1. Yoon S, Ostchega Y, Louis T. *Recent Trends in the Prevalence of High Blood Pressure and Its Treatment and Control, 1999–2008.* National Center for Health Statistics, Hyattsville, MD, 2010.
2. Ong KL, Cheung BM, Man YB, Lau CP, Lam KS. Prevalence, awareness, treatment, and control of hypertension among United States adults 1999–2004. *Hypertension.* 2007;49(1):69–75.
3. Egan BM, Zhao Y, Axon RN. US trends in prevalence, awareness, treatment, and control of hypertension, 1988–2008. *JAMA.* 2010;303(20):2043–2050.
4. Ford ES, Zhao G, Li C, Pearson WS, Mokdad AH. Trends in obesity and abdominal obesity among hypertensive and nonhypertensive adults in the United States. *Am J Hypertens.* 2008;21(10):1124–1128.
5. Mellen PB, Gao SK, Vitolins MZ, Goff DC Jr. Deteriorating dietary habits among adults with hypertension: DASH dietary accordance, NHANES 1988–1994 and 1999–2004. *Arch Intern Med.* 2008;168(3):308–314.
6. U.S. Department of Health and Human Services. *The Health Benefits of Smoking Cessation. A Report of the Surgeon General.* U.S. Department of Health and Human Services, Washington, DC, 1990.
7. Hypertension Prevention Collaborative Research Group. Effects of weight loss and sodium reduction intervention on blood pressure and hypertension incidence in overweight people with high-normal blood pressure. The Trials of Hypertension Prevention, phase II. *Arch Intern Med.* 1997;157(6):657–667.
8. Appel LJ, Moore TJ, Obarzanek E, et al. A clinical trial of the effects of dietary patterns on blood pressure. DASH Collaborative Research Group. *N Engl J Med.* 1997;336(16):1117–1124.
9. He J, Whelton PK, Appel LJ, Charleston J, Klag MJ. Long-term effects of weight loss and dietary sodium reduction on incidence of hypertension. *Hypertension.* 2000;35(2):544–549.
10. Centers for Disease Control and Prevention. Surgeon General's report on physical activity and health. *JAMA.* 1996;276(7):522.
11. Chobanian AV, Bakris GL, Black HR, et al. Seventh report of the Joint National Committee on Prevention, Detection, Evaluation, and Treatment of High Blood Pressure. *Hypertension.* 2003;42(6):1206–1252.
12. Khan NA, Hemmelgarn B, Herman RJ, et al. The 2009 Canadian Hypertension Education Program recommendations for the management of hypertension: Part 2—therapy. *Can J Cardiol.* 2009;25(5):287–298.

13. Appel LJ, Champagne CM, Harsha DW, et al. Effects of comprehensive lifestyle modification on blood pressure control: Main results of the PREMIER clinical trial. *JAMA.* 2003;289(16):2083–2093.
14. Phillips LS, Branch WT, Cook CB, et al. Clinical inertia. *Ann Intern Med.* 2001;135(9):825–834.
15. Berlowitz DR, Ash AS, Hickey EC, et al. Inadequate management of blood pressure in a hypertensive population. *N Engl J Med.* 1998;339(27):1957–1963.
16. Steinman MA, Fischer MA, Shlipak MG, et al. Clinician awareness of adherence to hypertension guidelines. *Am J Med.* 2004;117(10):747–754.
17. Oliveria SA, Lapuerta P, McCarthy BD, L'Italien GJ, Berlowitz DR, Asch SM. Physician-related barriers to the effective management of uncontrolled hypertension. *Arch Intern Med.* 2002;162(4):413–420.
18. Lin ND, Martins SB, Chan AS, et al. Identifying barriers to hypertension guideline adherence using clinician feedback at the point of care. *AMIA Annu Symp Proc.* 2006:494–498.
19. Viera AJ, Schmid D, Bostrom S, Yow A, Lawrence W, DuBard CA. Level of blood pressure above goal and clinical inertia in a Medicaid population. *J Am Soc Hypertension.* 2010;4(5):244–254.
20. Balas EA, Weingarten S, Garb CT, Blumenthal D, Boren SA, Brown GD. Improving preventive care by prompting physicians. *Arch Intern Med.* 2000;160(3):301–308.
21. Fahey T, Schroeder K, and Ebrahim S. Educational and organisational interventions used to improve the management of hypertension in primary care: A systematic review. *Br J Gen Pract.* 2005;55(520):875–882.
22. Krieger J, Collier C, Song L, Martin D. Linking community-based blood pressure measurement to clinical care: A randomized controlled trial of outreach and tracking by community health workers. *Am J Public Health.* 1999;89(6):856–861.
23. Barnett GO, Winickoff RN, Morgan MM, Zielstorff RD. A computer-based monitoring system for follow-up of elevated blood pressure. *Med Care.* 1983;21(4):400–409.
24. Bloom JR, Jordan SC. From screening to seeking care: Removing obstacles in hypertension control. *Prev Med.* 1979;8(4):500–506.
25. Cummings KM, Frisof KB, Demers P, Walsh D. An appointment reminder system's effect on reducing the number of hypertension patients who drop out from care. *Am J Prev Med.* 1985;1(5):54–60.
26. Fletcher SW, Appel FA, Bourgeois MA. Management of hypertension. Effect of improving patient compliance for follow-up care. *JAMA.* 1975;233(3):242–244.
27. Ahluwalia JS, McNagny SE, Kanuru NK. A randomized trial to improve follow-up care in severe uncontrolled hypertensives at an inner-city walk-in clinic. *J Health Care Poor Underserved.* 1996;7(4):377–389.
28. Glynn LG, Murphy AW, Smith SM, Schroeder K, Fahey T. Interventions used to improve control of blood pressure in patients with hypertension. *Cochrane Database Syst Rev.* 2010 (3):CD005182.
29. Tu K, Davis D. Can we alter physician behavior by educational methods? Lessons learned from studies of the management and follow-up of hypertension. *J Contin Educ Health Prof.* 2002;22(1):11–22.
30. Murray MD, Harris LE, Overhage JM, et al. Failure of computerized treatment suggestions to improve health outcomes of outpatients with uncomplicated hypertension: Results of a randomized controlled trial. *Pharmacotherapy.* 2004;24(3):324–337.
31. Goldstein, MK, Hoffman BB, Coleman RW, et al. Patient safety in guideline-based decision support for hypertension management: ATHENA DSS. *J Am Med Inform Assoc.* 2002;9:S11–S16.
32. Goldstein, MK, Coleman RW, Tu SW, et al. Translating research into practice: Organizational issues in implementing automated decision support for hypertension in three medical centers. *J Am Med Inform Assoc.* 2004;11(5):368–376.

33. Bosworth HB, Olsen MK, Dudley T, et al. Patient education and provider decision support to control blood pressure in primary care: A cluster randomized trial. *Am Heart J.* 2009;157:450–456. PMID 19249414.

34. Goldstein MK, Lavori P, Coleman R, Advani A, Hoffman BB. Improving adherence to guidelines for hypertension drug prescribing: Cluster-randomized controlled trial of general versus patient-specific recommendations. *Am J Manag Care.* 2005;11(11):677–685.

35. Bosworth HB, Olsen MK, Dudley T, et al. Patient education and provider decision support to control blood pressure in primary care: A cluster randomized trial. *Am Heart J.* 2009;157(3):450–456.

36. Rinfret S, Lussier MT, Peirce A, et al. The impact of a multidisciplinary information technology-supported program on blood pressure control in primary care. *Circ Cardiovasc Qual Outcomes.* 2009;2(3):170–177.

37. Roumie CL, Elasy TA, Greevy R, et al. Improving blood pressure control through provider education, provider alerts, and patient education: A cluster randomized trial. *Ann Intern Med, 2006*;145(3):165–175.

38. Svetkey LP, Pollak KI, Yancy WS Jr, et al. Hypertension improvement project: Randomized trial of quality improvement for physicians and lifestyle modification for patients. *Hypertension.* 2009;54(6):1226–1233.

39. Walsh JM, McDonald KM, Shojania KG, et al. Quality improvement strategies for hypertension management—A systematic review. *Med Care.* 2006;44(7):646–657.

40. Goldstein MK. Using health information technology to improve hypertension management. *Curr Hypertens Rep.* 2008;10(3):201–207.

41. Prochaska JO, Redding CA, Evers KE. The transtheoretical model and stages of change. In: *Health Behavior and Health Education: Theory, Research, and Practice.* K. Glanz, B.K. Rimer, F.M. Lewis (eds.). Jossey-Bass, San Francisco, CA, 2002:60–84.

42. Teutsch C. Patient-doctor communication. *Med Clin North Am.* 2003;87(5):1115–1145.

43. Barrier PA, Li JTC, Jensen NM. Two words to improve physician–patient communication: What else? *Mayo Clinic Proceedings.* 2003;78(2):211–214.

44. Rao JK, Anderson LA, Inui TS, Frankel RM. Communication interventions make a difference in conversations between physicians and patients: A systematic review of the evidence. *Med Care.* 2007;45(4):340–349.

45. Simkin-Silverman LR, Gleason KA, King WC, et al. Predictors of weight control advice in primary care practices: Patient health and psychosocial characteristics. *Prev Med.* 2005;40(1):71–82.

46. Sciamanna CN, Tate DF, Lang W, Wing RR. Who reports receiving advice to lose weight?: Results from a Multistate Survey. *Arch Intern Med.* 2000;160(15):2334–2339.

47. Kushner RF. Barriers to providing nutrition counseling by physicians: A survey of primary care practitioners. *Prev Med.* 1995;24(6):546–552.

48. Halm J, Amoako E. Physical activity recommendation for hypertension management: Does healthcare provider advice make a difference? *Ethn Dis.* 2008;18(3):278–282.

49. Valderrama AL, Tong X, Ayala C, Keenan NL. Prevalence of self-reported hypertension, advice received from health care professionals, and actions taken to reduce blood pressure among US adults—Health Styles, 2008. *J Clin Hypertens (Greenwich).* 2010;12(10):784–792.

50. Kreuter MW, Chheda SG, Bull FC. How does physician advice influence patient behavior? Evidence for a priming effect. *Arch Fam Med.* 2000;9(5):426–433.

51. Bull FC, Jamrozik K. Advice on exercise from a family physician can help sedentary patients to become active. *Am J Prev Med.* 1998;15(2):85–94.

52. Viera AJ, Kshirsagar AV, Hinderliter AL. Lifestyle modifications to lower or control high blood pressure: Is advice associated with action? The behavioral risk factor surveillance survey. *J Clin Hypertens (Greenwich).* 2008;10(2):105–111.

53. Murray DM, Kurth CL, Finnegan JR Jr, Pirie PL, Admire JB, Luepker RV. Direct mail as a prompt for follow-up care among persons at risk for hypertension. *Am J Prev Med.* 1988;4(6):331–335.

54. St George IM. Patient education leaflet for hypertension: A controlled study. *J R Coll Gen Pract.* 1983;33(253):508–510.

55. Laher M, O'Malley K, O'Brien E, O'Hanrahan M, O'Boyle C. Educational value of printed information for patients with hypertension. *Br Med J (Clin Res Ed).* 1981;282(6273):1360–1361.

56. Watkins CJ, Papacosta AO, Chinn S, Martin J. A randomized controlled trial of an information booklet for hypertensive patients in general practice. *J R Coll Gen Pract.* 1987;37(305):548–550.

57. Hunt JS, Siemienczuk J, Touchette D, Payne N. Impact of educational mailing on the blood pressure of primary care patients with mild hypertension. *J Gen Intern Med.* 2004;19(9):925–930.

58. Fahey T, Schroeder K, Ebrahim S. Interventions used to improve control of blood pressure in patients with hypertension. *Cochrane Database Syst Rev.* 2006;(2):CD005182.

59. Boulware LE, Daumit GL, Frick KD, Minkovitz CS, Lawrence RS, Powe NR. An evidence-based review of patient-centered behavioral interventions for hypertension. *Am J Prev Med.* 2001;21(3):221–232.

60. Erickson SR, Slaughter R, Halapy H. Pharmacists' ability to influence outcomes of hypertension therapy. *Pharmacotherapy.* 1997;17(1):140–147.

61. Logan AG, Milne BJ, Flanagan PT, Haynes RB. Clinical effectiveness and cost-effectiveness of monitoring blood pressure of hypertensive employees at work. *Hypertension.* 1983;5(6):828–836.

62. Park JJ, Kelly P, Carter BL, Burgess PP. Comprehensive pharmaceutical care in the chain setting. *J Am Pharm Assoc (Wash).* 1996;NS36(7):443–451.

63. Webb PA. Effectiveness of patient education and psychosocial counseling in promoting compliance and control among hypertensive patients. *J Fam Pract.* 1980;10(6):1047–1055.

64. Carnahan JE, Nugent, CA. The effects of self-monitoring by patients on the control of hypertension. *Am J Med Sci.* 1975;269(1):69–73.

65. Iso H, Shimamoto T, Yokota K, Sankai T, Jacobs DR Jr, Komachi Y. Community-based education classes for hypertension control. A 1.5-year randomized controlled trial. *Hypertension.* 1996;27(4):968–974.

66. Mühlhauser I, Sawicki PT, Didjurgeit U, Jörgens V, Trampisch HJ, Berger M. Evaluation of a structured treatment and teaching programme on hypertension in general practice. *Clin Exp Hypertens.* 1993;15(1):125–142.

67. Wyka-Fitzgerald C, Levesque P, Panciera T, Vendettoli D, Mattea E. Long-term evaluation of group education for high blood pressure control. *Cardiovasc Nurs.* 1984;20(3):13–18.

68. Bosworth HB, Olsen MK, Grubber JM, et al. Two self-management interventions to improve hypertension control: A randomized trial. *Ann Intern Med.* 2009;151(10):687–695.

69. Walsh JM, Sundaram V, McDonald K, Owens DK, Goldstein MK. Implementing effective hypertension quality improvement strategies: Barriers and potential solutions. *J Clin Hypertens (Greenwich).* 2008;10(4):311–316.

70. Borenstein JE, Graber G, Saltiel E, et al. Physician-pharmacist comanagement of hypertension: A randomized, comparative trial. *Pharmacotherapy.* 2003;23(2):209–216.

71. Carter BL, Rogers M, Daly J, Zheng S, James PA. The potency of team-based care interventions for hypertension: A meta-analysis. *Arch Intern Med.* 2009;69(19):1748–1755.

72. McLean DL, McAlister FA, Johnson JA, et al. A randomized trial of the effect of community pharmacist and nurse care on improving blood pressure management in patients

with diabetes mellitus: Study of cardiovascular risk intervention by pharmacists-hypertension (SCRIP-HTN). *Arch Intern Med*. 2008;168(21):2355–2361.

73. Carter BL, Bergus GR, Dawson JD, et al. A cluster randomized trial to evaluate physician/pharmacist collaboration to improve blood pressure control. *J Clin Hypertens (Greenwich)*. 2008;10(4):260–271.

74. Hunt JS, Siemienczuk J, Pape G, et al. A randomized controlled trial of team-based care: Impact of physician-pharmacist collaboration on uncontrolled hypertension. *J Gen Intern Med*. 2008;23(12): 1966–1972.

75. Green BB, Cook AJ, Ralston JD, et al. Effectiveness of home blood pressure monitoring, Web communication, and pharmacist care on hypertension control: A randomized controlled trial. *JAMA*. 2008;299(24):2857–2867.

76. Tobari H, Arimoto T, Shimojo N, et al. Physician-pharmacist cooperation program for blood pressure control in patients with hypertension: A randomized-controlled trial. *Am J Hypertens*. 2010;23(10):1144–1152.

77. Carter BL, Doucette WR, Franciscus CL, Ardery G, Kluesner KM, Chrischilles EA. Deterioration of blood pressure control after discontinuation of a physician-pharmacist collaborative intervention. *Pharmacotherapy*. 2010;30(3):228–235.

78. Rodriguez HP, Rogers WH, Marshall RE, Safran DG. Multidisciplinary primary care teams - Effects on the quality of clinician-patient interactions and organizational features of care. *Med Care*. 2007;45(1):19–27.

79. Hypertension Detection and Follow-up Program Cooperative Group. Therapeutic control of blood pressure in the hypertension detection and follow-up program. *Prev Med*. 1979;8(1):2–13.

80. Hypertension Detection and Follow-up Program Cooperative Group. Five-year findings of the hypertension detection and follow-up program. I. Reduction in mortality of persons with high blood pressure, including mild hypertension. *JAMA*. 1979;242(23):2562–2571.

81. Park MJ, Kim HS, Kim KS. Cellular phone and Internet-based individual intervention on blood pressure and obesity in obese patients with hypertension. *Int J Med Inform*. 2009;78(10):704–710.

82. McNeill LH, Puleo E, Bennett GG, Emmons KM. Exploring social contextual correlates of computer ownership and frequency of use among urban, low-income, public housing adult residents. *J Med Internet Res*. 2007;9(4):e35.

83. Houston TK, Allison JJ, Sussman M, et al. Culturally appropriate storytelling to improve blood pressure: A randomized trial. *Ann Intern Med*. 2011;154(2):77–84.

Section III

Special Considerations

Overview

Pao-Hwa Lin

Most researches on the association between nutrition, lifestyle factors, and blood pressure (BP) and relevant management plans have been conducted in adults with predetermined inclusion/exclusion criteria to minimize confounding of findings from other physiological or biological conditions. However, various physiological or biological factors may influence how nutrition and lifestyle relate to BP and/or how they can be used in managing BP, and thus are important to consider.

For example, nutritional needs in children and adolescents and during pregnancy are clearly different from those required during other life stages. Thus, the approach in nutrition and lifestyle interventions for BP control may also vary for these populations. Chapter 9 reviews the nutrition and lifestyle interventions in children and adolescents for BP control. Chapter 10 reviews the BP disorders during pregnancy and how nutrition and lifestyle factors may relate to the disorders and how they may be used in treatment of these disorders.

Diabetes often coexists with hypertension, and research shows that the coexistence of both the conditions greatly increases the risk for cardiovascular diseases and mortality. The BP control criteria for people with both hypertension and diabetes are thus lower than that for those with hypertension only. Chapter 11 reviews the evidence for tighter control of BP in the setting of coexistent diabetes. In addition, this chapter reviews how nutrition and lifestyle interventions can help control BP in this population.

Research has repeatedly shown that in the United States, certain racial/ethnic groups, such as African Americans, bear a disproportionate risk for hypertension prevalence and have a poor control. Although it is not clearly known why this disparity exists, many possible reasons have been suggested. African Americans as a group also seem to respond differently to certain lifestyle interventions. For example, the Dietary Approaches to Stop Hypertension (DASH) dietary pattern was more effective among the African American participants than in other racial subgroups. Chapter 12 reviews the possible reasons for the disparity in hypertension prevalence and control among different racial/ethnic groups and how nutrition and lifestyle interventions may be applied in controlling BP among minorities.

Besides race/ethnicity, other biological factors may also affect the response of BP to various lifestyle modifications. Many of these factors, such as age and body weight, have been well studied and can be easily identified in patients; others, such as genetic factors, are still evolving. Chapter 13 summarizes the BP-related effects of lifestyle modifications with a focus on evidence that biological factors influence the response of BP to various lifestyle changes. A closer understanding of the impact of these biological factors on responses of BP to lifestyle interventions may allow health care providers to target interventions to individuals who are most likely to benefit from them.

9 Lifestyle Interventions for Blood Pressure Control in Children and Adolescents

Diana H. Dolinsky and Sarah C. Armstrong
Duke University Medical Center

*Carissa M. Baker-Smith, Anna E. Czinn,
and Angelo S. Milazzo*
University of Maryland School of Medicine

CONTENTS

9.1 OVERVIEW

Currently, one-third of all children in the United States aged 2–19 years are over-weight, of which 16.9% are obese [1]. The onset of obesity in childhood confers a higher risk of adult cardiometabolic mortality due to diabetes, hypertension, isch-emic heart disease, and stroke [2]. Several longitudinal studies have linked early childhood weight gain and childhood obesity with adult obesity [3], and adolescent obesity is strongly predictive of adult obesity [4]. Obesity-related health conditions are the second leading cause of preventable death, following only tobacco use [5]. The dramatic rise in the prevalence of pediatric obesity over the past two decades has been predicted to lead to a decline in overall life expectancy in the United States [6].

Blood pressure (BP) elevation is a well-documented complication of obesity in children, and it is increasing in prevalence in parallel with the obesity epidemic [7]. In contrast, hypertension is rare in nonobese children [8]. The mechanisms for obesity-related hypertension are discussed in detail below, and they involve both increased fluid retention and inflammation [9]. Although no longitudinal data are currently able to link childhood-onset hypertension with adult cardiovascular dis-eases, emerging literature demonstrates the presence of a proatherosclerotic inflam-matory state and target-organ damage in children with hypertension [10]. In addition, children with obesity and hypertension usually possess multiple other metabolic risk factors for disease, and thus they form a group that merits evaluation and treatment.

Pharmacologic interventions are appropriate for hypertensive children who meet specific criteria as discussed below. Lifestyle interventions administered properly are effective and safe, and thus these should be utilized whenever indicated and available [11]. Exactly how much weight loss, or body mass index (BMI) reduction, is needed to achieve improvement in BP, lipid profiles, insulin sensitivity, and overall cardiovascular health in children is unknown. However, BP appears to be one of the earliest health outcomes to show improvement when lifestyle modification is suc-cessful [12].

In this chapter, we review the data on childhood obesity-related hypertension, screening and referral guidelines, and the most effective management strategies. Treatment options discussed here focus on evidence-based recommendations for lifestyle modifications. Options for a rational, yet comprehensive, treatment approach are presented. Many resources exist for the clinician to offer lifestyle modifications in his or her clinic- or hospital-based setting; this chapter provides references and resources as a guide to management of hypertension.

9.2 DEFINITION OF ELEVATED BP IN CHILDREN
AND ADOLESCENTS

In children and adolescents, hypertension is defined using BP reference tables provided by the National High Blood Pressure Education Program (NHBPEP) Working Group [13]. These tables provide standards for BP based on gender, height, and age (Tables 9.1 and 9.2). Hypertension is defined by an average systolic BP (SBP) and/or diastolic BP (DBP) that is greater than the 95th percentile for gender, age, and height based on

TABLE 9.1
Blood Pressure Reference Tables for Boys by Age and Height Percentile

Age (Year)	BP Percentile	Systolic BP (mmHg) Percentile of Height							Diastolic BP (mmHg) Percentile of Height						
		5th	10th	25th	50th	75th	90th	95th	5th	10th	25th	50th	75th	90th	95th
1	50th	80	81	83	85	87	88	89	34	35	36	37	38	39	39
	90th	94	95	97	99	100	102	103	49	50	51	52	53	53	54
	95th	98	99	101	103	104	106	106	54	54	55	56	57	58	58
	99th	105	106	108	110	112	113	114	61	62	63	64	65	66	66
2	50th	84	85	87	88	90	92	92	39	40	41	42	43	44	44
	90th	97	99	100	102	104	105	106	54	55	56	57	58	58	59
	95th	101	102	104	106	108	109	110	59	59	60	61	62	63	63
	99th	109	110	111	113	115	117	117	66	67	68	69	70	71	71
3	50th	86	87	89	91	93	94	95	44	44	45	46	47	48	48
	90th	100	101	103	105	107	108	109	59	59	60	61	62	63	63
	95th	104	105	107	109	110	112	113	63	63	64	65	66	67	67
	99th	111	112	114	116	118	119	120	71	71	72	73	74	75	75
4	50th	88	89	91	93	95	96	97	47	48	49	50	51	51	52
	90th	102	103	105	107	109	110	111	62	63	64	65	66	66	67
	95th	106	107	109	111	112	114	115	66	67	68	69	70	71	71
	99th	113	114	116	118	120	121	122	74	75	76	77	78	78	79
5	50th	90	91	93	95	96	98	98	50	51	52	53	54	55	55
	90th	104	105	106	108	110	111	112	65	66	67	68	69	69	70
	95th	108	109	110	112	114	115	116	69	70	71	72	73	74	74
	99th	115	116	118	120	121	123	123	77	78	79	80	81	81	82
6	50th	91	92	94	96	98	99	100	53	53	54	55	56	57	57
	90th	105	106	108	110	111	113	113	68	68	69	70	71	72	72
	95th	109	110	112	114	115	117	117	72	72	73	74	75	76	76
	99th	116	117	119	121	123	124	125	80	80	81	82	83	84	84

(continued)

TABLE 9.1 (continued)
Blood Pressure Reference Tables for Boys by Age and Height Percentile

Age (Year)	BP Percentile	Systolic BP (mmHg) Percentile of Height							Diastolic BP (mmHg) Percentile of Height						
		5th	10th	25th	50th	75th	90th	95th	5th	10th	25th	50th	75th	90th	95th
7	50th	92	94	95	97	99	100	101	55	55	56	57	58	59	59
	90th	106	107	109	111	113	114	115	70	70	71	72	73	74	74
	95th	110	111	113	115	117	118	119	74	74	75	76	77	78	78
	99th	117	118	120	122	124	125	126	82	82	83	84	85	86	86
8	50th	94	95	97	99	100	102	102	56	57	58	59	60	60	61
	90th	107	109	110	112	114	115	116	71	72	72	73	74	75	76
	95th	111	112	114	116	118	119	120	75	76	77	78	79	79	80
	99th	119	120	122	123	125	127	127	83	84	85	86	87	87	88
9	50th	95	96	98	100	102	103	104	57	58	59	60	61	61	62
	90th	109	110	112	114	115	117	118	72	73	74	75	76	76	77
	95th	113	114	116	118	119	121	121	76	77	78	79	80	81	81
	99th	120	121	123	125	127	128	129	84	85	86	87	88	88	89
10	50th	97	98	100	102	103	105	106	58	59	60	61	61	62	63
	90th	111	112	114	115	117	119	119	73	73	74	75	76	77	78
	95th	115	116	117	119	121	122	123	77	78	79	80	81	81	82
	99th	122	123	125	127	128	130	130	85	86	86	88	88	89	90
11	50th	99	100	102	104	105	107	107	59	59	60	61	62	63	63
	90th	113	114	115	117	119	120	121	74	74	75	76	77	78	78
	95th	117	118	119	121	123	124	125	78	78	79	80	81	82	82
	99th	124	125	127	129	130	132	132	86	86	87	88	89	90	90
12	50th	101	102	104	106	108	109	110	59	60	61	62	63	63	64
	90th	115	116	118	120	121	123	123	74	75	75	76	77	78	79
	95th	119	120	122	123	125	127	127	78	79	80	81	82	82	83
	99th	126	127	129	131	133	134	135	86	87	88	89	90	90	91

Age (Year)	BP Percentile	Systolic BP (mmHg) — Percentile of Height							Diastolic BP (mmHg) — Percentile of Height						
		5th	10th	25th	50th	75th	90th	95th	5th	10th	25th	50th	75th	90th	95th
13	50th	104	105	106	108	110	111	112	60	60	61	62	63	64	64
	90th	117	118	120	122	124	125	126	75	75	76	77	78	79	79
	95th	121	122	124	126	128	129	130	79	79	80	81	82	83	83
	99th	128	130	131	133	135	136	137	87	87	88	89	90	91	91
14	50th	106	107	109	111	113	114	115	60	61	62	63	64	65	65
	90th	120	121	123	125	126	128	128	75	76	77	78	79	79	80
	95th	124	125	127	128	130	132	132	80	80	81	82	83	84	84
	99th	131	132	134	136	138	139	140	87	88	89	90	91	91	92
15	50th	109	110	112	113	115	117	117	61	62	63	64	65	66	66
	90th	122	124	125	127	129	130	131	76	77	78	79	80	80	81
	95th	126	127	129	131	133	134	135	81	81	82	83	84	85	85
	99th	134	135	136	138	140	142	142	88	89	90	91	92	93	93
16	50th	111	112	114	116	118	119	120	63	63	64	65	66	67	67
	90th	125	126	128	130	131	133	134	78	78	79	80	81	82	82
	95th	129	130	132	134	135	137	137	82	83	83	84	85	86	87
	99th	136	137	139	141	143	144	145	90	90	91	92	93	94	94
17	50th	114	115	116	118	120	121	122	65	66	66	67	68	69	70
	90th	127	128	130	132	134	135	136	80	80	81	82	83	84	84
	95th	131	132	134	136	138	139	140	84	85	85	87	87	88	89
	99th	139	140	141	143	145	146	147	92	93	93	94	95	96	97

Source: Reproduced from NHLBI, Blood Pressure Tables for Children and Adolescents from the Fourth Report on the Diagnosis, Evaluation, and Treatment of High Blood Pressure in Children and Adolescents, http://www.nhlbi.nih.gov/guidelines/hypertension/child_tbl.htm (accessed September 5, 2011). With Permission.

BP means blood pressure.

The 90th percentile is 1.28 SD, 95th percentile is 1.64:5 SD, and the 99th percentile is 2.326 SD over the mean.

For research purposes, the standard deviations in Appendix Table B–1 in [67] allow one to compute BP Z-scores and percentiles for boys with height percentiles given in Table 3 in [67] (i.e., the 5th, 10th, 25th, 50th, 75th, 90th, and 95th percentiles). These height percentiles must be converted to height Z-scores given by 5% = -1.645; 10% = -1.28; 25% = -0.68; 50% = 0; 75% = 0.68; 90% = 1.28; 95% = 1.645 and then computed according to the methodology in steps 2–4 described in Appendix B in [67]. For children with height percentiles other than these, follow steps 1–4 as described in Appendix B.

TABLE 9.2

Blood Pressure Reference Tables for Girls by Age and Height Percentile

Age (Years)	BP Percentile	Systolic BP (mmHg) Percentile of Height							Diastolic BP (mmHg) Percentile of Height						
		5th	10th	25th	50th	75th	90th	95th	5th	10th	25th	50th	75th	90th	95th
1	50th	83	84	85	86	88	89	90	38	39	39	40	41	41	42
	90th	97	97	98	100	101	102	103	52	53	53	54	55	55	56
	95th	100	101	102	1047	105	106	107	56	57	57	58	59	59	60
	99th	108	108	109	111	112	113	114	64	64	65	65	66	67	67
2	50th	85	85	87	88	89	91	91	43	44	44	45	46	46	47
	90th	98	99	100	101	103	104	105	57	58	58	59	60	61	61
	95th	102	103	104	105	107	108	109	61	62	62	63	64	65	65
	99th	109	110	111	112	114	115	116	69	69	70	70	71	72	72
3	50th	86	87	89	89	91	92	93	47	48	48	49	50	50	51
	90th	100	100	102	103	104	106	106	61	62	62	63	64	64	65
	95th	104	104	105	107	108	109	110	65	66	66	67	68	68	69
	99th	111	111	113	114	115	116	117	73	73	74	74	75	76	76
4	50th	88	88	90	91	92	94	94	50	50	51	52	52	53	54
	90th	101	102	103	104	106	107	108	64	64	65	66	67	67	68
	95th	105	106	107	108	110	111	112	68	68	69	70	71	71	72
	99th	112	113	114	115	117	118	119	76	76	76	77	78	79	79
5	50th	89	90	91	93	94	95	96	52	53	53	54	55	55	56
	90th	103	103	105	106	107	109	109	66	67	67	68	69	69	70
	95th	107	107	108	110	111	112	113	70	71	71	72	73	73	74
	99th	114	114	116	117	118	120	120	78	78	79	79	80	81	81
6	50th	91	92	93	94	96	97	98	54	54	55	56	56	57	58
	90th	104	105	106	108	109	110	111	28	28	29	70	70	71	72
	95th	108	109	110	111	113	114	115	72	72	73	74	74	75	76
	99th	115	116	117	119	120	121	122	80	870	80	81	82	83	83

Age (Year)	BP Percentile	SBP (mmHg)							DBP (mmHg)						
7	50th	93	93	95	96	97	99	99	55	56	56	57	58	58	59
	90th	106	107	108	109	111	112	113	69	70	70	71	72	72	73
	95th	110	111	112	113	115	116	116	73	74	74	75	76	76	77
	99th	117	118	119	120	122	123	124	81	81	82	82	83	84	84
8	50th	95	95	96	98	99	100	101	57	57	57	58	59	60	60
	90th	108	109	110	111	113	114	114	71	71	71	72	73	74	74
	95th	112	112	114	115	116	118	118	75	75	75	76	77	78	78
	99th	119	120	121	122	123	125	125	82	82	83	83	84	85	86
9	50th	96	97	98	100	101	102	103	58	58	58	59	60	61	61
	90th	110	110	112	113	114	116	116	72	72	72	73	74	75	75
	95th	114	114	116	117	118	120	120	76	76	76	77	78	79	79
	99th	121	121	123	124	125	129	129	83	83	84	84	85	86	87
10	50th	98	99	100	102	103	104	105	59	59	59	60	61	62	62
	90th	112	112	114	115	116	118	118	73	73	73	74	75	76	76
	95th	116	116	117	119	120	121	122	77	77	77	78	79	80	80
	99th	123	123	125	126	127	129	129	84	84	85	86	86	87	88
11	50th	100	101	102	103	105	106	107	60	60	60	61	62	63	63
	90th	114	114	116	117	118	119	120	74	74	74	75	76	77	77
	95th	118	118	119	121	122	123	124	78	78	78	79	80	81	81
	99th	125	125	126	128	129	130	131	85	85	86	87	87	88	89
12	50th	102	103	104	105	107	108	109	61	61	61	62	63	64	64
	90th	116	116	117	119	120	121	122	75	75	75	76	77	78	78
	95th	119	120	121	123	124	125	126	79	79	79	80	81	82	82
	99th	127	127	128	130	131	132	133	86	86	87	88	88	89	90
13	50th	104	105	106	107	109	110	110	62	62	62	63	64	65	65
	90th	117	118	119	121	122	123	124	76	76	76	77	78	79	79
	95th	121	122	123	124	126	127	128	80	80	80	81	82	83	83
	99th	128	129	130	132	133	134	135	87	87	88	89	89	90	91
14	50th	106	106	107	109	110	111	112	63	63	63	64	65	66	66
	90th	119	120	121	122	124	125	125	77	77	77	78	79	80	80
	95th	123	123	125	126	127	129	129	81	81	81	82	83	84	84
	99th	130	131	132	133	135	136	136	88	88	89	90	90	91	92

(continued)

TABLE 9.2　(continued)
Blood Pressure Reference Tables for Girls by Age and Height Percentile

Age (Years)	BP Percentile	Systolic BP (mmHg) Percentile of Height							Diastolic BP (mmHg) Percentile of Height						
		5th	10th	25th	50th	75th	90th	95th	5th	10th	25th	50th	75th	90th	95th
15	50th	107	108	109	110	111	113	113	64	64	64	65	66	67	67
	90th	120	121	122	123	125	126	127	78	78	78	79	80	81	81
	95th	124	125	126	127	129	130	131	82	82	82	83	84	85	85
	99th	131	132	133	134	136	137	138	89	89	90	91	91	92	93
16	50th	108	108	110	111	112	114	114	64	64	65	66	66	67	68
	90th	121	122	123	124	126	127	128	78	78	79	80	81	81	82
	95th	125	126	127	128	130	131	132	82	82	83	84	85	85	86
	99th	132	133	134	135	137	138	139	90	90	90	91	92	93	93
17	50th	108	109	110	111	113	114	115	64	65	65	66	67	67	68
	90th	122	122	123	125	126	127	128	78	79	79	80	81	81	82
	95th	125	126	127	129	130	131	132	82	83	83	84	85	85	86
	99th	133	133	134	136	137	138	139	90	90	91	91	92	93	93

Source: Reproduced from NHLBI, Blood Pressure Tables for Children and Adolescents from the Fourth Report on the Diagnosis, Evaluation, and Treatment of High Blood Pressure in Children and Adolescents, http://www.nhlbi.nih.gov/guidelines/hypertension/child_tbl.htm, (accessed September 5, 2011).

BP means blood pressure

The 90th percentile is 1.28 SD, 95th percentile is 1.645 SD, and the 99th percentile is 2.326 SD over the mean.

For research purposes, the standard deviations in Appendix Table B–1 in [67] allow one to compute BP Z-scores and percentiles for girls with height percentiles given in Table 4 in [67] (i.e., the 5th, 10th, 25th, 50th, 75th, 90th, and 95th percentiles). These height percentiles must be converted to height Z-scores given by 5% = −1.645, 10% = −1.28, 25% = −0.68, 50% = 0, 75% = 0.68, 90% = 1.28%, 95% = 1.645 and then computed according to the methodology in steps 2–4 described in Appendix B in [67]. For children with height percentiles other than these, follow steps 1–5 as described in Appendix B.

three averaged BP measurements in a single encounter [14]. Prehypertension is defined by an average SBP or DBP that is greater than the 90th percentile but less than the 95th percentile or by a BP that is greater than 120/80 mmHg but less than the 95th percentile. Hypertension is stratified into stages to facilitate the organization of management strategies: stage 1 hypertension corresponds to a SBP or DBP between the 95th and 99th percentiles, plus 5 mmHg; and stage 2 hypertension corresponds to a SBP or DBP exceeding the 99th percentile, plus 5 mmHg. "White-coat hypertension" exists when a patient's BP is greater than the 95th percentile when measured in a physician's office or in other medical settings, but the patient's average BP is less than the 90th percentile when measured elsewhere. In contrast, the term "masked hypertension" describes the situation in which a patient is normotensive in a clinical setting but hypertensive otherwise [13,15].

9.3   ACCURATE MEASUREMENT OF BP

Children older than 3 years should have their BP measured annually. Accurate measurement of BP is necessary to quantify the degree of hypertension, both on individual and population levels. Accurate measurement of BP in children requires the use of an appropriately sized cuff and an appropriate technique. The width of the cuff's inflatable bladder should be at least 40% of the arm circumference at a point midway between the olecranon and the acromion [13].

BP measurements made in a pediatric office can often be inaccurate [15]. The data in the BP reference tables are based on auscultatory measurements [16], although measurement of BP in clinical settings is often performed by oscillometric devices [15]. A recent study evaluating the accuracy of BP measurements during standard vital sign measurements demonstrated a mean difference of >13 mmHg for SBP (>9 mmHg for DBP) when compared to pressures obtained by methods similar to those used for the BP reference tables. These measurement errors can lead to mis-identification of normotensive children as hypertensive [15].

Even when accurately measured, BP obtained in an outpatient clinical setting may not be the most accurate indicator of a patient's BP trend throughout the day. A technique utilized to overcome this limitation is the ambulatory blood pressure monitor (ABPM). The ABPM is a portable device worn by the patient, which measures and records BP over a specified period (typically 24 h) during the day [17]. Its usage is generally limited to children older than 5 years. The ABPM is being used more frequently by pediatric practitioners and can be especially useful in children with white-coat hypertension or masked hypertension. There are no outcome-based studies relating ABPM measurements (or BP measurements obtained in the clinic) and the sequelae of hypertension, such as myocardial infarction and stroke. Further research must be implemented to explore the utility of the ABPM in predicting future cardiovascular risks [18].

9.4   PREVALENCE AND PERSISTENCE OF PEDIATRIC HYPERTENSION

Both hypertension and obesity have been significantly increasing in children and adolescents over the past several decades [19]. Evidence from cross-sectional studies is important in determining the overall burden of disease and monitoring trends. Serial cross-sectional data analyzed from the National Health and Nutrition Examination Surveys (NHANES) demonstrated that there has been a significant increase in BP in children and adolescents aged 8–17 between 1988 and 2000. SBP was 1.4 mmHg higher and DBP was 3.3 mmHg higher in 1999–2000 than in 1988–1994. These differences were attenuated when adjusting for BMI, suggesting that the increase in BP is at least partially related to the increase in overweight and obesity. The prevalence of prehypertension was higher in non-Hispanic black girls than in non-Hispanic white girls [20]. However, data on the role of race and ethnicity in pediatric hypertension are incomplete and do not control for genetic and environmental factors [8].

Longitudinal cohort studies provide additional information regarding the tracking of childhood disease into adolescence and adulthood. A meta-analysis of 50 cohort studies from diverse populations shows strong evidence that BP tracks from childhood into adulthood [21]. Although no direct evidence is available to demonstrate that hypertension in childhood leads to cardiovascular events in adults, the persistence of elevated BP from childhood to adulthood demonstrates the importance of early intervention.

9.5   SECONDARY HYPERTENSION IN CHILDREN

It is important to distinguish between primary and secondary hypertension in children. Although adult hypertension is more likely to be primary, pediatric hypertension is more likely to be secondary, that is, related to an underlying cause. In general, the younger the child and the greater is the degree of BP elevation, it is more likely that there is an underlying cause [22]. Secondary causes of pediatric hypertension are most likely to be renal or renovascular diseases such as polycystic and multicystic dysplastic renal disease, hydronephrosis, chronic pyelonephritis, glomerulonephritis, chronic renal failure, and renal artery stenosis. Additional etiologies of secondary hypertension in children include cardiac (coarctation), medication and iatrogenic causes (caffeine, stimulant medications) and rare conditions such as Wilms tumor, neuroblastoma, and pheochromocytoma [22]. Children having elevated BP require consideration of secondary causes and further evaluation for suspected etiologies and target-organ damage.

Hypertension affects about 30% of adults in North America [23] and is notoriously difficult to treat or control. Primary or essential hypertension has origins in childhood, and it is directly related to the BMI and other factors that are coincident with childhood obesity. The increased prevalence of childhood hypertension with childhood obesity is suggestive of a unifying mechanism [8]. Sleep disorders, prevalent in obese children, are strongly associated with hypertension as well [24]. Genetic risk factors are associated with both hypertension and obesity. Both insulin resistance and markers of inflammation are associated with increased BMI and elevated BP [25]. In addition, lifestyle choices are directly related to the development of elevated BP. One study demonstrated higher BP associated with excessive BMI, carbohydrate intake, and sedentary lifestyle [26].

The mechanisms to explain the development of essential hypertension in the presence of excess adiposity are incompletely understood. Factors that are thought to be the major contributors to hypertension in obese children include disturbances in autonomic function, insulin resistance, and abnormalities in vascular function [27]. The sympathetic system is activated in obesity, and one mechanism for the resultant increase in BP is an increase in sodium resorption through the renal tubules. Renin, angiotensin, and aldosterone contribute to this process. The insulin-resistant state may promote elevation in BP through activation of the sympathetic nervous system and increases in related peptides [28]. Growing evidence suggests that hypertension is a proinflammatory state. Levels of C-reactive protein, interleukin-6, interleukin-1β, and intercellular cell adhesion molecule-1 correlate significantly with the ambulatory BP in obese children and adolescents, suggesting that inflammation may play a role in the modulation of BP relatively early in life [29]. Of all the markers of inflammation, uric acid has been of particular interest. Researchers evaluating data from the Bogalusa Heart study demonstrated that the uric acid level in childhood is correlated with BP during childhood and adulthood [30]. These data are suggestive that early elevation of uric acid could play an important role in BP throughout life, but the cause and effects have not been established. The emerging literature on the link between inflammation and hypertension suggests that closer attention to markers of inflammation should be considered in the pediatric hypertensive population.

9.6 IMPACT OF CHILDHOOD HYPERTENSION ON HEALTH

As discussed above, childhood hypertension tends to persist into adulthood, and adult hypertension is associated with significant morbidity. However, some complications of childhood hypertension develop during childhood. Left ventricular hypertrophy (LVH) is the most prominent evidence of target-organ damage. LVH is present anywhere between 8% and 38% of hypertensive children and in a greater proportion among obese children [31]. In general, the higher the BP, the more severe is the LVH. However, even among children with "white-coat" hypertension, the higher the BMI, the higher is the left ventricular (LV) volume [32]. LVH has been an established surrogate for associated cardiovascular damage [33]. Clinicians are advised to use the cutoffs for LV thickness for children established by NHBPEP in determining the treatment course [13].

Carotid intimal media thickness (CIMT) is a marker for end-organ damage as a result of hypertension. In a recent matched controlled study, examiners evaluated the CIMT in children closely matched for BMI. They found that hypertensive children had increased CIMT compared with matched controls and that higher CIMT correlated with more severe hypertension. This study provided evidence that CIMT is increased in childhood primary hypertension, independent of the effects of obesity [34]. However, unlike for LVH, there are no reference values of CIMT available to guide the practitioners for pediatric patients.

Studies investigating the effects of hypertension on renal disease in the pediatric population are limited. Recent studies suggest that the glomerular filtration rate can be affected even by mild levels of elevated BP [35]. Microalbuminuria has also been seen in children with essential hypertension, and interestingly, reducing microalbuminuria in these children appears to decrease the progression of or result in the improvement of LVH [36].

In adults, concerns about how the central nervous system affects hypertension have focused on gross pathological manifestations such as stroke. In contrast, recent studies have suggested that children with even mild to moderately elevated SBP are at risk for central nervous system damage as measured by decreased neuropsychological scores of attention and concentration [37]. This evidence highlights the potential effects on academic performance that may exist in pediatric patients with hypertension and prehypertension.

9.7 PHARMACOLOGIC MANAGEMENT OF PEDIATRIC HYPERTENSION

The NHBPEP has established guidelines for the management of pediatric hypertension. Recommendations for the initial management of hypertension in obese children include the institution of weight management through lifestyle modification, which includes establishing dietary changes, as well as increasing the level of physical activity [16]. The NHBPEP also recommends pharmacologic management for individuals with persistent stage 1 or stage 2 hypertension despite nonpharmacologic measures. The goal of any intervention is to reduce BP below the 95th percentile for age, gender, and height or below the 90th percentile in the presence of a severe chronic illness such as diabetes or renal disease. The presence of diabetes or end-organ damage is also an indication to begin treatment [13]. Guidelines for management, including the appropriate starting drugs, pediatric dosages, and monitoring, are well described elsewhere [38]. It is important to note, however, that long-term studies of safety and efficacy of these medications are lacking and that compliance is typically low [7,39].

9.8 LIFESTYLE MODIFICATIONS FOR PEDIATRIC HYPERTENSION

The impact of lifestyle modifications on BP, weight, and cardiometabolic markers has been well studied in the adult population [40–42]. In children, the evidence for improved health outcomes as a result of lifestyle modification programs is less robust. The HEALTHY study, a primary prevention trial conducted in 42 U.S. middle schools, modified the school nutrition and physical activity environments and provided targeted behavioral, educational, and promotional initiatives to the students [43]. Children attending intervention schools did not demonstrate a statistically different BMI change than control schools, however, improved their fruit, vegetable, and whole grain consumption and demonstrated significantly greater reductions in SBP [44].

In 2010, the U.S. Preventative Services Task Force (USPSTF) released a report updating its 2005 report on childhood obesity. In part due to the explosion of literature demonstrating the modest, yet important, effect of lifestyle intervention in these intervening years, the Task Force reversed its earlier position that data were insufficient to recommend routine screening for overweight in children and adolescents [45,46]. The updated report states that the evidence is now sufficient to recommend

BMI screening and referral to weight management programs for children aged 6 years and above [46].

The USPSTF recommendations were based on a targeted systematic review of childhood obesity lifestyle modification programs. Of over 2500 studies published, only 11 met the criteria for inclusion based on study design and quality. Hours of patient contact was used as a proxy for treatment intensity and was categorized as very low (<10), low (10–25), moderate (26–75), or high (>75). Weight outcomes were categorized as short-term (6–12 months after beginning the program) or mainte-nance (at least 2 years after starting the program and at least 1 year after ending the program). Comprehensive interventions included dietary counseling, physical activity counseling or program participation, and behavioral management counsel-ing [47]. All of the interventions demonstrated a short-term improvement in one or more weight-related measures (percentage overweight, BMI, BMI standard devia-tion score), with the three most-intense programs demonstrating the largest effects [48–50]. Health outcomes other than weight-related markers, such as BP, lipid pro-files, and insulin resistance, were not included in the analysis. Only two low-intensity programs that could potentially be initiated in a primary care office were included in the analysis [51,52]; challenges remain for determining how to provide lifestyle intervention to children.

Since obesity and hypertension in children are closely linked, it is worthwhile to review the current recommendations for identification and treatment of obesity. To assist medical providers who work with children, the American Academy of Pediatrics (AAP) gathered an expert panel whose revised recommendations were released in 2007. The report outlines screening of BMI and behavioral habits, identi-fying those at high risk for complications from overweight or obesity, frequency and content of follow-up visit with providers, and appropriate screening for comorbid health conditions. In particular, the report stresses the importance of using BMI to screen all children annually for overweight. This report redefined terminology, refer-ring to children at the 5th–85th percentile for BMI as "normal weight," 85th–95th percentile as "overweight" (formerly, "at risk for overweight"), and above the 95th percentile as "obese" (formerly, "overweight") [11].

Little pediatric data exist regarding the benefits of lifestyle modifications focused on BP reduction. However, recent data have suggested that improved BP levels and decreased levels of cardiometabolic markers follow structured exercise participa-tion. These studies suggest that regular, structured physical activity results in sig-nificant reductions in SBP by 3 months of participation, independent of weight loss [53]. However, additional studies have shown that the impact of structured activity is not sustained unless individuals remain physically active [54,55]. Torrance et al. [27] recently published a review of published studies examining the role of physical activity on BP in children. Similar to the above, this review states that the evidence was suggestive of a reduction in BP and improvement in endothelial function after physical activity in overweight children [27].

An important role exists not only for exercise but also for dietary changes in the management of children with obesity-related hypertension. In another study, 57 adolescents with prehypertension or hypertension who underwent 3 months of nutritional counseling emphasizing a diet high in fruits, vegetables, and low-fat dairy [Dietary Approaches to Stop Hypertension (DASH) intervention] demon-strated greater reductions in SBP than those in the standard care group (a reduction of −7.9% in the DASH intervention group compared with −1.5% in the standard care group) [56].

9.9 SPECIFIC DIETARY RECOMMENDATIONS

Dietary recommendations, as described by the NHBPEP Working Group on High Blood Pressure in Children and Adolescence and the American Heart Association (AHA; Table 9.3), include balancing diet and activity to achieve a healthy body weight. Both guidelines center on decreasing the amount of salt in one's diet, increasing the consumption of fresh fruits, vegetables, and fiber, decreasing the consumption of sugar-containing beverages, and consuming nonfat dairy. Both recommendations stress the importance of being physically active [13,57]. Additional dietary changes recommended by the AHA include consuming fish, especially oily fish, at least twice per week, limiting intake of saturated fat to <7% of energy, trans fat to <1% of energy, and cholesterol to <300 mg/dL by choos-ing lean meats and vegetable alternatives and by minimizing intake of partially hydrogenated fats [57].

Additional guidelines include the DASH diet as shown in Table 9.3. Institution of the DASH diet is based on the evidence that certain dietary patterns favorably affect the BP of adults with prehypertension or stage 1 hypertension. Specifically, the guidelines recommend including a diet rich in fruits, vegetables, and low-fat dairy products. Diets should also be low in saturated and total fat. The DASH diet is associated with a reported 5.5 mmHg reduction in SBP and 3 mmHg reduction in DBP in adults. Increasing fruits and vegetables alone lowered SBP to a lesser degree in the original DASH study [56,58]. The DASH study results have been rep-licated several times in adults [59,60], and there is limited evidence of its efficacy in children [56].

TABLE 9.3
Description of Dietary Recommendations by DASH, NHBEP, and AHA

Programs	Descriptions
DASH [56,58]	Eight servings per day of fruits and vegetables
	Three servings per day of nonfat or low-fat dairy foods
	Replace simple carbohydrates (e.g., white bread) with complex carbohydrates (e.g., whole grain bread)
	Reduce total and saturated fat
	Limited intake of meat, sweets, sugar-sweetened beverages
NHBEP and AHA [13,57]	Diet rich in vegetables and fruits
	Whole-grain, high-fiber foods
	Encourage physical activity
	Select nonfat dairy products
	Minimize intake of beverages and foods with added sugars
	Reduce amount of salt in diet

9.10   EXERCISE RECOMMENDATIONS

There is limited published information regarding exercise recommendations for the hypertensive pediatric population despite data supporting the important role of exercise in lowering BP as described above. To date, a general recommendation for children is that they participate in at least 60 min of moderate-to-vigorous physical activity per day [11]. Physical activity can vary in intensity. For example, walking is generally considered a low-intensity activity and jogging or running is considered to be of at least moderate intensity [61]. National pediatric hypertension guidelines are similar and recommend regular aerobic physical activity, which includes the following: (1) 30–60 min of moderate physical activity on most days of the week and (2) limitation of sedentary activities to <2 h per day. Current recommendations for physical activity do not include power lifting [13]. Besides the potential benefits for hypertension, exercise can result in physiologic changes that can lead to improved respiratory and cardiovascular conditioning, strength, and mental health [61].

9.11   COMPREHENSIVE APPROACH TO LIFESTYLE MODIFICATIONS

A comprehensive approach to pediatric lifestyle modification targets at-risk individuals, provides dietary and activity counseling in a culturally sensitive manner, and provides tools for sustained behavioral change with the goal of achieving a healthy diet, an active lifestyle, and a reduction in BMI or weight-related comorbid health conditions. Lifestyle modification programs with proven efficacy as discussed above can be time and resource consuming. It is not always reasonable to wait for such level of data when the need is great, the intervention is safe, and the potential for benefit is high. Providing nutrition, activity, and behavioral counseling in whatever capacity a provider is able to do is an acceptable option, and guidelines for these are provided by the AAP [11].

The National Institute for Children's Healthcare Quality (NICHQ) also provides a user-friendly approach to the AAP Expert Panel recommendations [62]. This guide, entitled "Expert Committee Recommendations on the Assessment, Prevention and Treatment of Child and Adolescent Overweight and Obesity—2007: An Implementation Guide from the Childhood Obesity Action Network" (see Appendix) does not provide advice specifically for BP control but instead for weight maintenance and weight loss, as appropriate. Step 1, "Obesity prevention at well care visits" provides resources for accurate measurement of BMI, identification of overweight and obesity, and both assessment and intervention tools for use in the office setting. Step 2, "Prevention plus visits" provides guidance for treatment visits. These treatment visits are analogous to the lifestyle interventions described above, yet modified for an outpatient setting. This step describes the personnel and training needed to provide quality dietary and exercise prescriptions. Step 3, "Going beyond your practice," provides information on advocacy for childhood obesity prevention in the wider community and policy-based changes. The three steps are useful in achieving the AAP standard of care. The guide is found in the

Appendix, as well as online at www.nichq.org/documents/coan-papers-and-publications/COANImplementationGuide62607FINAL.pdf. These and other resources may be accessed through the Childhood Obesity Action Network at www.nichq.org.

Another option is to use strategies such as "5-3-2-1-almost none" adopted by Eat Smart, Move More North Carolina as the statewide obesity prevention message [63]. The "5-3-2-1-almost none" strategy refers to consuming at least five fruits and vegetables a day, eating three structured meals daily, limiting screen time to 2 h or fewer per day, having at least 1 h of moderate-to-vigorous physical activity daily, and consuming almost no sugary beverages, which incorporate strategies recommended by the AAP Expert Panel [11,63]. The message is easy to remember and useful for both assessment of current behaviors and recommendations for behavior targets.

9.12 TECHNIQUES FOR IMPLEMENTING LIFESTYLE MODIFICATIONS

The AAP recommends using the motivational interviewing (MI) approach when providing lifestyle counseling for families and children [11]. MI is a tested communication style that values patient autonomy, collaborative approach to change, and support of self-efficacy, and supports the belief that human behavioral change results from motivation (internally driven) rather than information (externally driven). Active listening focusing on reflective listening is at the core of MI. Questions such as, "What goals do you have for your child's health" or "What, if anything, worries you about your child's weight?" can reveal the patient's and family's internal motivation. Subsequent questions such as, "What steps would you like to take toward achieving this goal?" raises the likelihood that the negotiated change will occur, as the actual changes are patient-driven. Helping the family formalize the goal, identify barriers, develop concrete steps, create methods to track the success of these steps, integrate rewards, and schedule follow-up physician visits will also increase the likelihood of change. Several studies have demonstrated that this technique is effective when used in a clinical setting, taking an average of 10–15 min per visit to achieve significant changes in smoking cessation, reductions in substance abuse, adherence to asthma medications, decreases in risky sexual behaviors, and improvements in alcoholism [64]. One study in children examined the effects of MI on childhood obesity and found a small but significant decrease in BMI percentile in the MI group versus the standard counseling group [65,66]. Continuing medical education (CME) resources are available to learn MI online. In addition, an extensive network of certified trainers (Motivational Interviewing Network of Trainers) offer in-person courses. More information about applying MI for lifestyle modification can be found in Chapter 6.

9.12.1 CASE EXAMPLE

Martha is a 10-year-old child who on screening at her annual pediatrician visit is noted to have both elevated BP and hypercholesterolemia. Her weight and height are both over the 95th percentile for gender and age, placing her BMI at the 96th percentile (obese). She has a family history of obesity, hypertension, and high cholesterol. She has not yet started her menses and has no other risk factors for cardiovascular diseases. You explain about BMI to her mother and inform her that Martha is overweight. You counsel her that if she adopts healthier habits and her BMI were in the normal range, her BP and lipids would likely return to normal. You schedule a follow-up visit with Martha in 1 month to recheck her BP and further discuss potential lifestyle modifications.

At the follow-up visit, her BMI remains above the 95th percentile, and her BP is 130/60, sitting and at rest. On exam, no acanthosis is present. She is in Tanner 3 stage and has not started menses. Given Martha's family history, you suspect essential hypertension and recommend lifestyle modifications including the DASH diet. You consider secondary causes of hypertension; however, since she has had only two elevations in the clinic, you wait to begin the workup.

Using "5-3-2-1-almost none," you learn that Martha eats a vegetable every other day, skips breakfast, watches 4 h of television (mostly on the television in her room), does not play outside, and has 45 min of physical education per week. She likes to drink a wide variety of beverages, including chocolate milk, Kool Aid, sports drinks, soda, and sweetened tea. You identify several areas for improvement:

1. Increasing consumption of fruits/vegetables to 5 daily
2. Eating breakfast daily
3. Decreasing screen time and possibly taking the television out of her room
4. Increasing the time Martha spends actively
5. Reducing the sugar levels in her beverages

Rather than telling the parent about everything that needs to change, you elect to use a patient-centered approach. You ask Martha's mom what concerns she has, how interested they are in changing, and how they would like to begin. She tells you that she is most concerned about Martha's heart health, given the family history. She knows they need to change but feels overwhelmed and is unsure where to begin. She notes that Martha's maternal grandmother cares for her in the afternoon, and she is not sure if her grandma sees her weight as a problem. Martha's mom thinks she could try buying bottled water instead of sugary drinks for Martha. She also plans on storing some water at grandma's house, so Martha would have a healthy drink option. You support Martha's mom in this goal and ask Martha what her concerns and goals are. She is more concerned about getting teased at school than she is about her future health. She thinks that she could drink more water but often turns to the sugary drinks for comfort when she feels sad, so Martha is not sure that the plan is going to work.

You provide information to the family and discuss the plan. You summarize the concerns: Martha's mom is concerned about Martha's heart, Martha is concerned about teasing, and you are concerned about Martha's overall health. You reiterate her mother's goal of buying water rather than sweet drinks and having those available at her grandma's house. You acknowledge the barrier of Martha's emotional state and her grandma's desire to show love through feeding. You suggest her mom to seek out counseling to help Martha develop healthier coping skills and suggest that Martha's grandma should attend the next visit. In addition, you suggest them to track the days in which Martha drinks at least four glasses of water and reward her (sticker chart, stars, etc). You schedule a follow-up visit in 2–3 months to recheck BP and assess success with their plan. You provide a handout on the sugar content of various sweetened beverages.

On return visit after 3 months, Martha's weight has remained unchanged, but she has grown by 3.5 cm, decreasing her BMI by 1.2 kg/m², placing her now in the "overweight" category, at the 92nd percentile. Martha's grandma has come to this visit and is engaged in the process. You recheck BP, which is still high but improved at 125/67 mmHg. You congratulate them on their success. You use "5-3-2-1-almost none" to reassess behaviors and find that the family has successfully limited sweet drinks to Friday nights only. You note that she still watches about 4 h of television per day. You discuss her progress with grandma and Martha, and they decide that they would like to continue improving their lifestyle. With your assistance, the family decides to reduce Martha's television time. Since the family seems motivated and Martha remains overweight, you schedule another follow-up visit in 3 months.

9.13   CONCLUSION

Childhood hypertension is strongly linked with childhood obesity and is a problem all providers face, from primary care to surgical to subspecialty fields. The tracking of elevated BP from childhood to adulthood necessitates monitoring and early recognition of hypertension in children. Care must be taken so that BP is appropriately measured and appropriate follow-up of an elevated BP is performed by the physician. Lifestyle modifications for hypertensive obese children are a valuable treatment modality, and physicians' comfort with discussing dietary and physical activity recommendations is crucial. Despite barriers, providers now have a wide array of resources to increase knowledge, confidence, and efficacy in providing this much-needed intervention to parents, children, and adolescents (Table 9.4).

TABLE 9.4
Summary: Take-Home Messages

Key Evidences	Recommendations for Health Care Practitioners
• Approximately, one-third of children and adolescents are overweight or obese, a major risk factor for hypertension	• Regular screening of weight status and provide intervention as needed
• BP tracks from childhood to adulthood	• Regular screening of BP
• Complications of hypertension can occur in children	• Follow-up visits to reassess elevated BP
• Accurate diagnosis of hypertension requires the use of appropriately sized BP cuffs and comparison to standardized tables	• MI should be used to encourage lifestyle modifications
• Lifestyle modification is a core treatment strategy for obese hypertensive children	• Pharmacologic management should be considered in hypertensive children unresponsive to lifestyle management

APPENDIX

NICHQ Implementation Guide

Expert Committee Recommendations on the Assessment, Prevention and Treatment of Child and Adolescent Overweight and Obesity—2007: An Implementation Guide from the Childhood Obesity Action Network

Overview

In 2005, the American Medical Association (AMA), Health Resources and Services Administration (HRSA), and Center for Disease Control (CDC) convened an Expert Committee to revise the 1997 childhood obesity recommendations. Representatives from 15 health-care organizations submitted nominations for the experts who would compose the three writing groups (assessment, prevention, treatment). The initial recommendations were released on June 6, 2007 in a document titled "Appendix: Expert Committee Recommendations on the Assessment, Prevention and Treatment of Child and Adolescent Overweight and Obesity" (www.ama-assn.org/ama/pub/category/11759.html).

In 2006, the National Initiative for Children's Healthcare Quality (NICHQ) launched the Childhood Obesity Action Network (COAN). With more than 40 health-care organizations and 600 health professionals, the network is aimed at rapidly sharing knowledge, successful practices, and innovation. This Implementation Guide is the first of a series of products designed for health-care professionals by COAN to accelerate improvement in the prevention and treatment of childhood obesity.

The Implementation Guide combines key aspects of the Expert Committee Recommendations summary released on June 6, 2007 and practice tools identified in 2006 by NICHQ from primary care groups that have successfully developed obesity care strategies (www.NICHQ.org). These tools were developed before the 2007 Expert Recommendations and there may be some inconsistencies such as the *overweight* instead of *obesity* for BMI ≥ 95th percentile. The tools are intended as a source of ideas to facilitate implementation. As tools are updated or new tools are developed based on the Expert Recommendations, the Implementation Guide will be updated. The Implementation Guide defines three key steps to the implementation of the 2007 Expert Committee Recommendations:

- Step 1—Obesity Prevention at Well Care Visits (Assessment and Prevention)
- Step 2—Prevention Plus Visits (Treatment)
- Step 3—Going Beyond Your Practice (Prevention and Treatment)

Step 1—Obesity Prevention at Well Care Visits (Assessment and Prevention)

Action Steps	Expert Recommendations	Action Network Tips and Tools
Assess all children for obesity at all well care visits from 2 to 18 years	Physicians and allied health professionals should perform, at a minimum, a yearly assessment	A *presentation* for your staff and colleagues can help implement obesity prevention in your practice

(continued)

Step 1—(continued)

Action Steps	Expert Recommendations	Action Network Tips and Tools
Use body mass index (BMI) to screen for obesity	• **Accurately measure height and weight** • **Calculate BMI** 　BMI (English) [weight (lb) ÷ height (in) ÷ height (in)] × 703 　BMI (metric) [weight (kg) ÷ height (cm) ÷ height (cm)] × 10,000 • **Plot BMI on BMI growth chart** • Not recommended: skinfold thickness, waist circumference	BMI is very sensitive to measurement errors, particularly height. Having a standard measurement protocol and training can improve accuracy. *BMI calculation* tools are also helpful. Use the CDC BMI percentile-for-age growth charts
Make a weight category diagnosis using BMI percentile	• 5th percentile: underweight • 5–84th percentile: healthy weight • 85–94th percentile: Overweight • 95–98th percentile: Obesity • ≥99th percentile	Until the BMI percentile is added to the growth charts, *Table A.1* can be used to determine the 99th percentile cut points. Physicians should exercise judgment when choosing how to inform the family. Using more neutral terms such as *weight, excess weight, BMI, or risk for diabetes and heart disease* can reduce the risk of stigmatization or harm to self-esteem
Measure blood pressure	• Use a cuff large enough to cover 80% of the upper arm • Measure pulse in the standard manner	Diagnose hypertension using *NHLBI tables*. An abbreviated table is shown below (*Table A.2*)
Take a focused family history	• Obesity • Type 2 diabetes • Cardiovascular disease (hypertension, cholesterol) • Early deaths from heart disease or stroke	A child with one obese parent has a threefold increased risk of becoming obese. This risk increases to 13-fold with two obese parents. Using a *clinical documentation* tool can be helpful
Take a focused review of systems	Take a focused review of systems	See *Table A.3*. Using a *clinical documentation* tool can be helpful
Assess behaviors and attitudes	**Diet behaviors** • Sweetened-beverage consumption • Fruit and vegetable consumption • Frequency of eating out and family meals • Consumption of excessive portion sizes • Daily breakfast consumption	Using behavioral risk assessment tools can facilitate history taking and save clinicians' time

Step 1—(continued)

Action Steps	Expert Recommendations	Action Network Tips and Tools
	Physical activity behaviors • Amount of moderate physical activity • Level of screen time and other sedentary activities **Attitudes** • Self-perception or concern about weight • Readiness to change • Successes, barriers, and challenges	
Perform a thorough physical examination Order the appropriate laboratory tests	Perform a thorough physical examination BMI 85–94th percentile *without* risk factors • Fasting lipid profile • MI 85–94th percentile age 10 years and other *with* risk factors • Fasting lipid profile • Alanine aminotransferase (ALT) and aspartate aminotransferase (AST) • Fasting glucose BMI ≥ 95th percentile age 10 years and above • Fasting lipid profile • ALT and AS • Fasting glucose • Other tests as indicated by health risks	See *Table A.3*. Using a *clinical documentation* tool can be helpful Consider ordering ALT, AST, and glucose tests beginning at 10 years of age and then periodically (every 2 years). Provider decision support tools can be helpful when choosing assessment and treatment options Delivering lab results can be one way to open the conversation about weight and health with a family
Give consistent evidence-based messages for all children regardless of weight	• Limit sugar-sweetened beverages • Eat at least five servings of fruits and vegetables • Moderate to vigorous physical activity for at least 60 min a day • Limit screen time to no more than 2 h/day • Remove television from children's bedrooms • Eat breakfast everyday • Limit eating out, especially at fast food • Have regular family meals • Limit portion sizes	An example from the Maine collaborative: • Five fruits and vegetables • Two hours or less of TV per day • One hour or more physical activity • Zero servings of sweetened beverages Exam and waiting room *posters* and family *education materials* can help deliver these messages and facilitate dialogue. Encourage an authoritative parenting style in support of increased physical activity and reduced TV viewing. Discourage a restrictive parenting style regarding child eating

(continued)

Step 1—(continued)

Action Steps	Expert Recommendations	Action Network Tips and Tools
		Encourage parents to be good role models and address as a family issue rather than the child's problem
Use *empathize/elicit*, *provide*, and *elicit* to improve the effectiveness of your counseling	Assess self-efficacy and readiness to change. Use *empathize/elicit*, *provide*, and *elicit* to improve the effectiveness of your counseling **Empathize/Elicit** • Reflect • What is your understanding? • What do you want to know? • How ready are you to make a change (1–10 scale)? **Provide** • Advice or information • Choices or options **Elicit** • What do you make of that? • Where does that leave you?	A possible dialogue: *empathize/ elicit* "Yours child's height and weight may put him/her at increased risk for developing diabetes and heart diseases at a very early age" "What do you make of this?" "Would you be interested in talking more about ways to reduce your child's risk?" **Provide** "Some different ways to reduce your child's risk are ... " "Do any of these seem like something your family could work or do you have other ideals?" **Elicit** "Where does that leave you?" "What might you need to be successful!" Communication guidelines can be helpful when developing communication skills

Step 2—Prevention Plus Visits (Treatment)

Action Steps	Expert Recommendations	Action Network Tips and Tools
Develop an office-based approach for follow-up of overweight and obese children	A staged approach to treatment is recommended for ages 2–19 whose BMI is 85–64th percentile with risk factors and all whose BMI is ≥ 95th percentile In general, treatment beings with stage 1 Prevention Plus (Table A. 4) and progresses to the next stage if there has been no improvement in weight/BMI or velocity after 3–6 months and the family is willing/ready The recommended weight loss targets are shown in Table A. 5	Prevention Plus visits may include the following: • Health education materials • Behavioral risk assessment and self-monitoring tools • Action planning and goal-setting tools • Clinical documentation tools • Counseling protocols • Other health professionals such as dietitians, psychologists, and health educators

Step 2—(continued)

Action Steps	Expert Recommendations	Action Network Tips and Tools
	Stage 1—Prevention Plus	Besides behavioral and weight goals, improving self-esteem and self-efficacy (confidence) are important outcomes. Although weight maintenance is a good goal, more commonly, a slower weight gain reflected in a decreased BMI velocity is the outcome seen in lower intensity behavioral interventions such as Prevention Plus. Measuring and plotting BMI after 3–6 months in an important step to determine the effectiveness of obesity treatment
	Family visits with physician or health professionals who have had some training in pediatric weight management/ behavioral counseling	
	Can be individual or group visits	
	Frequency—individualized to family needs and risk factors; consider monthly	
	Behavioral Goals	
	Decrease screen time to 2 h/day or fewer	
	No sugar-sweetened beverages	
	Consume at least five servings of fruits and vegetables daily	
	Be physically active 1 h or more daily	
	Prepare more meals at home as a family (the goal is 5–6 times a week)	
	Limit meals outside the home	
	Eat a healthy breakfast daily	
	Involve the whole family in lifestyle changes	
	More focused attention to lifestyle changes and more frequent follow-up distinguishes Prevention Plus from Prevention Counseling	
	Weight Goal—weight maintenance or a decrease in BMI velocity. The long-term BMI goal is <85th percentile although some children can be healthy with a BMI 85–94th percentile.	
	Advance to stage 2 (structure weight management) if no improvement in weight/BMI or velocity in 3–6 months and the family is willing/ready to make changes	
Use motivational interviewing at Prevention Plus visits for ambivalent families and to improve the success of action planning	Use patient-centered counseling— motivational interviewing	Research suggests that motivational interviewing may be an effective approach to address childhood obesity prevention and treatment. Motivational interviewing is particularly effective for ambivalent families but can also be used for action planning. Instead of telling patients what changes to make, you elicit "change talk" from them, taking their ideas, strengths, and barriers into account. Communication guidelines and communication training can be helpful with skill development

(continued)

Step 2—(continued)

Action Steps	Expert Recommendations	Action Network Tips and Tools
Develop a reimbursement strategy for Prevention Plus visits		Coding strategies can help with reimbursement for Prevention Plus visits. Advocacy through professional organizations to address reimbursement policies is another strategy

Step 3—Going Beyond Your Practice (Prevention and Treatment)

Action Steps	Expert Recommendations	Action Network Tips and Tools
Advocate for improved access to fresh fruits and vegetables and safe physical activity in your community and schools	The Expert Committee recommends that physicians, allied health-care professionals, and professional organizations advocate for • the federal government to increase physical activity at school through intervention programs as early as grade I through the end of high school and college and through creating school environments that support physical activity in general • supporting efforts to preserve and enhance parks as areas for physical activity, informing local development initiatives regarding the inclusion of walking and bicycle paths, and promoting families' use of local physical activity options by making information and suggestions about physical activity alternatives available in doctors' offices	Physicians and health professionals can play a key role in advocating for policy and built environment changes to support healthy eating and physical activity in communities, child-care settings, and schools (including after-school programs). Advocacy tools and resources can be helpful in advocacy efforts Partnering with others and using evidence-based strategies are also critical to the success of multifaceted community interventions
Identify and promote community services that encourage healthy eating and physical activity	Promote physical activity at school and in child-care setting (including after-school programs) by asking children and parents about activity in these settings during routine office visits	Public health departments and parks and recreation are good places to start looking for community programs and resources
Identify or develop more intensive weight management interventions for the families that do not respond to Prevention Plus	The Expert Committee recommends the following staged approach for children between the ages of 2 and 19, whose BMI is 85–94th percentile with risk factors and all whose BMI is ≥ 95th percentile • Stage 2—Structured Weight Management (Family visits with physician or health professional specifically trained in weight management. Monthly visits can be individual or group)	Stage 2 could be done without a tertiary care center if community professionals from different disciplines collaborate, for example, if a physician provided the medical assessment, a dietitian provided classes, and the local YMCA provided an exercise program.
Identify or develop more intensive weight management interventions for the families that do not respond to Prevention Plus	• Stage 3—Comprehensive, Multidisciplinary Intervention (Multidisciplinary team with experience in childhood obesity. Frequency is often weekly for 8–12 weeks with follow-up.) • Stage 4—Tertiary Care Intervention (medications: sibutramine and orlistat; very-low-calorie diets; weight control	Partnering with your community tertiary care center can be an effective strategy to develop or link to more intensive weight management interventions (Stages 3 and 4) as well as referral protocols to care for

Step 3—(continued)

Action Steps	Expert Recommendations	Action Network Tips and Tools
	surgery: gastric bypass or banding) recommended for select patients only when provided by experienced programs with established clinical or research protocols. Gastric banding is in clinical trials and not currently FDA approved	families who do not respond to Prevention Plus visits. Provider decision support tools can be helpful when choosing appropriate treatment and referral options. Weight management protocols and curriculum can also be helpful when getting started
Join the Childhood Obesity Action Network to learn from your colleagues and accelerate progress		The Childhood Obesity Action Network has launched "Join the network" (*www.NICHO. org*) to learn from our national obesity experts, share what you have learned, and access the tools in this guide. Together we can make a difference!

Implementation Guide Authors: Scott Gee, MD; Victoria Rogers, MD; Lenna Liu, MD, MPH; and Jane McGrath, MD.

Implementation Guide Contact: obesity@nichq.org

TABLE A.9.1
BMI 99th Percentile Cut–Points (kg/m²)

Age (Years)	Boys	Girls
5	20.1	21.5
6	21.6	23.0
7	23.6	24.6
8	25.6	26.4
9	27.6	28.2
10	29.3	29.9
11	30.7	31.5
12	31.8	33.1
13	32.6	34.6
14	33.2	36.0
15	33.6	37.5
16	33.9	39.1
17	34.4	40.8

TABLE A.9.2
Abbreviated NHLBI Blood Pressure Table by Age, Sex, and Height Percentile

Age (Years)	Boys Height (Percentile)		Girls Height (Percentile)	
	50th Percentile	90th Percentile	50th Percentile	90th Percentile
2	106/61	109/63	105/63	108/65
5	112/72	115/74	110/72	112/73
8	116/78	119/79	115/76	118/78
11	121/80	124/82	121/79	123/81
14	128/82	132/84	126/82	129/84
17	136/87	139/88	129/84	131/85

Source: Adapted from National High Blood Pressure Education Program Working Group on High Blood Pressure in Children and Adolescents, *Pediatrics*, 114, 555–576, August 2004.

TABLE A.9.3
Symptoms and Signs of Conditions Associated with Obesity

Symptoms

- Anxiety, school avoidance, social isolation (depression)
- Polyuria, polydipsia, weight loss (type 2 diabetes mellitus)
- Headaches (pseudotumor cerebri)

- Night breathing difficulties (sleep apnea, hyperventilation syndrome, asthma)
- Daytime sleepiness (sleep apnea, hyperventilation syndrome, depression)
- Abdominal pain (gastroesophageal reflux, gall bladder disease, constipation)
- Hip or knee pain (slipped capital femoral epiphysis)
- Oligomenorrhea or amenorrhea (polycystic ovary syndrome)

Signs

- Poor linear growth (hyperthyroidism, Cushing's Prader–Willi syndrome)
- Dysmorphic features (genetic disorders, including Prader–Willi syndrome)
- Acanthosis nigricans (NIDDM, insulin resistance)
- Hirsutism and excessive acne (polycystic ovary syndrome)
- Violaceous striae (Cushing's syndrome)

- Papilledema, cranial nerve VI paralysis (pseudotumor cerebri)
- Tonsillar hypertrophy (sleep apnea)

- Abdominal tenderness (gall bladder disease, GERD, NAFLD)
- Hepatomegaly [nonalcoholic fatty liver disease (NAFLD)]
- Undescended testicle (Prader–Willi syndrome)
- Limited hip range of motion (slipped capital femoral epiphysis)
- Lower leg bowing (Blount's disease)

TABLE A.9.4
A Staged Approach to Obesity Treatment

Age (Years)	BMI 85–94th Percentile No Risks	BMI 85–94th Percentile with Risks	BMI 95–98th Percentile	BMI ≥ 99th Percentile
2–5	prevention counseling	Initial: Stage 1 Highest: Stage 2	Initial: Stage 1 Highest: Stage 3	Initial: Stage 1 Highest: Stage 3
6–11	prevention counseling	Initial: Stage 1 Highest: Stage 2	Initial: Stage 1 Highest: Stage 3	Initial: Stages 1–3 Highest: Stage 3
12–18	prevention counseling	Initial: Stage 1 Highest: Stage 3	Initial: Stage 1 Highest: Stage 4	Initial: Stages 1–3 Highest: Stage 4

Stage 1	Prevention plus	Primary care office
Stage 2	Structured weight management	Primary care office with support
Stage 3	Comprehensive, multidisciplinary (Intervention)	(Pediatric Weight Management Center)
Stage 4	Tertiary care (Intervention)	Tertiary care center

TABLE A.9.5
Weight Loss Targets

Age (Years)	BMI 85–94th Percentile with No Risks	BMI 85–94th Percentile with Risks	BMI 95–98th Percentile	BMI ≥ 99 Percentile
2–5	Maintain weight velocity	Decrease weight velocity or weight maintenance	Weight maintenance	Gradual weight loss of up to 1 lb a month if BMI is very high (>21 or 22 kg/m^2)
6–11	Maintain weight velocity	Decrease weight velocity or weight maintenance	Weight maintenance or gradual loss (1 lb/month)	Weight loss (average is 2 lb/week)[a]
12–18	Maintain weight velocity. After linear growth is complete, maintain weight	Decrease weight velocity or weight maintenance	Weight loss (average is 2 lb/week)[a]	Weight loss (average is 2 lb/week)[a]

Source: NICHQ, Expert Committee Recommendations on the Assessment, Prevention and Treatment of Child and Adolescent Overweight and Obesity—2007: An Implementation Guide from the Childhood Obesity Action Network, http://www.nichq.org/documents/coan-papers-and-publications/COANImplementationGuide62607FINAL.pdf (accessed September 5, 2011). With permission.

[a] Excessive weight loss should be evaluated for high risk behaviors.

REFERENCES

1. Ogden CL, Carroll MD, Curtin LR, Lamb MM, Flegal KM. Prevalence of high body mass index in US children and adolescents, 2007–2008. *JAMA.* 2010;303(3):242–249.
2. Reilley KJ, Giulianotti M, Dooley CT, Nefzi A, McLaughlin JP, Houghten RA. Identification of two novel, potent, low-liability antinociceptive compounds from the direct in vivo screening of a large mixture-based combinatorial library. *AAPS J.* 2010;12(3):318–329.
3. Silventoinen K, Kaprio J. Genetics of tracking of body mass index from birth to late middle age: Evidence from twin and family studies. *Obes Facts.* 2009;2(3):196–202.
4. The NS, Suchindran C, North KE, Popkin BM, Gordon-Larsen P. Association of adolescent obesity with risk of severe obesity in adulthood. *JAMA.* 2010;304(18):2042–2047.
5. U.S. Public Health Service. Office of the Surgeon General., United States. Office of Disease Prevention and Health Promotion, Centers for Disease Control and Prevention (U.S.), National Institutes of Health (U.S.). *The Surgeon General's Call to Action to Prevent and Decrease Overweight and Obesity.* Rockville, MD, Washington, DC: U.S. Department of Health and Human Services, Public Health Service, For sale by the Supt. of Docs., U.S. G.P.O.; 2001.
6. Olshansky SJ, Passaro DJ, Hershow RC, et al. A potential decline in life expectancy in the United States in the 21st century. *N Engl J Med.* 2005;352(11):1138–1145.
7. Flynn JT. Pediatric hypertension: Recent trends and accomplishments, future challenges. *Am J Hypertens.* 2008;21(6):605–612.
8. Ostchega Y, Carroll M, Prineas RJ, McDowell MA, Louis T, Tilert T. Trends of elevated blood pressure among children and adolescents: Data from the National Health and Nutrition Examination Survey1988–2006. *Am J Hypertens.* 2009;22(1):59–67.
9. Kotsis V, Stabouli S, Papakatsika S, Rizos Z, Parati G. Mechanisms of obesity-induced hypertension. *Hypertens Res.* 2010;33(5):386–393.
10. Berenson GS, Srinivasan SR, Bao W, Newman WP 3rd, Tracy RE, Wattigney WA. Association between multiple cardiovascular risk factors and atherosclerosis in children and young adults. The Bogalusa Heart Study. *N Engl J Med. 1*998;338(23):1650–1656.
11. Barlow SE. Expert committee recommendations regarding the prevention, assessment, and treatment of child and adolescent overweight and obesity: Summary report. *Pediatrics.* 2007;120 Suppl 4:S164–S192.
12. Ford AL, Hunt LP, Cooper A, Shield JP. What reduction in BMI SDS is required in obese adolescents to improve body composition and cardiometabolic health? *Arch Dis Child.* 2010;95(4):256–261.
13. National High Blood Pressure Education Program Working Group on High Blood Pressure in Children and Adolescents. The fourth report on the diagnosis, evaluation, and treatment of high blood pressure in children and adolescents. *Pediatrics.* 2004;114(2 Suppl 4th Report):555–576.
14. Expert Panel on Integrated Guidelines for Cardiovascular Health and Risk Reduction in Children and Adolescents; National Heart, Lung, and Blood Institute. Expert panel on integrated guidelines for cardiovascular health and risk reduction in children and adolescents: Summary Report. *Pediatrics.* 2011;128:S213. DOI: 10.1542/peds.2009-2107C.
15. Podoll A, Grenier M, Croix B, Feig DI. Inaccuracy in pediatric outpatient blood pressure measurement. *Pediatrics.* 2007;119(3):e538–e543.
16. Gordon-Larsen P, Adair LS, Nelson MC, Popkin BM. Five-year obesity incidence in the transition period between adolescence and adulthood: The National Longitudinal Study of Adolescent Health. *Am J Clin Nutr.* 2004;80(3):569–575.
17. Berenson GS, Dalferes E, Jr., Savage D, Webber LS, Bao W. Ambulatory blood pressure measurements in children and young adults selected by high and low casual blood pressure levels and parental history of hypertension: The Bogalusa Heart Study. *Am J Med Sci.* 1993;305(6):374–382.

18. Feber J, Ahmed M. Hypertension in children: New trends and challenges. *Clin Sci.* 2010;119:151–161.
19. Must A, Spadano J, Coakley EH, Field AE, Colditz G, Dietz WH. The disease burden associated with overweight and obesity. *JAMA.* 27 1999;282(16):1523–1529.
20. Muntner P, He J, Cutler JA, Wildman RP, Whelton PK. Trends in blood pressure among children and adolescents. *JAMA.* 2004;291(17):2107–2113.
21. Chen X, Wang Y. Tracking of blood pressure from childhood to adulthood: A systematic review and meta-regression analysis. *Circulation.* 2008;117(25):3171–3180.
22. McCrindle BW. Assessment and management of hypertension in children and adolescents. *Nat Rev Cardiol.* 2010;7(3):155–163.
23. Keenan NL, Rosendorf KA. Prevalence of hypertension and controlled hypertension—United States, 2005–2008. *MMWR Surveill Summ.* 2011;60 Suppl:94–97.
24. Amin RS, Carroll JL, Jeffries JL, et al. Twenty-four-hour ambulatory blood pressure in children with sleep-disordered breathing. *Am J Respir Crit Care Med.* 2004;169(8):950–956.
25. Maffeis C, Banzato C, Brambilla P, et al. Insulin resistance is a risk factor for high blood pressure regardless of body size and fat distribution in obese children. *Nutr Metab Cardiovasc Dis.* 2010;20(4):266–273.
26. Robinson RF, Batisky DL, Hayes JR, Nahata MC, Mahan JD. Body mass index in primary and secondary pediatric hypertension. *Pediatr Nephrol.* 2004;19(12):1379–1384.
27. Torrance B, McGuire KA, Lewanczuk R, McGavock J. Overweight, physical activity and high blood pressure in children: A review of the literature. *Vasc Health Risk Manag.* 2007;3(1):139–149.
28. Rahmouni K, Correia ML, Haynes WG, Mark AL. Obesity-associated hypertension: New insights into mechanisms. *Hypertension.* 2005;45(1):9–14.
29. Muntner P, He J, Cutler J. Trends in blood pressure among children and adolescents. *JAMA.* 2004;291:2107–2113.
30. Alper AB Jr, Chen W, Yau L, Srinivasan SR, Berenson GS, Hamm LL. Childhood uric acid predicts adult blood pressure: The Bogalusa Heart Study. *Hypertension.* 2005;45(1):34–38.
31. Hanevold C, Waller, Daniels S, Portman R, Sorof J. The effects of obesity, gender, and ethnic group on left ventricular hypertrophy and geometry in hypertensive children: A collaborative study of the International Pediatric Hypertension Association. *Pediatrics.* 2004;113:328–333.
32. McNiece KL, Gupta-Malhotra M, Samuels J, et al. Left ventricular hypertrophy in hypertensive adolescents: Analysis of risk by 2004 National High Blood Pressure Education Program Working Group staging criteria. *Hypertension.* 2007;50(2):392–395.
33. Daniels SR, Loggie JM, Khoury P, Kimball TR. Left ventricular geometry and severe left ventricular hypertrophy in children and adolescents with essential hypertension. *Circulation.* 1998;97(19):1907–1911.
34. Lande MB, Carson NL, Roy J, Meagher CC. Effects of childhood primary hypertension on carotid intima media thickness: A matched controlled study. *Hypertension.* 2006;48(1):40–44.
35. Lubrano R, Travasso E, Raggi C, Guido G, Masciangelo R, Elli M. Blood pressure load, proteinuria and renal function in pre-hypertensive children. *Pediatr Nephrol.* 2009;24(4):823–831.
36. Assadi F. Effect of microalbuminuria lowering on regression of left ventricular hypertrophy in children and adolescents with essential hypertension. *Pediatr Cardiol.* 2007;28(1):27–33.
37. Lande MB, Kaczorowski JM, Auinger P, Schwartz GJ, Weitzman M. Elevated blood pressure and decreased cognitive function among school-age children and adolescents in the United States. *J Pediatr.* 2003;143(6):720–724.

38. Flynn JT, Daniels SR. Pharmacologic treatment of hypertension in children and adolescents. *J Pediatr.* 2006;149(6):746–754.

39. Benjamin DK Jr, Smith PB, Jadhav P, et al. Pediatric antihypertensive trial failures: Analysis of end points and dose range. *Hypertension.* 2008;51(4):834–840.

40. Appel LJ, Champagne CM, Harsha DW, et al. Effects of comprehensive lifestyle modification on blood pressure control: Main results of the PREMIER clinical trial. *JAMA.* 2003;289(16):2083–2093.

41. Stevens VJ, Obarzanek E, Cook NR, et al. Long-term weight loss and changes in blood pressure: Results of the Trials of Hypertension Prevention, phase II. *Ann Intern Med.* 2001;134(1):1–11.

42. Appel LJ, Espeland MA, Easter L, Wilson AC, Folmar S, Lacy CR. Effects of reduced sodium intake on hypertension control in older individuals: Results from the Trial of Nonpharmacologic Interventions in the Elderly (TONE). *Arch Intern Med.* 2001;161(5):685–693.

43. Foster GD, Linder B, Baranowski T, et al. A school-based intervention for diabetes risk reduction, The HEALTHY Study Group. *N Engl J Med.* July 29, 2010;363(5):443–453.

44. Siega-Riz AM, El Ghormli L, Mobley C, et al. The effects of the HEALTHY study intervention on middle school student dietary intakes. *Int J Behav Nutr Phys Act.* February 4, 2011;8:7.

45. Mahler DA, Fierro-Carrion G, Mejia-Alfaro R, Ward J, Baird JC. Responsiveness of continuous ratings of dyspnea during exercise in patients with COPD. *Med Sci Sports Exerc.* 2005;37(4):529–535.

46. Barton M. Screening for obesity in children and adolescents: U.S. Preventive Services Task Force recommendation statement. *Pediatrics.* 2010;125(2):361–367.

47. Whitlock EP, O'Connor EA, Williams SB, Beil TL, Lutz KW. Effectiveness of weight management interventions in children: A targeted systematic review for the USPSTF. *Pediatrics.* 2010;125(2):e396–e418.

48. Savoye M, Shaw M, Dziura J, et al. Effects of a weight management program on body composition and metabolic parameters in overweight children: A randomized controlled trial. *JAMA.* 2007;297(24):2697–2704.

49. Reinehr T, de Sousa G, Toschke AM, Andler W. Long-term follow-up of cardiovascular disease risk factors in children after an obesity intervention. *Am J Clin Nutr.* 2006;84(3):490–496.

50. Nemet D, Barkan S, Epstein Y, Friedland O, Kowen G, Eliakim A. Short- and long-term beneficial effects of a combined dietary-behavioral-physical activity intervention for the treatment of childhood obesity. *Pediatrics.* 2005;115(4):e443–e449.

51. McCallum Z, Wake M, Gerner B, et al. Outcome data from the LEAP (Live, Eat and Play) trial: A randomized controlled trial of a primary care intervention for childhood overweight/mild obesity. *Int J Obes (Lond).* 2007;31(4):630–636.

52. Saelens BE, Sallis JF, Wilfley DE, Patrick K, Cella JA, Buchta R. Behavioral weight control for overweight adolescents initiated in primary care. *Obes Res.* 2002;10(1):22–32.

53. Farpour-Lambert NJ, Aggoun Y, Marchand LM, Martin XE, Herrmann FR, Beghetti M. Physical activity reduces systemic blood pressure and improves early markers of atherosclerosis in pre-pubertal obese children. *J Am Coll Cardiol.* 2009;54(25):2396–2406.

54. Paffenbarger RS Jr, Hyde RT, Wing AL, Steinmetz CH. A natural history of athleticism and cardiovascular health. *JAMA.* 1984;252(4):491–495.

55. Woo KS, Chook P, Yu CW, et al. Effects of diet and exercise on obesity-related vascular dysfunction in children. *Circulation.* 2004;109(16):1981–1986.

56. Couch SC, Saelens BE, Levin L, Dart K, Falciglia G, Daniels SR. The efficacy of a clinic-based behavioral nutrition intervention emphasizing a DASH-type diet for adolescents with elevated blood pressure. *J Pediatr.* 2008;152(4):494–501.

57. Gidding SS, Lichtenstein AH, Faith MS, et al. Implementing American Heart Association pediatric and adult nutrition guidelines: A scientific statement from the American Heart Association Nutrition Committee of the Council on Nutrition, Physical Activity and Metabolism, Council on Cardiovascular Disease in the Young, Council on Arteriosclerosis, Thrombosis and Vascular Biology, Council on Cardiovascular Nursing, Council on Epidemiology and Prevention, and Council for High Blood Pressure Research. *Circulation.* 3 2009;119(8):1161–1175.

58. Appel LJ, Moore TJ, Obarzanek E, et al. A clinical trial of the effects of dietary patterns on blood pressure. DASH Collaborative Research Group. *N Engl J Med.* 1997;336(16):1117–1124.

59. Conlin PR, Erlinger TP, Bohannon A, et al. The DASH diet enhances the blood pressure response to losartan in hypertensive patients. *Am J Hypertens.* 2003;16(5 Pt 1):337–342.

60. Sacks FM, Svetkey LP, Vollmer WM, et al. Effects on blood pressure of reduced dietary sodium and the Dietary Approaches to Stop Hypertension (DASH) diet. DASH-Sodium Collaborative Research Group. *N Engl J Med.* 2001;344(1):3–10.

61. Sharkey BJ. *NetLibrary Inc. Fitness and Health*, 4th ed. Champaign, IL: Human Kinetics, 1997. Available at: http://eresources.lib.unc.edu/external_db/external_database_auth.html?A=P%7CF=N%7CID=328%7CREL=AAL%7CURL=http://libproxy.lib.unc.edu/login?url=http://www.netLibrary.com/urlapi.asp?action=summary&v=1&bookid=28690.

62. Homer CJ. Responding to the childhood obesity epidemic: From the provider visit to health care policy—Steps the health care sector can take. *Pediatrics.* 2009;123 Suppl 5:S253–257.

63. Eat Smart MMNC. *Pediatric Obesity: Assessment, Prevention & Treatment Guide For Clinicians.* Available at: http://www.eatsmartmovemorenc.com/PediatricObesityTools/Texts/ClinicianRefGuide.pdf (accessed November 29, 2010).

64. Rubak S, Sandbaek A, Lauritzen T, Christensen B. Motivational interviewing: A systematic review and meta-analysis. *Br J Gen Pract.* 2005;55(513):305–312.

65. Schwartz RP, Hamre R, Dietz WH, et al. Office-based motivational interviewing to prevent childhood obesity: A feasibility study. *Arch Pediatr Adolesc Med.* 2007;161(5):495–501.

66. Schwartz RP. Motivational interviewing (patient-centered counseling) to address childhood obesity. *Pediatr Ann.* 2010;39(3):154–158.

67. NHLBI. Blood Pressure Tables for Children and Adolescents from the Fourth Report on the Diagnosis, Evaluation, and Treatment of High Blood Pressure in Children and Adolescents. Available at: http://www.nhlbi.nih.gov/guidelines/hypertension/child_tbl.htm (accessed September 5, 2011).

68. NICHQ. Expert Committee Recommendations on the Assessment, Prevention and Treatment of Child and Adolescent Overweight and Obesity-2007: An Implementation Guide from the Childhood Obesity Action Network. Available at: http://www.nichq.org/documents/coan-papers-and-publications/COANImplementationGuide62607FINAL.pdf (accessed September 5, 2011).

10 Lifestyle, Nutrition, and Hypertensive Disorders during Pregnancy

Chang-Ching Yeh
Yale University and Taipei Veterans General Hospital

*Zhen-Ming Wu**
Yale University and Shanghai Jiao Tong University

Deborah Day
Amity Regional High School

S. Joseph Huang
Yale University

CONTENTS

* Zhen-Ming Wu and Chang-Ching Yeh have equally contributed to this work.

10.1 INTRODUCTION

Hypertension is the most common medical problem encountered during pregnancy, complicating 6%–8% of pregnancies [1], and hypertensive disorders in pregnancy remain a leading source of maternal mortality and morbidity. The National High Blood Pressure Education Program Working Group on High Blood Pressure in Pregnancy classifies hypertensive disorders during pregnancy into four categories: (1) chronic hypertension, (2) preeclampsia–eclampsia, (3) preeclampsia superimposed on chronic hypertension, and (4) gestational hypertension (Table 10.1) [1].

Chronic hypertension in a pregnant woman is defined as hypertension that existed before pregnancy or that was diagnosed for the first time before 20 weeks of gestation. It also includes hypertension diagnosed during pregnancy that persists postpartum. Chronic hypertension affects 3% of pregnant women in the United States [2,3], with a higher prevalence seen in black women and older women [4,5]. As with nonpregnant women, the etiology of chronic hypertension in pregnant women is usually essential hypertension, but other causes such as renal diseases (e.g., glomerulonephritis, renal artery stenosis), connective tissue diseases (e.g., lupus erythematosus, systemic sclerosis), or endocrine disorders (e.g., hyperaldosteronism, pheochromocytoma) should also be considered [6]. Chronic hypertension is a known risk factor for preeclampsia [6]. Superimposed preeclampsia is seen in approximately 10%–25% of women with preexisting hypertension [5,7].

Preeclampsia develops in approximately 25%–50% of women with hypertension diagnosed during pregnancy. The later is the gestational age at the onset of hypertension, the higher is the rate of progression of hypertension to preeclampsia [8–10] and eclampsia. Eclampsia usually follows preeclampsia as patients suffer from seizures unrelated to preexisting brain conditions. However, up to 10% of eclampsia may occur in the absence of overt proteinuria or other symptoms associated with preeclampsia [11]. Thus, it is important for pregnant women with hypertension to always receive further evaluation, close monitoring, and proper treatment.

Preeclampsia superimposed on chronic hypertension is diagnosed when there is a new onset of proteinuria in women with hypertension before 20 weeks of gestation or there is a sudden worsening of hypertension and proteinuria in women with

TABLE 10.1

Classification of Hypertensive Disorders in Pregnancy

Hypertensive Disorders	Description
Chronic hypertension[a]	Hypertension present before pregnancy or diagnosed before 20 weeks of gestation or hypertension first diagnosed during pregnancy and persisting postpartum
Preeclampsia–eclampsia	Hypertension detected after 20 weeks of gestation in previously normotensive women, along with proteinuria, defined as urinary protein excretion $\geq$300 mg in a 24-h specimen (preferable) or $\geq$1+ reading on dipstick; occurrence of seizures in women with preeclampsia is not attributed to other causes
Preeclampsia superimposed on chronic hypertension	Diagnosis is highly likely in the following: (1) New onset of proteinuria in women with hypertension before 20 weeks of gestation (2) Sudden worsening of high blood pressure (BP) and proteinuria, presence of thrombocytopenia (<100,000 cells/mm^3), or elevated liver enzyme levels in women with hypertension and proteinuria before 20 weeks of gestation
Gestational hypertension	Hypertension diagnosed for the first time after 20 weeks of gestation without proteinuria, which normalizes postpartum (transient hypertension of pregnancy)

Source: Adapted and modified from National Heart, Lung, and Blood Institute, Report of the National High Blood Pressure Education Program Working Group on High Blood Pressure in Pregnancy, *Am. J. Obstet. Gynecol.,* 183, S1–S22, 2000.

[a] Hypertension is defined as systolic blood pressure (SBP) $\geq$ 140 mmHg and/or diastolic blood pressure (DBP) $\geq$ 90 mmHg.

hypertension and proteinuria before 20 weeks of gestation. All the chronic hypertensive disorders, despite their origins, may predispose to superimposed preeclampsia [6]. The onset of superimposed preeclampsia in chronic hypertensive women tends to be earlier than the onset of "pure" preeclampsia [12]. The severity of the disease is often more intense when preeclampsia is superimposed on chronic hypertension. Among women with chronic hypertension, those who have preeclampsia superimposed on chronic hypertension have a higher risk in the delivery of small-for-gestation baby and preterm birth than those who do not have such superimposition [12]. Intervention-related events including delivery at less than 34 weeks, cesarean delivery, and admission to neonatal intensive care unit are significantly higher in pregnant women with superimposed preeclampsia than in pregnant women with preeclampsia [13]. The underlying vasculopathy in chronic hypertensive disorders is proposed to deteriorate the complications found in superimposed preeclampsia [14]. Thus, target-organ damages, such as ventricular dysfunction, retinopathy, and nephropathy, should be closely monitored. To date, limited evidence regarding the nutrition and lifestyle prevention or management specific for this high-risk group is available.

Gestational hypertension refers to hypertension diagnosed for the first time after 20 weeks of gestation, without proteinuria, which resolves after delivery. Therefore, gestational hypertension is usually diagnosed postpartum, that is, it can be determined if blood pressure (BP) returns to normal in the postpartum period and if proteinuria does not develop either before or after delivery. Gestational hypertension is associated with intrauterine growth restriction and iatrogenic prematurity [15]. The etiology of gestational hypertension is unclear. Prepregnancy body mass index (BMI) and high altitude have been shown to be the risk factors [16,17]. In women with gestational hypertension, their risks for hypertension, diabetes, and cardiovascular diseases in later life are increased, which suggests the need for further follow-up and preventive lifestyle interventions postpartum [18–21].

The lifestyle approach to chronic hypertension in pregnant women is the same as that for adults in general, and it has been covered in other chapters of this book. Even though gestational hypertension and preeclampsia might share some lifestyle risk factors, very little is known about how lifestyle factors are related to gestational hypertension. Nevertheless, clinical management of BP is similar for all hypertensive disorders during pregnancy. Thus, this chapter mainly focuses on the association between various lifestyle and dietary factors and preeclampsia. Evidence on gestational hypertension is also discussed whenever data are available.

10.2 PREECLAMPSIA

Preeclampsia, manifested by hypertension and proteinuria after 20 weeks of gestation, is a systemic disorder of human pregnancy, which is a major cause of maternal and fetal morbidity and mortality. It complicates 5%–10% of pregnancies [22,23] and usually leads to intrauterine growth restriction and preterm delivery. Preeclampsia may result in adverse outcomes to both the mother and the fetus. Accumulated evidence indicates that fetal development in the uterus may also influence lifetime health of the baby [24–27], besides genetic influences, postpartum environment, or acquired factors. Prematurity plays a major role in the occurrence of major long-term morbid conditions such as chronic lung diseases [28], cardiovascular diseases [29], and intellectual and behavioral problems during postnatal development [30]. Several impacts of preeclampsia on mother's later life have been demonstrated. Similar to the impact of gestational hypertension, the risk of cardiovascular and cerebrovascular diseases in later life is doubled in women with preeclampsia compared with age-matched controls [31]. The risk of later renal disease in women with preeclampsia is 4- to 17-fold compared with that in uncomplicated pregnancies [32]. About 20% of women with preeclampsia develop hypertension or microalbuminuria within 7 years of their pregnancies compared with 2% of women with uncomplicated pregnancies [31]. Consequently, preeclampsia is a major cause of stress and financial burden for the affected families and the society.

The physiology of pregnancy and the pathophysiology of preeclampsia involving immune maladaptation, endothelial dysfunction, and aberrant oxidative stress suggest the potential for lifestyle and nutritional interventions to modify the incidence and course of preeclampsia. Following human implantation, blastocyst-derived extravillous trophoblasts invade the decidua where they surround, breach, and transform the spiral arteries to produce large-caliber, high-capacitance vessels. The resulting increased uterine blood flow to the intervillous space fulfills the requirements of development and survival of the fetoplacental unit [33,34]. Like other mucosal surfaces, the human uterus protects itself and the fetoplacental unit against pathogens. However, it is poised to mediate immune tolerance of the invading extravillous trophoblasts, thereby preventing rejection of the semiallogeneic embryo [35,36]. Fetal–maternal immune maladaptation perturbing this equilibrium may lead to preeclampsia [37]. Invasion of the decidua by shallow extravillous trophoblasts elicits incomplete remodeling of the decidual blood vessels [34,38] and a severely reduced uteroplacental blood flow. The resulting hypoxic placenta [39] releases an array of circulating factors that initiate systemic endothelial cell activation and dysfunction. Ultimately, the maternal syndrome of preeclampsia develops. In addition, an imbalance of pro- and antioxidants results in oxidative stress characterized by an accumulation of free radicals or reactive oxygen/nitrogen species. This oxidative stress is believed to underlie the maternal endothelial activation and extravillous trophoblasts apoptosis.

The pathophysiology of preeclampsia mediated through inflammatory responses [40], endothelial function [41], and oxidative stress may be modulated by nutrient intake, and thus prescribing multinutrient supplementation including antioxidants is a common practice by obstetricians. In this chapter, we review the evidence concerning the association of various nutrients, foods, and dietary patterns with preeclampsia. Since preeclampsia is a disorder manifested by cardiovascular involvements, lifestyle interventions aimed at reducing cardiovascular disease risk factors have been suggested for the prevention of preeclampsia. Thus, we review the evidence of other lifestyle factors also associated with the risk of preeclampsia [42,43].

10.3 LIFESTYLE

10.3.1 Obesity

According to the National Heart, Lung, and Blood Institute, obesity is defined as a condition characterized by a BMI ≥ 30.0. The other categories classified based on BMI are underweight (BMI < 18.5), normal ($18.5 \leq$ BMI ≤ 24.9), and overweight ($25.0 \leq$ BMI ≤ 29.9). The prevalence of obesity is increasing and has become a worldwide public health issue [44,45]. Consequently, the incidence of prepregnancy obesity is elevated each year [46–48]. Obesity usually leads to chronic, often fatal, health conditions, such as cardiovascular diseases, diabetes, and cancer. It is also related to increased risks in a variety of adverse pregnancy outcomes worldwide, such as gestational hypertension, preeclampsia, gestational diabetes mellitus, delivery of large-for-gestational-age (LGA) infants, and the overall incidence of fetal congenital defects in obese women compared with pregnant women with normal BMI [49–54]. Furthermore, an increasing body of evidence suggests that the adversity of maternal obesity on a fetus developing in such a suboptimal *in utero* environment may predispose it to chronic lung and cardiovascular diseases, as well as learning and behavioral problems, in the neonate's later life [55,56]. A positive correlation between the occurrence of increased BMI and the preeclampsia has been demonstrated by many studies [57–61]. In contrast, the risk of preeclampsia seems to be decreased in underweight women [62]. Moreover, controlling weight gain during pregnancy significantly reduces the risk of preeclampsia in overweight and obese women [63,64]. The risk of preeclampsia is increased with a higher rate of weight gain during pregnancy in each BMI category [65]. The alterations in lipid levels and the activation of an inflammatory state with the resulting oxidative stress and endothelial cell dysfunction in obesity have been proposed to be the underlying mechanisms of preeclampsia associated with obesity [66–68].

Although data from randomized trials are lacking, observational data suggest that preeclampsia may be prevented by avoiding or minimizing obesity prior to conception and avoiding excessive weight gain during pregnancy.

10.3.2 CIGARETTE SMOKING

The prevalence of cigarette smoking during pregnancy varies from 15% to 30% across countries [69–72], and it is rising in developing countries [73]. Smoking is associated with a number of adverse pregnancy outcomes, including significantly higher BP in the offspring [74]. Paradoxically, smoking has repeatedly been shown to be associated with an overall 30%–40% reduction in the risk of preeclampsia [75,76]. Interestingly, the relative risk of preeclampsia decreased with an increased number of daily cigarettes smoked at the onset of pregnancy. The protective effect of smoking on preeclampsia was even stronger for women who continued to smoke after 20 weeks of pregnancy [43,77,78]. Recent studies suggest that smoking in the first trimester only does not reduce the risk of preeclampsia [79]. Thus, smoking in the middle or late pregnancy may also play a major role in reducing the risk of preeclampsia [80]. The beneficial effects of cigarette smoking on preeclampsia and gestational hypertension were suggested to be mediated by nicotine through its inhibition of IL-2, the production of TNF-α [81] and thromboxane A2 [82], and the induction of antioxidants [83]. Furthermore, smoking is believed to affect proangiogenic mechanisms, which are important in successful pregnancies. Antiangiogenic factors such as soluble fms-like tyrosine kinase 1 (sFlt-1) and soluble endoglin (sEng) were found to be lower, and a proangiogenic factor such as placental growth factor (PlGF) was found to be higher in smokers during pregnancy [84,85]. The tobacco combustion product carbon monoxide (CO) was demonstrated to inhibit production of sFlt-1 and sEng [86] and trophoblast apoptosis [87], and it was found to be exhaled less by preeclamptic women [88]. A recent *in vitro* study showed that nicotine recovers the endothelial dysfunction resulting from excess sFlt-1 and sEng, suggesting its protective role against preeclampsia [89].

Interestingly, prepregnancy BMI does not affect the decreased risk of preeclampsia in smokers, suggesting that smoking is the dominant factor, while obesity and smoking act independently in affecting the occurrence of preeclampsia [90,91].

It is worth noting that any potential benefit of cigarette smoking on preeclampsia is overshadowed by its considerable detrimental effects on fetal growth and BP in the offspring, risk of placental abruption and placenta previa, risk of preterm birth and neonatal morbidity, as well as the risk to maternal health [92,93]. Nonetheless, understanding the mechanisms by which smoking apparently protects from preeclampsia may ultimately lead to new therapies that do not carry the considerable risks of smoking.

Early cessation of smoking is evidently beneficial to pregnancy outcomes, including reducing low-birth-weight infants and preterm birth [78,94], and is clearly indicated for the health of the mother regardless of the pregnancy status. Thus, pregnant women should be encouraged to quit smoking as early as possible.

10.3.3 Physical Activity

Physical activity has been proposed to affect pregnancy by stimulation of placental growth and angiogenesis, as well as reduction of oxidative stress and endothelial dysfunction [95], which play crucial roles in the pathogenesis of preeclampsia. In addition, epidemiological studies show that the incidence of preeclampsia is reduced by occupational [96] and leisure-time physical activity [42,97,98]. Thus, preventive measures, such as increased leisure-time activity in the year before pregnancy, have been hypothesized to be a beneficial strategy of proactively decreasing the incidence of preeclampsia. An early study showed that leisure-time physical activity during the first half of pregnancy is associated with reduced risk of both preeclampsia and gestational hypertension [97]. Consistently, combined work place and leisure-time activity was shown to reduce the risk of preeclampsia regardless of caloric expenditure, employment status, or level of physical activity [98]. On the other hand, another study showed that leisure-time physical activity during the year before pregnancy apparently does not protect against preeclampsia [99]. Both studies were observational; there are currently no clinical trial data to determine a causal relationship between physical activity and risk of preeclampsia. Thus, despite the promising potential of physical activity in protecting against preeclampsia, more studies are needed to draw definitive conclusions.

Pending additional data, pregnant women are encouraged to follow the national guideline on physical activity for pregnant women (www.health.gov/paguidelines). In brief, healthy women who are not already highly active or doing vigorous-intensity activity should get at least 150 min (2 h and 30 min) of moderate-intensity aerobic activity per week during pregnancy and the postpartum period. Preferably, this activity should be spread throughout the week. Pregnant women who habitually engage in vigorous-intensity aerobic activity or are highly active can continue physical activity during pregnancy and the postpartum period, provided that they remain healthy and discuss with their health care provider how and when the activity should be adjusted over time.

10.3.4 Alcohol

The placenta is essential for the maternal–fetal vascular supply and nutrition exchange. It plays important roles in the fetal development and the maintenance of a successful pregnancy. Alcohol consumption during pregnancy is known to result in dose-dependent placental vasoconstriction [100], which may lead to adverse pregnancy outcomes, including gestational hypertension. However, conflicting results were shown in the studies of alcohol consumption and individual adverse pregnancy outcomes, including preeclampsia [101–103]. Thus, existing research evidence is inconclusive regarding alcohol and hypertensive disorders during pregnancy. It is, nevertheless, prudent for pregnant women to avoid the potential negative impact of alcohol by limiting alcohol consumption during pregnancy. In addition, health care providers should inform pregnant women of the potential health risk from alcohol drinking.

10.3.5 Caffeine

Caffeine may be the most commonly consumed stimulant [104]. The major sources (96%) of caffeine are coffee and tea; others (4%) include caffeinated soft drinks, cocoa, chocolate, or medications [105]. Epidemiological studies suggest that coffee might be associated with high BP and plasma homocysteine levels [106]. Nonetheless, restriction of caffeine intake is not recommended in nonpregnant individuals. However, during pregnancy, caffeine intake has been demonstrated to increase the risks of spontaneous abortion, fetal growth restriction, low birth weight, and preterm delivery [106–110]. High consumption of caffeine may increase SBP, but not DBP, in the first and third trimester, but the evidence is not conclusive and further investigations are required [111]. According to the committee opinion of American College of Obstetricians and Gynecologists (ACOG) 2010, moderate caffeine intake (200 mg/day—roughly the amount in two cups of coffee) does not appear to lead to miscarriage or preterm birth [112]. Unexpectedly, caffeine consumption after 20 weeks of pregnancy was suggested to reduce the risk of preeclampsia in women with type I diabetes [113]. Chocolate is also reported to reduce the likelihood of preeclampsia [114,115]. Nonetheless, individual variation in caffeine metabolism due to various activities of enzymes including cytochrome p450 1A2 or N-acetyltransferase [116,117] and the accuracy of different methods in measuring caffeine intake should be taken into consideration. Future studies with a large cohort and more precise measurement of caffeine intake are needed to understand the effect of caffeine on preeclampsia and BP in pregnancy.

Until further evidence is available, it is advisable for pregnant women to limit coffee consumption to 3 cups/day (<300 mg caffeine/day) during pregnancy to avoid the possibility of adverse pregnancy outcomes [118] (Table 10.2).

10.4 MACRONUTRIENTS

Maternal factors such as infection, obesity, diabetes, and microvascular diseases are proposed to increase the risk of preeclampsia. Although it is still controversial, maternal nutritional status is also proposed to contribute to the occurrence of preeclampsia. Micronutrient intake during pregnancy is necessary not only for fetal development but also for preventing the development of preeclampsia. Thus, in recent decades, more attention has been paid to the role of several micronutrients and dietary components in the development of preeclampsia.

10.4.1 Calorie Intake

A balanced maternal calorie intake is required for the development of the fetus during pregnancy [119]. The study of wartime famine illustrates the association between

TABLE 10.2
Relationship between Lifestyle and Preeclampsia and Recommendations for Prevention

Lifestyle	Relationship with Preeclampsia	Recommendations
Obesity	Known risk factor for preeclampsia	Control weight gain (to within 25–40 lb) during pregnancy
		Reduce weight before pregnancy in overweight/obese women to a realistic goal
Smoking	Reduces risk of preeclampsia, but the benefit does not outweigh other adverse pregnancy outcomes caused by smoking	Smoking cessation
Physical activity	May reduce risk of preeclampsia	Healthy women who are not already highly active should get at least 150 min of moderate-intensity aerobic activity per week during pregnancy and postpartum
		Pregnant women who are habitually highly active should continue physical activity during pregnancy and postpartum
Alcohol	May be associated with placenta-associated syndromes such as placental abruption and placenta previa. However, no direct evidence in the pathogenesis of preeclampsia. May contribute to fetal alcohol syndrome	Avoid during pregnancy
Caffeine	No direct evidence of relationship with preeclampsia. High dosage may result in other adverse pregnancy outcomes	Limit daily consumption to three cups

maternal diet and the pregnancy outcome in humans. A low food intake during widespread hunger in Holland during World War II (Dutch Hunger) reduced the nutrition supply from the mother to the fetus and resulted in a smaller baby at birth [120]. A high-calorie diet has been shown to induce endothelial dysfunction, oxidative stress, and inflammatory responses [121,122], and hence lead to hypertension [123], suggesting the association of high-calorie intake and the risk of preeclampsia [124,125] (see Section 10.3.1). Although an increased BMI seems to correlate with the susceptibility of pregnant women to preeclampsia, the restriction of calorie intake in obese pregnant women has been shown to have no effect on the development of preeclampsia [126]. Therefore, the effects of calorie intake on the development of preeclampsia still need to be scrutinized.

The ACOG suggests an extra calorie intake of 300 kcal/day during pregnancy for women of normal weight. Similarly, the Dietary References Intakes (DRI) recommends an extra intake of about 400 kcal/day during the second and third trimesters [127].

10.4.2 Protein

The severity of hypertension is affected by the intake of various nutrients. Proteins are biochemical compounds consisting of polypeptides containing amino acids, which are essential for fetal growth and development. The fetoplacental unit consumes approximately 1 kg of protein during pregnancy, with the majority of this requirement in the last 6 months. To fulfill this need, pregnant women are suggested to ingest 1.1 g/kg/day of protein, which is moderately higher than the 0.8 g/kg/day recommended for nonpregnant adult women [128]. It has been suggested that some amino acids such as arginine, citrulline, glycine, and histidine may scavenge free oxygen radicals to maintain the normal endothelial function [41,129,130]. Epidemiological studies indicate that higher protein intake is associated with lower BP levels [131], and relatively higher protein intake is a component of the BP-lowering Dietary Approaches to Stop Hypertension (DASH) dietary pattern [132]. However, there is no direct evidence to show the relationship between low protein intake and the pathogenesis of preeclampsia [125,133]. Similarly, recent studies found that a high-protein diet (protein providing at least 25% of total energy content) does not reduce the risk of preeclampsia [126], and protein restriction might only prevent deterioration of chronic renal insufficiency [134].

Thus, the effect of protein intake on the development of preeclampsia remains unclear [133]. Protein intake of 1.1 g/kg/day is recommended during pregnancy to meet the physiological demands.

10.4.3 Sugar

In observational data, high sugar intake is related to an increased risk of preeclampsia [125]. Hyperglycemia after sugar loading suppresses endothelium-dependent vasodilation [135], which may contribute to the development of preeclampsia. In addition, high intake of sucrose may exacerbate existing dyslipidemia in women with preeclampsia. Similarly, a study of dietary pattern during pregnancy suggests that high consumption of cake and soft drinks increases the risk of preeclampsia [136]. Although higher sugar intake is associated with a higher prevalence of preeclampsia, whether the higher risk of preeclampsia is due to higher sugar intake per se or due to an increased maternal BMI as a result of increased caloric intake needs to be further investigated [137]. Thus, it is inconclusive if sugar intake is associated with preeclampsia or not; however, it is prudent for pregnant women to follow the national dietary guidelines of reducing added sugar intake (http://www.cnpp.usda. gov/DGAs2010-PolicyDocument.htm).

10.4.4 Salt Intake

In the early twentieth century, edema was believed to lead to hypertension in preeclampsia, and a low-salt diet was often recommended as a treatment of edema to reduce the development of high BP. However, edema is now recognized as a common symptom observed in normal pregnancy. Thus, this recommendation has not been valid since 1950s. Strict dietary sodium restriction during pregnancy was found to result in the reduction of the intake of energy, protein, and calcium, which limited normal maternal weight gain [138]. An observation in a pregnant mouse model showed that an increase in sodium intake could reverse the gestation-associated vasopressor resistance via modulating the activity of potassium and calcium channels and consequently inducing hypertension [139]. This observation suggests that salt intake affects maternal BP [139]. However, epidemiological studies suggest that the reduction of salt intake is not associated with the development of preeclampsia [140].

Therefore, whether salt restriction is beneficial for the prevention and the treatment of preeclampsia is undetermined. Nevertheless, pregnant women should follow the national guidelines and limit sodium intake to <2300 mg/day, or to <1500 mg/day if any hypertensive disorder is diagnosed (http://www.cnpp.usda.gov/DGAs2010-PolicyDocument.htm).

10.4.5 LIPID AND FISH OIL

Metabolic syndrome is characterized by maternal obesity, diabetes mellitus, hypertriglyceridemia, hyperleptinemia, and chronic hypertension. Evidences of chronic systemic inflammation, insulin resistance, oxidative stress, hypercoagulopathy, and diffuse endothelial dysfunction can be detected in patients with metabolic syndrome [141,142]. Since endothelial dysfunction resulting from impaired spiral artery remodeling is known to be responsible for the development of preeclampsia, hypertriglyceridemia is proposed to be a potential risk factor for preeclampsia [143]. Moreover, women with preeclampsia have higher levels of both circulating free fatty acids and markers of low-density lipoprotein (LDL) oxidation, an essential step in lipid-mediated endothelial dysfunction [143]. Further clinical studies are required to determine whether prepregnancy weight reduction and dietary modification of lipid intake can lower the risk of preeclampsia.

Fish oils are a rich source of the n-3 long-chain polyunsaturated fatty acids (PUFA), eicosapentaenoic acid (EPA), and docosahexaenoic acid (DHA). These fatty acids are precursors to the 3-series prostaglandins and have been shown to modulate inflammatory and vascular functions. Since preeclampsia and gestational hypertension are associated with vasoconstriction and endothelial damage, it is plausible that fish oil fatty acids, especially EPA, may inhibit detrimental effects on the endothelium through direct competition with thromboxane A2 precursor, that is, arachidonic acid. Also, fish oil fatty acids have been shown to decrease platelet aggregation. Thus, fish oil was believed to be beneficial for the prevention of preeclampsia [144]. However, according to many epidemiological studies, the effect of fish oil supplementation on the reduction of preeclampsia is still controversial [145–147].

Hyperlipidemia is speculated to be involved in the pathogenesis of preeclampsia. Further studies are required to demonstrate the causal effects. Pregnant women are recommended to consume omega-3 fatty acids from sources including vegetable oils, seafood (2 servings/week), and omega-3 fatty acid supplements containing EPA and DHA or DHA alone [148]. However, existing evidence does not support the recommendation to modify fat or fish oil intake for the prevention of preeclampsia.

10.5 MICRONUTRIENTS

Micronutrients are vitamins and minerals required in minute amounts for normal functioning, growth, and development during pregnancy. Micronutrient status may play an important role in normal and pathological pregnancies [149]. An increasing body of evidence indicates that certain micronutrient deficiencies are involved in the occurrence of endothelial dysfunction, oxidative stress, and inflammatory response, which can lead to the development of preeclampsia [150].

10.5.1 VITAMIN A

Vitamin A is a lipid-soluble molecule that can be found in two principal forms, such as retinoids and carotenoids, in foods. Retinoids, retinol and retinoic acid, are found in animal-derived foods, including liver, kidney, eggs, and dairy products. Carotenoids, such as beta-carotene, are found in plants, including dark or yellow vegetables and carrots [151]. Beta-carotene can be converted to vitamin A in the liver where vitamin A is stored. In pregnancy, an additional amount of vitamin A is required for fetal growth and maternal metabolism; hence, ACOG recommends a dietary intake of 770 μg/day during pregnancy. Patients with vitamin A deficiency have been shown to be more vulnerable to infections [152], and vitamin A supplement may enhance antibody production through its role in immune protection [153]. Moreover, beta-carotene was shown to decrease endothelial cell damage via its antioxidant activity [152]. All these findings suggest that vitamin A may help in the prevention of preeclampsia; however, clinical studies have shown inconsistent association between preeclampsia and vitamin A levels [151,154–156]. Thus, more research is needed to clarify the role of vitamin A in prevention of preeclampsia.

10.5.2 VITAMIN B AND FOLATE

Folate, vitamin B6, and vitamin B12 are essential for homocysteine metabolism [157], and elevated homocysteine level is considered a risk factor for cardiovascular diseases [158]. Abnormal maternal and fetal homocysteine metabolism is believed to be associated with fetal neural tube defect coexisting with various conditions characterized by placental vasculopathy, including preeclampsia. ACOG suggests a dietary intake of 600 μg/day of folate, 1.9 mg/day of vitamin B6, and 2.6 μg/day of vitamin B12 during pregnancy. In normal pregnancy, homocysteine level declines as pregnancy progresses [159]. Homocysteine level is elevated in patients with preeclampsia than in women with normal pregnancy [160,161]. Clinically, hyperhomocysteinemia induces oxidative stress and endothelial dysfunction that ultimately lead to hypertension and proteinuria during gestation [162]. Although vitamin B6, vitamin B12, and folate are implicated in the regulation of homocysteine levels [163], the plasma levels of vitamin B12 and folate are not significantly different between normal pregnant women and women with preeclampsia [164]. Furthermore, folate deficiency, not hyperhomocysteinemia, has lead to the development of hypertension and proteinuria in a mouse model [162].

Thus, a direct association between vitamin B6, vitamin B12, and folate deficiency and the occurrence of preeclampsia has not been made [157,163,164]. Therefore, the benefit of vitamin B6, vitamin B12, and folate, in food or as supplementation, in the prevention of preeclampsia cannot be determined yet [157,159,164].

10.5.3 Vitamin D

Vitamin D is not only obtained from food, but it is also derived from the synthesis of a steroid precursor. The main dietary sources of vitamin D are oily fish, cod liver oil, and fortified margarine and milk [165]. During pregnancy, maternal serum concentrations of 25-hydroxyvitamin D (25-(OH)D), the circulating form of vitamin D, are highly correlated with dietary vitamin D intake and vitamin D obtained from exposure to sun [166].

In nonpregnant individuals, vitamin D is essential for calcium homeostasis, bone mineralization, immune function, and cell proliferation [167]. The classical function of vitamin D is found in kidneys, liver, and intestine to facilitate calcium and phosphate absorption, as well as bone synthesis and metabolism. Recent data indicate that vitamin D functions in nonclassical ways as well. In general, $1,25(OH)_2D$ reduces the activity of the adaptive immune system while enhancing the activity of the innate immune system. $1,25(OH)_2D$ also plays a critical role in modulating cell-cycle progression, cell differentiation, and the induction of apoptosis.

During pregnancy, synthesis of $24,25(OH)_2D$ occurs in human decidua and placenta, whereas $1,25(OH)_2D$ is found only in the decidua. The active form of vitamin D, $1,25(OH)_2D$, is elevated in the maternal circulation during pregnancy [167]. Placental gene expression involved in normal placentation, including extravillous trophoblast invasion and angiogenesis, is possibly controlled by $1,25(OH)D$ [168]. Vitamin D deficiency was shown to increase BP. Vitamin D deficiency during pregnancy is potentially associated with the occurrence of preeclampsia, insulin resistance, and gestational diabetes mellitus, relating to its nonclassical functions [169]. Interestingly, impaired vitamin D metabolism is found in preeclampsia. Low serum vitamin D in early pregnancy was demonstrated to predispose women to preeclampsia [170]. This observation is supported by reduced incidence of preeclampsia with vitamin D supplementation in one study [165], but there are contradictory results in other studies [171]. The immunomodulatory properties of vitamin D may also be relevant to the pathogenesis of preeclampsia.

DRI recommends daily dietary intake of 15-µg vitamin D during pregnancy. Taken together, vitamin D supplementation is recommended during pregnancy mainly for other reasons (e.g., to prevent hypocalcemic seizure [172] and bone weakness in babies [173,174]), but it is unclear if it prevents preeclampsia.

10.5.4 Vitamin C and Vitamin E

Impaired uterine spiral artery remodeling can result in oxidative stress and subsequent inflammatory responses, as well as endothelial activation, which account for the characteristics of preeclampsia, including vascular vasospasm, capillary leakage, and coagulopathy. Preeclamptic placenta was found to have lower levels of antioxidants [175] and higher lipid oxidative stress compared with control placenta [176]. Vitamins C and E are two essential nutrients that scavenge free radicals and inhibit reactive oxygen species (ROS)-induced cellular damage. Based on the biological actions of these antioxidants, supplementation of these vitamins during pregnancy is believed to prevent or delay the onset of preeclampsia but direct evidence of such an effect is lacking [177].

Vitamin C or ascorbic acid is an essential water-soluble micronutrient involved in the synthesis of collagen, and it also functions as an antioxidant. Unlike most animals, humans are unable to synthesize vitamin C; therefore, they need to maintain an adequate dietary intake of vitamin C. ACOG suggests dietary intake of 85 mg/day of vitamin C during pregnancy. Vitamin C is found in many fruits and vegetables, with high levels noted in guava, blackcurrants, citrus fruits, strawberries, tomatoes, and broccoli [177]. During pregnancy, vitamin C is actively transported across the placenta [178]. As an antioxidant, vitamin C protects tissues from damage by harmful free radicals. Women with preeclampsia have lower levels of circulating vitamin C [179]. Studies have also showed that the risk of preeclampsia was increased in women with elevated levels of plasma-oxidized LDL and low levels of circulating vitamin C [122] or in women with less than 85 mg of vitamin C consumption daily [180]. Although there may be a potential benefit of vitamin C supplementation in preventing preeclampsia, the safety and effectiveness of high-dose vitamin C supplementation in preventing preeclampsia still needs to be clarified [178].

Vitamin E is the major lipid-soluble and plant-derived antioxidant in the body, including four tocopherols and four tocotrienols. Besides its antioxidant function, vitamin E enhances the release of prostacyclin, a metabolite of arachidonic acid that inhibits platelet aggregation, suppresses uterine contractility, increases vasodilation, and hence increases blood flow from mother to the fetoplacental unit [181]. Daily dietary consumption of 15 mg of vitamin E is recommended during pregnancy.

Natural alpha-tocopherol is the most biologically active form of vitamin E. A high level of tocopherol is found in some plant oils, including wheat germ oil, nuts, some cereals, and some leafy green vegetables. Vitamin E deficiency, rarely seen in healthy adults, can be aggravated by iron overload and high dietary intake of PUFA. During pregnancy, transfer of vitamin E to the fetus are believed to be minimal [178]. Vitamin E protects phospholipid fatty acids from oxidation by harmful free radicals, thereby stabilizing cell membranes. The link between oxidative stress and the development of adult diseases, including cardiovascular diseases, cancer, and chronic inflammation, implicates its role in the development of preeclampsia. A reduced level of vitamin E in patients with severe preeclampsia has been consistently reported [182], but there is no clear evidence that vitamin E supplementation prevents the development of preeclampsia.

The synergistic effect between vitamins C and E makes the coadministration of these two vitamins more effective in promoting their antioxidation effects. Nevertheless, outcomes of clinical trials yield conflicting results concerning the efficacy of these vitamins in reducing the incidence or severity of preeclampsia [177,183–186]. Some recent studies found that excessive amount of combined vitamin C (1000 mg/day) and vitamin E (400 IU/day) supplement during pregnancy not only fails to prevent preeclampsia but also relates to increased risks of preterm rupture of membranes and low birth weight [187,188]. Thus, the role of vitamin C and E supplements and the role of their antioxidant properties in the prevention of preeclampsia remain inconclusive.

10.5.5 IRON

Iron is an essential micronutrient for the formation of hemoglobin to transport oxygen, and it is required for the synthesis of enzymes involved in aerobic reactions to provide energy [120]. Iron-rich foods include liver, meat, fish, poultry, and non-animal-derived foods, such as legumes, green-leafy vegetables, nut, oilseeds, and dried fruits. In general, animal-derived foods tend to have higher iron content than non-animal-derived foods [189]. Iron absorption may be inhibited by the mixed intake of some other elements, such as cereal grains, milk products, coffee and cocoa, or phosphates in egg yolk.

Body iron is mainly stored in the reticuloendothelial cells in the bone marrow, liver, and spleen. The demand for iron during pregnancy gradually increases from 0.8 mg/day in the first trimester to 7.5 mg/day in the third trimester [190]. The iron intake during pregnancy is predominantly used to expand the woman's erythrocyte mass, fulfill the iron requirements of the fetus, and compensate for iron loss at delivery. Dietary iron is insufficient to fulfill the iron requirement during pregnancy. ACOG recommends dietary intake of 27 mg/day during pregnancy.

Epidemiological studies showed that the mean serum iron level in women with preeclampsia is significantly higher than that in normal pregnant women, whereas the total iron-binding capacity is significantly lower in preeclamptic patients [191]. Serum transferrin levels (a measure of iron storage) are significantly decreased only in women with severe preeclampsia. These observations suggest that oxidative stress can be induced by excess amounts of free iron, which may play a role in the development of preeclampsia. However, there is no association between iron supplementation and the incidence of preeclampsia [190].

10.5.6 CALCIUM

Calcium plays crucial roles in bone metabolism, signal transduction, release of neurotransmitter from neurons, muscle contraction, maintaining cell membrane potential, blood coagulation, and fertilization. Calcium also functions as a cofactor for many enzymes. Such factors associated with calcium homeostasis as membrane stability of vascular smooth muscle cells, the production and secretion of endothelium-derived relaxing factor, neuronal function, vascular relaxation, and calcium-regulating hormones (parathyroid hormone and calcitonin) have been proposed to be involved in the regulation of BP [192].

ACOG recommends dietary intake of 1000 mg/day calcium during pregnancy. Low calcium intake induces either parathyroid hormone or renin secretion, which increases intracellular calcium in vascular smooth muscle cells and ultimately leads to vasoconstriction [193]. Given these observations, calcium supplementation can potentially reduce smooth muscle contractility and lower BP. Moreover, calcium supplementation reduces vascular angiotensin II sensitivity, prolongs the mean duration of gestation, reduces the incidence of premature delivery, lowers BP, and reduces the incidence of gestational hypertension [138,194]. A fluctuation of calcium levels in red blood cells, platelets, immune cells, endothelial cells, vascular smooth muscle cells, and extracellular matrix was also detected in the patients with preeclampsia [195]. Hence, calcium supplementation is proposed as a potential intervention to reduce the risk of preeclampsia. Unfortunately, the role of calcium supplementation in preventing preeclampsia is still undetermined due to inconsistency among clinical studies [150,192,194,196].

10.5.7 Magnesium

Magnesium is an essential mineral for bone metabolism, neurotransmission, cardiac excitability, neuromuscular conduction, muscle contraction, vasomotor tone, and maintenance of BP. Chronic magnesium deficiency has been detected in many chronic diseases, including diabetes mellitus, hypertension, coronary heart disease, and osteoporosis [197].

Parenteral magnesium sulfate prevents recurrent seizures in patients with preeclampsia [198] and in pregnant women with varying degrees of hypertension. Such success suggests that magnesium might be deficient in women with preeclampsia. Indeed, a reduction in magnesium levels in serum, intracellular compartments, and erythrocytes was detected in some patients with preeclampsia [199]. Therefore, the potential role of magnesium in the pathogenesis of preeclampsia and the preventive effect of its supplementation have been proposed. Nonetheless, increasing dietary magnesium during pregnancy does not seem to be beneficial [200]. Thus, further investigation is needed to define the role of magnesium and preeclampsia and other hypertensive disorders during pregnancy.

10.5.8 Selenium

The trace element selenium is an essential component of the antioxidant selenoproteins, such as glutathione peroxidase (GPx) and thioredoxin reductase [201]. Reduced GPx is associated with the generation of toxic lipid peroxides and leads to endothelial dysfunction and hypertension. Selenium plays critical roles in regulating antioxidation, adjustment of immune function, and cell growth.

Selenium levels in maternal sera decrease as gestation proceeds, presumably due to an increasing metabolic demand [202]. The selenium level is further decreased in women with preeclampsia [201]. Low selenium was found to correlate with the severity of preeclampsia [203,204]. Thus, low maternal selenium may predispose to preeclampsia. In a rat model, it was found that selenium deficiency was associated with preeclampsia [205]. In a pilot study in humans, selenium supplementation tended to reduce the incidence of preeclampsia, but the results were not statistically significant [206]. Thus, the clinical relevance of selenium supplementation for the prevention of preeclampsia is still uncertain. Since high selenium levels may potentially induce cancerous diseases and type II diabetes [207,208], the risks versus benefits of selenium supplementation in pregnant women at high risk of preeclampsia remain questionable [203,209].

TABLE 10.3

Relationship between Nutrient Intake and Preeclampsia and Recommendations for Prevention

Nutrients	Relationship with Preeclampsia	Recommendations
Protein	Unclear. Limited clinical evidence available	DRI: 71 g/day
Sugar	Inconclusive. High sugar intake may be associated with increased risk of preeclampsia	National dietary guideline: reduce added sugar intake
Salt	Inconclusive. Limited clinical evidence available	National dietary guideline: limit sodium intake to ≤2300 mg/day in non-hypertensive women and 1500 mg/day in hypertensive pregnant women
Lipid and fish oil	Inconclusive	Control weight gain during pregnancy. Consume omega-3 fatty acids from vegetable oils, seafood, and omega-3 fatty acid supplements
Vitamin A	Inconclusive	DRI: 770 µg/day
Vitamin B and folate	Inconclusive	DRI: Vitamin B6: 1.9 mg/day, vitamin B12: 2.6 µg/day, and folate: 600 µg/day
Vitamin D	Vitamin D deficiency is associated with preeclampsia. Inconclusive clinical evidence on supplementation of vitamin D and the prevention of preeclampsia.	DRI: 15 µg/day
Vitamin C and E	Low circulating levels of vitamin C and E are associated with preeclampsia. Inconclusive evidence on supplementation of vitamin C and E and prevention of preeclampsia. Some studies even show that excessive combined supplement of vitamin C and E increases the risks of adverse pregnancy outcomes	DRI: Vitamin C: 85 mg/day and vitamin E: 15 mg/day
Iron	Unclear. Limited clinical evidence available	DRI: 27 mg/day
Calcium	Calcium supplementation may reduce the risk of preeclampsia	DRI: 1000 mg/day
Magnesium	Unclear. Limited clinical evidence available	DRI: 350–360 mg/day
Selenium	Selenium deficiency was found in preeclampsia. Inconclusive clinical evidence on supplementation of selenium and the prevention of preeclampsia	DRI: 60 mg/day
Zinc	Unclear. Limited clinical evidence available	DRI: 11 mg/day

10.5.9 ZINC

Zinc is required for normal cell function and metabolism and for maintaining the function of free radical-scavenging enzymes, such as superoxide dismutase [210]. Since oxidative stress may play an important role in the development of preeclampsia, impaired antioxidation by a decrease in the activity of superoxide dismutase due to zinc deficiency may be related to the pathogenesis of preeclampsia. However, conflicting data regarding zinc level and preeclampsia were reported [199,211]. Therefore, the benefit of zinc supplementation in the prevention of preeclampsia remains an unresolved issue [211] (Table 10.3).

10.6 SUMMARY

Preeclampsia is a life-threatening hypertensive disorder that occurs during pregnancy, which increases the maternal and the perinatal morbidity and mortality. Although our understanding of preeclampsia and other hypertensive disorders in pregnancy has dramatically increased in the past decades, the actual pathophysiology of such pregnancy complications remains unclear. Although delivery is the only effective treatment for preeclampsia and the treatment for hypertensive disorders in pregnancy is limited, early identification of high-risk groups, adequate monitoring, and timely intervention are crucial in managing and reducing adverse outcomes.

Although many potential lifestyle and dietary factors may be responsible in the development of hypertensive disorders in pregnancy, many questions remain to be answered (Figure 10.1). Obesity is a known risk factor for preeclampsia and

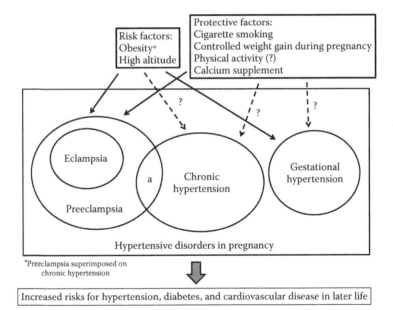

FIGURE 10.1 Factors affecting hypertensive disorders in pregnancy. Obesity and high altitude are related to increased risk of preeclampsia and gestational hypertension, whereas cigarette smoking, controlled weight gain during pregnancy, and calcium supplement may have protective effect against preeclampsia. Hypertensive disorders in pregnancy are associated with increased risks of hypertension, diabetes, and cardiovascular diseases in mother's later life. *Note*: Obesity is a known risk factor for essential hypertension, gestational hypertension, and preeclampsia. However, current evidence is insufficient to clarify its relationship with chronic hypertension in pregnancy.

gestational hypertension, and hence adequate weight control may be a preventive measure. Physical activity may also be beneficial in preventing preeclampsia; however, conflicting results exist. Recommendations for intake of micro- and macronutrients are even less evidence-based.

Despite the evidence of association between various nutrients and preeclampsia, the causative role of various nutrients has not been thoroughly studied, and there is very little clinical trial evidence to establish the efficacy of supplementing or restricting various nutrients to prevent or treat preeclampsia. Sodium restriction apparently does not prevent preeclampsia. High sugar intake may promote obesity, a risk factor for preeclampsia, but it probably does not affect preeclampsia risk directly [150]. Supplementation with calcium, vitamin D, n-3 fatty acids, vitamin C, and vitamin E in high-risk women seems to be promising in the prevention of preeclampsia, but there are no conclusive clinical trials. High daily intake of fiber has been shown to reduce the risk of hypertension and insulin resistance, suggesting a possible protective role against preeclampsia. Additional evidence is needed for all these dietary factors. In addition, it is unlikely that preeclampsia is caused by or can be prevented by a single nutrient, and evidence concerning combinations of nutrients or dietary patterns is lacking. In the absence of evidence, a prudent approach to lifestyle in the pregnant woman involves screening for the lifestyle risk factors, assessing nutritional status, recommending general healthy lifestyle guidelines, and providing supplements that are clearly effective in promoting maternal and fetal health.

REFERENCES

1. National Heart, Lung, and Blood Institute. Report of the National High Blood Pressure Education Program Working Group on High Blood Pressure in Pregnancy. *Am J Obstet Gynecol* 2000;183: S1–S22.
2. Wolz M, Cutler J, Roccella EJ, et al. Statement from the National High Blood Pressure Education Program: Prevalence of hypertension. *Am J Hypertens* 2000;13: 103–104.
3. Walther T, Wessel N, Baumert M, et al. Longitudinal analysis of heart rate variability in chronic hypertensive pregnancy. *Hypertens Res* 2005;28: 113–118.
4. Wallis AB, Saftlas AF, Hsia J, Atrash HK. Secular trends in the rates of preeclampsia, eclampsia, and gestational hypertension, United States, 1987–2004. *Am J Hypertens* 2008;21: 521–526.
5. Jim B, Sharma S, Kebede T, Acharya A. Hypertension in pregnancy: A comprehensive update. *Cardiol Rev* 2010;18: 178–189.
6. Sibai BM. Chronic hypertension in pregnancy. *Obstet Gynecol* 2002;100: 369–377.
7. Gilbert WM, Young AL, Danielsen B. Pregnancy outcomes in women with chronic hypertension: A population-based study. *J Reprod Med* 2007;52: 1046–1051.
8. Barton JR, O'Brien JM, Bergauer NK, Jacques DL, Sibai BM. Mild gestational hypertension remote from term: Progression and outcome. *Am J Obstet Gynecol* 2001;184: 979–983.
9. Saudan P, Brown MA, Buddle ML, Jones M. Does gestational hypertension become pre-eclampsia? *Br J Obstet Gynaecol* 1998;105: 1177–1184.
10. Magee LA, von Dadelszen P, Bohun CM, et al. Serious perinatal complications of nonproteinuric hypertension: An international, multicentre, retrospective cohort study. *J Obstet Gynaecol Can* 2003;25: 372–382.

11. Chesley LC. Diagnosis of preeclampsia. *Obstet Gynecol* 1985;65: 423–425.
12. Chappell LC, Enye S, Seed P, et al. Adverse perinatal outcomes and risk factors for preeclampsia in women with chronic hypertension: A prospective study. *Hypertension* 2008;51: 1002–1009.
13. Tuuli MG, Rampersad R, Stamilio D, Macones G, Odibo AO. Perinatal outcomes in women with preeclampsia and superimposed preeclampsia: Do they differ? *Am J Obstet Gynecol* 2011;204: 508 e1–e7.
14. Sibai BM, Lindheimer M, Hauth J, et al. Risk factors for preeclampsia, abruptio placentae, and adverse neonatal outcomes among women with chronic hypertension. National Institute of Child Health and Human Development Network of Maternal-Fetal Medicine Units. *N Engl J Med* 1998;339: 667–671.
15. Sibai BM, Gordon T, Thom E, et al. Risk factors for preeclampsia in healthy nulliparous women: A prospective multicenter study. The National Institute of Child Health and Human Development Network of Maternal-Fetal Medicine Units. *Am J Obstet Gynecol* 1995;172: 642–648.
16. Ehrenthal DB, Jurkovitz C, Hoffman M, Jiang X, Weintraub WS. Prepregnancy body mass index as an independent risk factor for pregnancy-induced hypertension. *J Womens Health* (Larchmt) 2011;20: 67–72.
17. Moore LG, Hershey DW, Jahnigen D, Bowes W, Jr. The incidence of pregnancy-induced hypertension is increased among Colorado residents at high altitude. *Am J Obstet Gynecol* 1982;144: 423–429.
18. Lykke JA, Langhoff-Roos J, Sibai BM, et al. Hypertensive pregnancy disorders and subsequent cardiovascular morbidity and type 2 diabetes mellitus in the mother. *Hypertension* 2009;53: 944–951.
19. Magnussen EB, Vatten LJ, Smith GD, Romundstad PR. Hypertensive disorders in pregnancy and subsequently measured cardiovascular risk factors. *Obstet Gynecol* 2009;114: 961–970.
20. Garovic VD, Bailey KR, Boerwinkle E, et al. Hypertension in pregnancy as a risk factor for cardiovascular disease later in life. *J Hypertens* 2010;28: 826–833.
21. Robbins CL, Dietz PM, Bombard J, Valderrama AL. Gestational hypertension: A neglected cardiovascular disease risk marker. *Am J Obstet Gynecol* 2011;203: e1–e9.
22. Duley L. Maternal mortality associated with hypertensive disorders of pregnancy in Africa, Asia, Latin America and the Caribbean. *Br J Obstet Gynaecol* 1992;99: 547–553.
23. Duley L. The global impact of pre-eclampsia and eclampsia. *Semin Perinatol* 2009;33: 130–137.
24. Barker DJ. The fetal and infant origins of adult disease. *BMJ* 1990;301: 1111.
25. Barker DJ. Fetal nutrition and cardiovascular disease in later life. *Br Med Bull* 1997;53: 96–108.
26. Lucas A, Fewtrell MS, Cole TJ. Fetal origins of adult disease-the hypothesis revisited. *BMJ* 1999;319: 245–249.
27. Alexander BT. Fetal programming of hypertension. *Am J Physiol Regul Integr Comp Physiol* 2006;290: R1–R10.
28. Correa-Villasenor A, Ferencz C, Boughman JA, Neill CA. Total anomalous pulmonary venous return: Familial and environmental factors. The Baltimore-Washington Infant Study Group. *Teratology* 1991;44: 415–428.
29. Levent E, Atik T, Darcan S, et al. The relation of arterial stiffness with intrauterine growth retardation. *Pediatr Int* 2009;51: 807–811.
30. Hack M, Taylor HG, Klein N, et al. School-age outcomes in children with birth weights under 750 g. *N Engl J Med* 1994;331: 753–759.
31. Nisell H, Lintu H, Lunell NO, Mollerstrom G, Pettersson E. Blood pressure and renal function seven years after pregnancy complicated by hypertension. *Br J Obstet Gynaecol* 1995;102: 876–881.

32. Vikse BE, Irgens LM, Bostad L, Iversen BM. Adverse perinatal outcome and later kidney biopsy in the mother. *J Am Soc Nephrol* 2006;17: 837–845.
33. Moffett-King A. Natural killer cells and pregnancy. *Nat Rev Immunol* 2002;2: 656–663.
34. Kaufmann P, Black S, Huppertz B. Endovascular trophoblast invasion: Implications for the pathogenesis of intrauterine growth retardation and preeclampsia. *Biol Reprod* 2003;69: 1–7.
35. Miyazaki S, Tsuda H, Sakai M, et al. Predominance of Th2-promoting dendritic cells in early human pregnancy decidua. *J Leukoc Biol* 2003;74: 514–522.
36. Piccinni MP, Romagnani S. Regulation of fetal allograft survival by a hormone-controlled Th1- and Th2-type cytokines. *Immunol Res* 1996;15: 141–150.
37. Sibai B, Dekker G, Kupferminc M. Pre-eclampsia. *Lancet* 2005;365: 785–799.
38. van den Brule F, Berndt S, Simon N, et al. Trophoblast invasion and placentation: Molecular mechanisms and regulation. *Chem Immunol Allergy* 2005;88: 163–180.
39. Caniggia I, Winter J, Lye SJ, Post M. Oxygen and placental development during the first trimester: Implications for the pathophysiology of pre-eclampsia. *Placenta* 2000;21 Suppl A: S25–S30.
40. De Caterina R, Massaro M. Omega-3 fatty acids and the regulation of expression of endothelial pro-atherogenic and pro-inflammatory genes. *J Membr Biol* 2005;206: 103–116.
41. Cuevas AM, Germain AM. Diet and endothelial function. *Biol Res* 2004;37: 225–230.
42. Sorensen TK, Williams MA, Lee IM, et al. Recreational physical activity during pregnancy and risk of preeclampsia. *Hypertension* 2003;41: 1273–1280.
43. Marcoux S, Brisson J, Fabia J. The effect of cigarette smoking on the risk of preeclampsia and gestational hypertension. *Am J Epidemiol* 1989;130: 950–957.
44. Caballero B. The global epidemic of obesity: An overview. *Epidemiol Rev* 2007;29: 1–5.
45. Murakami Y, Miura K, Ueshima H. Comparison of the trends and current status of obesity between Japan and other developed countries. *Nihon Rinsho* 2009;67: 245–252.
46. Yeh J, Shelton JA. Increasing prepregnancy body mass index: Analysis of trends and contributing variables. *Am J Obstet Gynecol* 2005;193: 1994–1998.
47. Chu SY, Kim SY, Bish CL. Prepregnancy obesity prevalence in the United States, 2004–2005. *Matern Child Health J* 2009;13: 614–620.
48. Alexandra P, Vassilios B, Alexandra V, et al. Population-based trends of pregnancy outcome in obese mothers: What has changed over 15 years. *Obesity* (Silver Spring) 2011;19: 1861–1865.
49. Heslehurst N, Simpson H, Ells LJ, et al. The impact of maternal BMI status on pregnancy outcomes with immediate short-term obstetric resource implications: A meta-analysis. *Obes Rev* 2008;9: 635–683.
50. Birdsall KM, Vyas S, Khazaezadeh N, Oteng-Ntim E. Maternal obesity: A review of interventions. *Int J Clin Pract* 2009;63: 494–507.
51. Stothard KJ, Tennant PW, Bell R, Rankin J. Maternal overweight and obesity and the risk of congenital anomalies: A systematic review and meta-analysis. *JAMA* 2009;301: 636–650.
52. Athukorala C, Rumbold AR, Willson KJ, Crowther CA. The risk of adverse pregnancy outcomes in women who are overweight or obese. *BMC Pregnancy Childbirth* 2010;10: 56.
53. Liu X, Du J, Wang G, et al. Effect of pre-pregnancy body mass index on adverse pregnancy outcome in north of China. *Arch Gynecol Obstet* 2011;283: 65–70.
54. Schneider S, Freerksen N, Maul H, et al. Risk groups and maternal-neonatal complications of preeclampsia—Current results from the national German Perinatal Quality Registry. *J Perinat Med* 2011 May;39(3):257–65. Epub 2011 Feb 10.
55. Catalano PM, Ehrenberg HM. The short- and long-term implications of maternal obesity on the mother and her offspring. *BJOG* 2006;113: 1126–1133.

56. Oken E. Maternal and child obesity: The causal link. *Obstet Gynecol Clin North Am* 2009;36: 361–377, ix–x.
57. Sibai BM, Ewell M, Levine RJ, et al. Risk factors associated with preeclampsia in healthy nulliparous women. The Calcium for Preeclampsia Prevention (CPEP) Study Group. *Am J Obstet Gynecol* 1997;177: 1003–1010.
58. Odegard RA, Vatten LJ, Nilsen ST, Salvesen KA, Austgulen R. Risk factors and clinical manifestations of pre-eclampsia. *BJOG* 2000;107: 1410–1416.
59. Duckitt K, Harrington D. Risk factors for pre-eclampsia at antenatal booking: Systematic review of controlled studies. BMJ 2005;330: 565.
60. Bianco AT, Smilen SW, Davis Y, et al. Pregnancy outcome and weight gain recommendations for the morbidly obese woman. *Obstet Gynecol* 1998;91: 60–64.
61. Bodnar LM, Ness RB, Markovic N, Roberts JM. The risk of preeclampsia rises with increasing prepregnancy body mass index. *Ann Epidemiol* 2005;15: 475–482.
62. Sebire NJ, Jolly M, Harris J, Regan L, Robinson S. Is maternal underweight really a risk factor for adverse pregnancy outcome? A population-based study in London. *BJOG* 2001;108: 61–66.
63. Kiel DW, Dodson EA, Artal R, Boehmer TK, Leet TL. Gestational weight gain and pregnancy outcomes in obese women: How much is enough? *Obstet Gynecol* 2007;110: 752–758.
64. Flick AA, Brookfield KF, de la Torre L, et al. Excessive weight gain among obese women and pregnancy outcomes. *Am J Perinatol* 2010;27: 333–338.
65. Mbah AK, Kornosky JL, Kristensen S, et al. Super-obesity and risk for early and late pre-eclampsia. *BJOG* 2010;117: 997–1004.
66. Ramsay JE, Ferrell WR, Crawford L, et al. Maternal obesity is associated with dys-regulation of metabolic, vascular, and inflammatory pathways. *J Clin Endocrinol Metab* 2002;87: 4231–4237.
67. Stewart FM, Freeman DJ, Ramsay JE, et al. Longitudinal assessment of maternal endo-thelial function and markers of inflammation and placental function throughout pregnancy in lean and obese mothers. *J Clin Endocrinol Metab* 2007;92: 969–975.
68. Zavalza-Gomez AB. Obesity and oxidative stress: A direct link to preeclampsia? *Arch Gynecol Obstet* 2011;283: 415–422.
69. Cnattingius S, Haglund B. Decreasing smoking prevalence during pregnancy in Sweden: The effect on small-for-gestational-age births. *Am J Public Health* 1997;87: 410–413.
70. Cnattingius S, Lambe M. Trends in smoking and overweight during pregnancy: Prevalence, risks of pregnancy complications, and adverse pregnancy outcomes. *Semin Perinatol* 2002;26: 286–295.
71. Janakiraman V, Gantz M, Maynard S, El-Mohandes A. Association of cotinine levels and preeclampsia among African-American women. *Nicotine Tob Res* 2009;11: 679–684.
72. Aliyu MH, Lynch O, Wilson RE, et al. Association between tobacco use in pregnancy and placenta-associated syndromes: A population-based study. *Arch Gynecol Obstet.* 2011 April;283(4):729–734. Epub 2010 March 31.
73. Cnattingius S. The epidemiology of smoking during pregnancy: Smoking prevalence, maternal characteristics, and pregnancy outcomes. *Nicotine Tob Res* 2004;6 Suppl 2: S125–S140.
74. Wen X, Triche EW, Hogan JW, Shenassa ED, Buka SL. Prenatal factors for childhood blood pressure mediated by intrauterine and/or childhood growth? *Pediatrics* 2011;127: e713–e721.
75. Conde-Agudelo A, Althabe F, Belizan JM, Kafury-Goeta AC. Cigarette smoking during pregnancy and risk of preeclampsia: A systematic review. *Am J Obstet Gynecol* 1999;181: 1026–1035.
76. England L, Zhang J. Smoking and risk of preeclampsia: A systematic review. *Front Biosci* 2007;12: 2471–2483.

77. Pipkin FB. Smoking in moderate/severe preeclampsia worsens pregnancy outcome, but smoking cessation limits the damage. *Hypertension* 2008;51: 1042–1046.
78. Xiong X, Zhang J, Fraser WD. Quitting smoking during early versus late pregnancy: The risk of preeclampsia and adverse birth outcomes. *J Obstet Gynaecol Can* 2009;31: 702–707.
79. Bakker R, Steegers EA, Mackenbach JP, Hofman A, Jaddoe VW. Maternal smoking and blood pressure in different trimesters of pregnancy: The Generation R study. *J Hypertens* 2010;28: 2210–2218.
80. Wikstrom AK, Stephansson O, Cnattingius S. Tobacco use during pregnancy and preeclampsia risk: Effects of cigarette smoking and snuff. *Hypertension* 2010;55: 1254–1259.
81. Madretsma GS, Donze GJ, van Dijk AP, et al. Nicotine inhibits the in vitro production of interleukin 2 and tumour necrosis factor-alpha by human mononuclear cells. *Immunopharmacology* 1996;35: 47–51.
82. Ylikorkala O, Viinikka L, Lehtovirta P. Effect of nicotine on fetal prostacyclin and thromboxane in humans. *Obstet Gynecol* 1985;66: 102–105.
83. Srivastava ED, Hallett MB, Rhodes J. Effect of nicotine and cotinine on the production of oxygen free radicals by neutrophils in smokers and non-smokers. *Hum Toxicol* 1989;8: 461–463.
84. Jeyabalan A, Powers RW, Durica AR, et al. Cigarette smoke exposure and angiogenic factors in pregnancy and preeclampsia. *Am J Hypertens* 2008;21: 943–947.
85. Levine RJ, Lam C, Qian C, et al. Soluble endoglin and other circulating antiangiogenic factors in preeclampsia. *N Engl J Med* 2006;355: 992–1005.
86. Cudmore M, Ahmad S, Al-Ani B, et al. Negative regulation of soluble Flt-1 and soluble endoglin release by heme oxygenase-1. *Circulation* 2007;115: 1789–1797.
87. Bainbridge SA, Belkacemi L, Dickinson M, Graham CH, Smith GN. Carbon monoxide inhibits hypoxia/reoxygenation-induced apoptosis and secondary necrosis in syncytiotrophoblast. *Am J Pathol* 2006;169: 774–783.
88. Kreiser D, Baum M, Seidman DS, et al. End tidal carbon monoxide levels are lower in women with gestational hypertension and pre-eclampsia. *J Perinatol* 2004;24: 213–217.
89. Mimura K, Tomimatsu T, Sharentuya N, et al. Nicotine restores endothelial dysfunction caused by excess sFlt1 and sEng in an in vitro model of preeclamptic vascular endothelium: A possible therapeutic role of nicotinic acetylcholine receptor (nAChR) agonists for preeclampsia. *Am J Obstet Gynecol* 2010;202: 464. e1–e6.
90. Stone CD, Diallo O, Shyken J, Leet T. The combined effect of maternal smoking and obesity on the risk of preeclampsia. *J Perinat Med* 2007;35: 28–31.
91. Voigt M, Jorch G, Briese V, et al. The combined effect of maternal body mass index and smoking status on perinatal outcomes—An analysis of the German perinatal survey. *Z Geburtshilfe Neonatol* 2011;215: 23–28.
92. Dekker G, Sibai B. Primary, secondary, and tertiary prevention of pre-eclampsia. *Lancet* 2001;357: 209–215.
93. Miller EC, Cao H, Wen SW, et al. The risk of adverse pregnancy outcomes is increased in preeclamptic women who smoke compared with nonpreeclamptic women who do not smoke. *Am J Obstet Gynecol* 2010;203: 334. e331–338.
94. Lumley J, Chamberlain C, Dowswell T, et al. Interventions for promoting smoking cessation during pregnancy. *Cochrane Database Syst Rev* 2009: CD001055.
95. Weissgerber TL, Wolfe LA, Davies GA. The role of regular physical activity in pre-eclampsia prevention. *Med Sci Sports Exerc* 2004;36: 2024–2031.
96. Irwin DE, Savitz DA, St Andre KA, Hertz-Picciotto I. Study of occupational risk factors for pregnancy-induced hypertension among active duty enlisted Navy personnel. *Am J Ind Med* 1994;25: 349–359.

97. Marcoux S, Brisson J, Fabia J. The effect of leisure time physical activity on the risk of pre-eclampsia and gestational hypertension. *J Epidemiol Community Health* 1989;43: 147–152.

98. Saftlas AF, Logsden-Sackett N, Wang W, Woolson R, Bracken MB. Work, leisure-time physical activity, and risk of preeclampsia and gestational hypertension. *Am J Epidemiol* 2004;160: 758–765.

99. Hegaard HK, Ottesen B, Hedegaard M, et al. The association between leisure time physical activity in the year before pregnancy and pre-eclampsia. *J Obstet Gynaecol* 2010;30: 21–24.

100. Burd L, Roberts D, Olson M, Odendaal H. Ethanol and the placenta: A review. *J Matern Fetal Neonatal Med* 2007;20: 361–375.

101. Aliyu MH, Wilson RE, Zoorob R, et al. Alcohol consumption during pregnancy and the risk of early stillbirth among singletons. *Alcohol* 2008;42: 369–374.

102. Henderson J, Gray R, Brocklehurst P. Systematic review of effects of low-moderate prenatal alcohol exposure on pregnancy outcome. *BJOG* 2007;114: 243–252.

103. Yang Q, Witkiewicz BB, Olney RS, et al. A case-control study of maternal alcohol consumption and intrauterine growth retardation. *Ann Epidemiol* 2001;11: 497–503.

104. Nawrot P, Jordan S, Eastwood J, et al. Effects of caffeine on human health. *Food Addit Contam* 2003;20: 1–30.

105. Clausson B, Granath F, Ekbom A, et al. Effect of caffeine exposure during pregnancy on birth weight and gestational age. *Am J Epidemiol* 2002;155: 429–436.

106. Kuczkowski KM. Caffeine in pregnancy. *Arch Gynecol Obstet* 2009;280: 695–698.

107. Cnattingius S, Signorello LB, Anneren G, et al. Caffeine intake and the risk of first-trimester spontaneous abortion. *N Engl J Med* 2000;343: 1839–1845.

108. Boylan SM, Cade JE, Kirk SF, et al. Assessing caffeine exposure in pregnant women. *Br J Nutr* 2008;100: 875–882.

109. Weng X, Odouli R, Li DK. Maternal caffeine consumption during pregnancy and the risk of miscarriage: A prospective cohort study. *Am J Obstet Gynecol* 2008;198: 279 e271–e278.

110. Bakker R, Steegers EA, Obradov A, et al. Maternal caffeine intake from coffee and tea, fetal growth, and the risks of adverse birth outcomes: The Generation R Study. *Am J Clin Nutr* 2010;91: 1691–1698.

111. Bakker R, Steegers EA, Raat H, Hofman A, Jaddoe VW. Maternal caffeine intake, blood pressure, and the risk of hypertensive complications during pregnancy. The generation R study. *Am J Hypertens* 2011;24: 421–428.

112. American College of Obstetricians and Gynecologists. ACOG CommitteeOpinion No. 462: Moderate caffeine consumption during pregnancy. *Obstet Gynecol* 2010;116: 467–468.

113. Khoury JC, Miodovnik M, Buncher CR, et al. Consequences of smoking and caffeine consumption during pregnancy in women with type 1 diabetes. *J Matern Fetal Neonatal Med* 2004;15: 44–50.

114. Triche EW, Grosso LM, Belanger K, et al. Chocolate consumption in pregnancy and reduced likelihood of preeclampsia. *Epidemiology* 2008;19: 459–464.

115. Saftlas AF, Triche EW, Beydoun H, Bracken MB. Does chocolate intake during pregnancy reduce the risks of preeclampsia and gestational hypertension? *Ann Epidemiol* 2010;20: 584–591.

116. Grosso LM, Bracken MB. Caffeine metabolism, genetics, and perinatal outcomes: A review of exposure assessment considerations during pregnancy. *Ann Epidemiol* 2005;15: 460–466.

117. Zusterzeel PL, te Morsche RH, Raijmakers MT, et al. N-acetyl-transferase phenotype and risk for preeclampsia. *Am J Obstet Gynecol* 2005;193: 797–802.

118. Higdon JV, Frei B. Coffee and health: A review of recent human research. *Crit Rev Food Sci Nutr* 2006;46: 101–123.

119. Hoet JJ, Hanson MA. Intrauterine nutrition: Its importance during critical periods for cardiovascular and endocrine development. *J Physiol* 1999;514 (Pt 3):617–627.

120. Scholl TO. Maternal nutrition before and during pregnancy. *Nestle Nutr Workshop Ser Pediatr Program* 2008;61:79–89.

121. Mayret-Mesquiti M, Perez-Mendez O, Rodriguez ME, et al. Hypertriglyceridemia is linked to reduced nitric oxide synthesis in women with hypertensive disorders of pregnancy. *Hypertens Pregnancy* 2007;26:423–431.

122. Qiu C, Phung TT, Vadachkoria S, et al. Oxidized low-density lipoprotein (Oxidized LDL) and the risk of preeclampsia. *Physiol Res* 2006;55:491–500.

123. Ijarotimi OS, Keshinro OO. Nutritional knowledge, nutrients intake and nutritional status of hypertensive patients in Ondo State, Nigeria. *Tanzan J Health Res* 2008;10: 59–67.

124. Lauro V, Pisani C, Ngoyi V, Fabbris M. Pre-eclampsia: Role of excessive caloric intake. *Acta Biomed Ateneo Parmense* 2000;71 Suppl 1:593–596.

125. Clausen T, Slott M, Solvoll K, et al. High intake of energy, sucrose, and polyunsaturated fatty acids is associated with increased risk of preeclampsia. *Am J Obstet Gynecol* 2001;185:451–458.

126. Kramer MS, Kakuma R. Energy and protein intake in pregnancy. *Cochrane Database Syst Rev* 2003:CD000032.

127. American Congress of Obstetricians and Gynecologists (ACOG). Nutrition During Pregnancy: American College of Obstetrics and Gynecology Patient education pamphlets #AP001. 2010.

128. Imdad A, Bhutta ZA. Effect of balanced protein energy supplementation during pregnancy on birth outcomes. *BMC public health* 2011;11 Suppl 3:S17.

129. Wu G, Meininger CJ. Regulation of nitric oxide synthesis by dietary factors. *Annu Rev Nutr* 2002;22: 61–86.

130. Scholl TO, Leskiw M, Chen X, Sims M, Stein TP. Oxidative stress, diet, and the etiology of preeclampsia. *Am J Clin Nutr* 2005;81: 1390–1396.

131. Savica V, Bellinghieri G, Kopple JD. The effect of nutrition on blood pressure. *Annu Rev Nutr* 2010;30: 365–401.

132. Appel LJ, Moore TJ, Obarzanek E, et al. A clinical trial of the effects of dietary patterns on blood pressure. DASH Collaborative Research Group. *N Eng J Med* 1997;336: 1117–1124.

133. Morris CD, Jacobson SL, Anand R, et al. Nutrient intake and hypertensive disorders of pregnancy: Evidence from a large prospective cohort. *Am J Obstet Gynecol* 2001;184: 643–651.

134. Kaysen GA, Gambertoglio J, Jimenez I, Jones H, Hutchison FN. Effect of dietary protein intake on albumin homeostasis in nephrotic patients. *Kidney Int.* 1986;29: 572–577.

135. Williams SB, Goldfine AB, Timimi FK, et al. Acute hyperglycemia attenuates endothelium-dependent vasodilation in humans in vivo. *Circulation* 1998;97: 1695–1701.

136. Brantsaeter AL, Haugen M, Samuelsen SO, et al. A dietary pattern characterized by high intake of vegetables, fruits, and vegetable oils is associated with reduced risk of preeclampsia in nulliparous pregnant Norwegian women. *J Nutr* 2009;139: 1162–1168.

137. HAPO Study Cooperative Research Group. Hyperglycaemia and Adverse Pregnancy Outcome (HAPO) Study: Associations with maternal body mass index. *BJOG* 2010;117: 575–584.

138. van Buul BJ, Steegers EA, Jongsma HW, et al. Dietary sodium restriction in the prophylaxis of hypertensive disorders of pregnancy: Effects on the intake of other nutrients. *Am J Clin Nutr* 1995;62: 49–57.

139. Auger K, Beausejour A, Brochu M, St-Louis J. Increased Na⁺ intake during gestation in rats is associated with enhanced vascular reactivity and alterations of K⁺ and Ca2⁺ function. *Am J Physiol Heart Circ Physiol* 2004;287: H1848–H1856.

140. Duley L, Henderson-Smart D, Meher S. Altered dietary salt for preventing pre-eclampsia, and its complications. *Cochrane Database Syst Rev* 2005: CD005548.

141. Ray JG, Diamond P, Singh G, Bell CM. Brief overview of maternal triglycerides as a risk factor for pre-eclampsia. *BJOG* 2006;113: 379–386.

142. Esmaillzadeh A, Kimiagar M, Mehrabi Y, et al. Dietary patterns, insulin resistance, and prevalence of the metabolic syndrome in women. *Am J Clin Nutr* 2007;85: 910–918.

143. Villa PM, Laivuori H, Kajantie E, Kaaja R. Free fatty acid profiles in preeclampsia. *Prostaglandins Leukot Essent Fatty Acids* 2009; 81: 17–21.

144. Saldeen P, Saldeen T. Women and omega-3 Fatty acids. *Obstet Gynecol Surv* 2004;59: 722–730; quiz 745–726.

145. Horvath A, Koletzko B, Szajewska H. Effect of supplementation of women in high-risk pregnancies with long-chain polyunsaturated fatty acids on pregnancy outcomes and growth measures at birth: A meta-analysis of randomized controlled trials. *Br J Nutr* 2007;98: 253–259.

146. Oken E, Ning Y, Rifas-Shiman SL, et al. Diet during pregnancy and risk of preeclampsia or gestational hypertension. *Ann Epidemiol* 2007;17: 663–668.

147. Makrides M, Duley L, Olsen SF. Marine oil, and other prostaglandin precursor, supplementation for pregnancy uncomplicated by pre-eclampsia or intrauterine growth restriction. *Cochrane Database Syst Rev* 2006;3: CD003402.

148. Greenberg JA, Bell SJ, Ausdal WV. Omega-3 fatty acid supplementation during pregnancy. *Rev Obstet Gynecol* 2008;1: 162–169.

149. Haider BA, Bhutta ZA. Multiple-micronutrient supplementation for women during pregnancy. *Cochrane Database Syst Rev* 2006: CD004905.

150. Roberts JM, Balk JL, Bodnar LM, et al. Nutrient involvement in preeclampsia. *J Nutr* 2003;133: 1684S–1692S.

151. van den Broek N, Dou L, Othman M, et al. Vitamin A supplementation during pregnancy for maternal and newborn outcomes. *Cochrane Database Syst Rev* 2010;11: CD008666.

152. Faisel H, Pittrof R. Vitamin A and causes of maternal mortality: Association and biological plausibility. *Public Health Nutr* 2000;3: 321–327.

153. Stephensen CB. Vitamin A, infection, and immune function. *Annu Rev Nutr* 2001;21: 167–192.

154. Williams MA, Woelk GB, King IB, Jenkins L, Mahomed K. Plasma carotenoids, retinol, tocopherols, and lipoproteins in preeclamptic and normotensive pregnant Zimbabwean women. *Am J Hypertens* 2003;16: 665–672.

155. Kolusari A, Kurdoglu M, Yildizhan R, et al. Catalase activity, serum trace element and heavy metal concentrations, and vitamin A, D and E levels in pre-eclampsia. *J Int Med Res* 2008;36: 1335–1341.

156. Bakheit KH, Ghebremeskel K, Zaiger G, Elbashir MI, Adam I. Erythrocyte antioxidant enzymes and plasma antioxidant vitamins in Sudanese women with pre-eclampsia. *J Obstet Gynaecol* 2010;30: 147–150.

157. Makedos G, Papanicolaou A, Hitoglou A, et al. Homocysteine, folic acid and B12 serum levels in pregnancy complicated with preeclampsia. *Arch Gynecol Obstet* 2007;275: 121–124.

158. Dionisio N, Jardin I, Salido GM, Rosado JA. Homocysteine, intracellular signaling and thrombotic disorders. *Curr Med Chem* 2010;17: 3109–3119.

159. Hague WM. Homocysteine and pregnancy. *Best Pract Res Clin Obstet Gynaecol* 2003;17: 459–469.

160. Rajkovic A, Mahomed K, Malinow MR, et al. Plasma homocyst(e)ine concentrations in eclamptic and preeclamptic African women postpartum. *Obstet Gynecol* 1999;4: 355–360.

161. Powers RW, Evans RW, Majors AK, et al. Plasma homocysteine concentration is increased in preeclampsia and is associated with evidence of endothelial activation. *Am J Obstet Gynecol* 1989;179: 1605–1611.
162. Falcao S, Bisotto S, Gutkowska J, Lavoie JL. Hyperhomocysteinemia is not sufficient to cause preeclampsia in an animal model: The importance of folate intake. *Am J Obstet Gynecol* 2009;200: 198 e191–195.
163. Thaver D, Saeed MA, Bhutta ZA. Pyridoxine (vitamin B6) supplementation in pregnancy. *Cochrane Database Syst Rev* 2006: CD000179.
164. Guven MA, Coskun A, Ertas IE, et al. Association of maternal serum CRP, IL-6, TNF-alpha, homocysteine, folic acid and vitamin B12 levels with the severity of preeclampsia and fetal birth weight. *Hypertens Pregnancy* 2009;28: 190–200.
165. Haugen M, Brantsaeter AL, Trogstad L, et al. Vitamin D supplementation and reduced risk of preeclampsia in nulliparous women. *Epidemiology* 2009;20: 720–726.
166. Salle BL, Delvin EE, Lapillonne A, Bishop NJ, Glorieux FH. Perinatal metabolism of vitamin D. *Am J Clin Nutr* 2000;71: 1317S–1324S.
167. Shin JS, Choi MY, Longtine MS, Nelson DM. Vitamin D effects on pregnancy and the placenta. *Placenta* 2010;31: 1027–1034.
168. Li YC, Kong J, Wei M, et al. 1,25-Dihydroxyvitamin D(3) is a negative endocrine regulator of the renin–angiotensin system. *J Clin Invest* 2002;110: 229–238.
169. Lapillonne A. Vitamin D deficiency during pregnancy may impair maternal and fetal outcomes. *Med Hypotheses* 2010;74: 71–75.
170. Bodnar LM, Catov JM, Simhan HN, et al. Maternal vitamin D deficiency increases the risk of preeclampsia. *J Clin Endocrinol Metab* 2007;92: 3517–3522.
171. Powe CE, Seely EW, Rana S, et al. First trimester vitamin D, vitamin D binding protein, and subsequent preeclampsia. *Hypertension* 2010;56: 758–763.
172. Camadoo L, Tibbott R, Isaza F. Maternal vitamin D deficiency associated with neonatal hypocalcaemic convulsions. *Nutr J* 2007;6: 23.
173. Javaid MK, Crozier SR, Harvey NC, et al. Maternal vitamin D status during pregnancy and childhood bone mass at age 9 years: A longitudinal study. *Lancet* 2006;367: 36–43.
174. Sayers A, Tobias JH. Estimated maternal ultraviolet B exposure levels in pregnancy influence skeletal development of the child. *J Clin Endocrinol Metab* 2009;94: 765–771.
175. Wang Y, Walsh SW. Antioxidant activities and mRNA expression of superoxide dismutase, catalase, and glutathione peroxidase in normal and preeclamptic placentas. *J Soc Gynecol Investig* 1996;3: 179–184.
176. Hubel CA, Kagan VE, Kisin ER, McLaughlin MK, Roberts JM. Increased ascorbate radical formation and ascorbate depletion in plasma from women with preeclampsia: Implications for oxidative stress. *Free Radic Biol Med* 1997;23: 597–609.
177. Rumbold A, Duley L, Crowther CA, Haslam RR. Antioxidants for preventing preeclampsia. *Cochrane Database Syst Rev* 2008: CD004227.
178. Rumbold A, Crowther CA. Vitamin C supplementation in pregnancy. *Cochrane Database Syst Rev* 2005: CD004072.
179. Llurba E, Gratacos E, Martin-Gallan P, Cabero L, Dominguez C. A comprehensive study of oxidative stress and antioxidant status in preeclampsia and normal pregnancy. *Free Radic Biol Med* 2004;37: 557–570.
180. Zhang C, Williams MA, King IB, et al. Vitamin C and the risk of preeclampsia—Results from dietary questionnaire and plasma assay. *Epidemiology* 2002;13: 409–416.
181. Herrera E, Barbas C. Vitamin E: Action, metabolism and perspectives. *J Physiol Biochem* 2001;57: 43–56.
182. Xu H, Shatenstein B, Luo ZC, Wei S, Fraser W. Role of nutrition in the risk of preeclampsia. *Nutr Rev* 2009;67: 639–657.
183. Chappell LC, Seed PT, Briley AL, et al. Effect of antioxidants on the occurrence of preeclampsia in women at increased risk: A randomised trial. *Lancet* 1999;354: 810–816.

184. Polyzos NP, Mauri D, Tsappi M, et al. Combined vitamin C and E supplementation during pregnancy for preeclampsia prevention: A systematic review. *Obstet Gynecol Surv* 2007;62: 202–206.

185. Spinnato JA, 2nd, Freire S, Pinto ESJL, et al. Antioxidant therapy to prevent preeclampsia: A randomized controlled trial. *Obstet Gynecol* 2007;110: 1311–1318.

186. Villar J, Purwar M, Merialdi M, et al. World Health Organisation multicentre randomised trial of supplementation with vitamins C and E among pregnant women at high risk for pre-eclampsia in populations of low nutritional status from developing countries. *BJOG* 2009;116: 780–788.

187. Poston L, Briley AL, Seed PT, Kelly FJ, Shennan AH. Vitamin C and vitamin E in pregnant women at risk for pre-eclampsia (VIP trial): Randomised placebo-controlled trial. *Lancet* 2006;367: 1145–1154.

188. Xu H, Perez-Cuevas R, Xiong X, et al. An international trial of antioxidants in the prevention of preeclampsia (INTAPP). *Am J Obstet Gynecol* 2010;202: 239. e231–239. e210.

189. Gautam CS, Saha L, Sekhri K, Saha PK. Iron deficiency in pregnancy and the rationality of iron supplements prescribed during pregnancy. *Medscape J Med* 2008;10: 283.

190. Milman N. Iron and pregnancy—A delicate balance. *Ann Hematol* 2006;85: 559–565.

191. Serdar Z, Gur E, Develioglu O. Serum iron and copper status and oxidative stress in severe and mild preeclampsia. *Cell Biochem Funct* 24: 209–215.

192. Trumbo PR, Ellwood KC. Supplemental calcium and risk reduction of hypertension, pregnancy-induced hypertension, and preeclampsia: An evidence-based review by the US Food and Drug Administration. *Nutr Rev* 2007.65: 78–87.

193. Briceno-Perez C, Briceno-Sanabria L, Vigil-De Gracia P. Prediction and prevention of preeclampsia. *Hypertens Pregnancy* 2009;28: 138–155.

194. Hofmeyr GJ, Duley L, Atallah A. Dietary calcium supplementation for prevention of pre-eclampsia and related problems: A systematic review and commentary. *BJOG* 2007; 114: 933–943.

195. Adamova Z, Ozkan S, Khalil RA. Vascular and cellular calcium in normal and hypertensive pregnancy. *Curr Clin Pharmacol* 2009;4: 172–190.

196. Buppasiri P, Lumbiganon P, Thinkhamrop J, Ngamjarus C, Laopaiboon M. Calcium supplementation (other than for preventing or treating hypertension) for improving pregnancy and infant outcomes. *Cochrane Database of Syst Rev* 2011: CD007079.

197. Swaminathan R. Magnesium metabolism and its disorders. *Clin Biochem Rev* 2003;24: 47–66.

198. Sibai BM. Magnesium sulfate prophylaxis in preeclampsia: Lessons learned from recent trials. *Am J Obstet Gynecol* 2004;190: 1520–1526.

199. Jain S, Sharma P, Kulshreshtha S, Mohan G, Singh S. The role of calcium, magnesium, and zinc in pre-eclampsia. *Biol Trace Elem Res* 2010;133: 162–170.

200. Makrides M, Crowther CA. Magnesium supplementation in pregnancy. *Cochrane Database Syst Rev* 2001: CD000937.

201. Mistry HD, Wilson V, Ramsay MM, Symonds ME, Broughton Pipkin F. Reduced selenium concentrations and glutathione peroxidase activity in preeclamptic pregnancies. *Hypertension* 2008;52: 881–888.

202. Mihailovic M, Cvetkovic M, Ljubic A, et al. Selenium and malondialdehyde content and glutathione peroxidase activity in maternal and umbilical cord blood and amniotic fluid. *Biol Trace Elem Res* 2000;73: 47–54.

203. Rayman MP. Selenoproteins and human health: Insights from epidemiological data. *Biochim Biophys Acta* 2009;1790: 1533–1540.

204. Maleki A, Fard MK, Zadeh DH, et al. The relationship between plasma level of Se and preeclampsia. Hypertension in pregnancy: Official journal of the International Society for the Study of Hypertension in Pregnancy 2011;30: 180–187.

205. Vanderlelie J, Venardos K, Perkins AV. Selenium deficiency as a model of experimental pre-eclampsia in rats. *Reproduction.* 2004;128: 635–641.
206. Tara F, Maamouri G, Rayman MP, et al. Selenium supplementation and the incidence of preeclampsia in pregnant Iranian women: A randomized, double-blind, placebo-controlled pilot trial. *Taiwan J Obstet Gynecol* 2010;49: 181–187.
207. Steinbrenner H, Speckmann B, Pinto A, Sies H. High selenium intake and increased diabetes risk: Experimental evidence for interplay between selenium and carbohydrate metabolism. *J Clin Biochem Nutrit* 2011;48: 40–45.
208. Stranges S, Galletti F, Farinaro E, et al. Associations of selenium status with cardiometabolic risk factors: An 8-year follow-up analysis of the Olivetti Heart Study. *Atherosclerosis.* 2011 July;217(1):274–278. Epub 2011 Mar 30.
209. Brozmanova J, Manikova D, Vlckova V, Chovanec M. Selenium: A double-edged sword for defense and offence in cancer. *Arch Toxicol* 2010;84: 919–938.
210. Salle A, Demarsy D, Poirier AL, et al. Zinc deficiency: A frequent and underestimated complication after bariatric surgery. *Obes Surg* 2010;20: 1660–1670.
211. Harma M, Kocyigit A. Correlation between maternal plasma homocysteine and zinc levels in preeclamptic women. *Biol Trace Elem Res* 2005;104: 97–105.

11 Lifestyle Treatment of Hypertension in Patients with Type II Diabetes

Bryan C. Batch and Lauren Gratian
Duke University Medical Center

CONTENTS

11.1 EPIDEMIOLOGY OF DIABETES MELLITUS

Type II diabetes has become one of the most significant contributors to morbidity and mortality among the U.S. population. The Centers for Disease Control (CDC) estimated that 23.6 million (7.8%) people in the United States had either diagnosed or undiagnosed diabetes in 2007 [1]. Diabetes-related costs to U.S. health care systems are substantial. In 2007, the total direct and indirect costs were estimated at 174 billion dollars [1]. Patients with diabetes are at an increased risk of developing cardiovascular diseases such as myocardial infarction (MI), stroke, and heart failure [2]. Furthermore, compared with patients without diabetes, patients with type II diabetes have a significantly higher mortality rate after an MI or stroke [3,4]. In general, death rates are twice as high among patients with diabetes, making diabetes one of the top 10 causes of death in the United States [1]. Besides increasing the risk of cardiovascular diseases, diabetes is also the leading cause of blindness, end-stage renal disease, and nontraumatic amputations in the United States [1,5]. Please note that for the remainder of the chapter, the use of diabetes will refer to patients with type II diabetes unless otherwise indicated.

11.2 CORRELATION BETWEEN HYPERTENSION AND DIABETES

There appears to be a concordance between hypertension and diabetes in the adult population. Hypertension is approximately twice as common in persons with diabetes as in those without [6]. Conversely, persons with hypertension are 2.5 times more likely to develop type II diabetes than their nonhypertensive counterparts [7]. When both conditions are present, the result is an increased risk of diabetic complications and death. Data obtained from death certificates indicate that hypertensive disease is implicated in 4.4% of deaths coded to diabetes, and diabetes is implicated in 10% of deaths coded to hypertensive disease [6].

11.3 BENEFITS OF BLOOD PRESSURE CONTROL IN PATIENTS WITH DIABETES

An estimated 35%–75% of diabetic complications can be attributed to the coexistence of hypertension and diabetes [6]. The association of hypertension with increased diabetic complications is supported by the results of a cross-sectional analysis of 950 patients with type II diabetes mellitus. The results indicate a strong association between the presence of hypertension and multiple diabetic complications such as nephropathy, cardiovascular diseases, retinopathy, peripheral vascular disease, and left ventricular hypertrophy [8].

Several large-scale, randomized controlled trials have confirmed that lowering blood pressure (BP) in patients with diabetes reduces the rate of complications. These trials comprise the bulk of evidence supporting BP control in diabetic patients and are discussed below.

The Systolic Hypertension in China (Syst-China) trial was a multicenter, double-blind, placebo-controlled trial designed to determine the effect of antihypertensive-drug treatment on stroke and other cardiovascular end points including fatal and nonfatal heart failure, fatal and nonfatal MI, and sudden death in older Chinese patients with isolated systolic hypertension. Patients were stratified by sex and cardiovascular complications and then were alternately assigned to receive either active treatment or placebo. Active treatment was initiated with nitrendipine, with the possible addition of captopril, hydrochlorothiazide, or both drugs. Of the 2394 persons enrolled in the study, 98 had diabetes at baseline (47 in the placebo group and 51 in the active treatment group). Wang et al. [9] conducted a subgroup analysis of this population. Within the treatment group, patients were treated similarly regardless of whether the patients had diabetes or not, and their BP decreased to a similar extent. In the placebo group, the cardiovascular event rates in patients with diabetes were approximately twice as high as that in patients without diabetes. In the patients with diabetes of the active treatment group, the excess cardiovascular risk was reduced to the rates observed in the patients without diabetes. Active treatment in patients with diabetes showed a consistent trend in reducing the total mortality (59%; $p = .15$), the cardiovascular mortality (57%; $p = .22$), all cardiovascular end points (74%; $p = .03$), the fatal and nonfatal stroke (45%; $p = .42$), and all cardiac end points (90%; $p = .08$). These results suggest that the control of BP confers substantial benefits to the patients with diabetes. However, the statistical significance was limited by the small sample size of the subgroup with diabetes [9].

These findings were confirmed in the Systolic Hypertension in Europe (Syst-Europe) trial. This trial enrolled 4695 patients with isolated systolic hypertension, of which 492 (10.5%) had diabetes. The patients were randomized either to an active treatment with nitrendipine or to placebo. A subgroup analysis of the patients with diabetes showed that after 2 years of treatment with nitrendipine, the average systolic BP (SBP) was reduced by 8.6 mmHg, which was similar to that in the patients without diabetes. Among the patients with diabetes, the active treatment group experienced statistically significant relative risk reductions in overall mortality by 55%, mortality from cardiovascular diseases by 76%, all cardiovascular events combined by 69%, fatal and nonfatal strokes by 73%, and all cardiac events combined by 63%, compared with the control group. Interestingly, although patients with and without diabetes in the active treatment group achieved the same degree of lowering of SBP, the group with diabetes experienced significantly larger reductions in overall mortality and in the mortality from cardiovascular diseases and all cardiovascular events [10].

The increased benefits obtained due to reduction of BP identified in patients with diabetes compared with patients without diabetes were also reported in the Systolic Hypertension in the Elderly Program (SHEP). This study enrolled 4736 adults with isolated systolic hypertension, including 583 patients with noninsulin-dependent diabetes. The patients were randomly assigned to either active treatment or placebo. Active treatment consisted of low-dose chlorthalidone with a step-up to atenolol or reserpine if needed. After 5 years, the rate of major cardiovascular diseases decreased by 34% in the active treatment group compared with the placebo group, both for patients with diabetes (95% confidence interval [CI], 6%–54%) and for patients without diabetes (95% CI, 21%–45%). However, because of the higher incidence of cardiovascular events in patients with diabetes, absolute risk reduction with active treatment compared with the placebo was twice as great for the patients with diabetes compared with the patients without diabetes (101/1000 vs. 51/1000). These data indicate that we would need to treat 19 patients without diabetes as compared to 10 patients with diabetes to prevent one major cardiovascular disease event [11].

11.4 EVIDENCE FOR TIGHTER BP CONTROL IN PATIENTS WITH DIABETES

The trials discussed above clearly demonstrate that reduction of BP in patients with diabetes decreases the risk of adverse cardiovascular outcomes and mortality. Additional trials have addressed the following questions: (1) Does more intensive reduction of BP result in greater benefit with regard to cardiovascular outcomes? (2) What is the optimal BP-reduction goal for a patient with diabetes?

The United Kingdom Prospective Diabetes Study (UKPDS) was a large prospective observational study including 3642 adults with diabetes. The study demonstrated that each 10 mmHg decrease in SBP was associated with a relative risk reduction of 12% in the rates of any complication associated with diabetes, 15% in diabetes-related mortality, 11% in MI, and 13% in the microvascular complications of retinopathy or nephropathy. As an observational study, these findings were limited in their ability to evaluate causation. However, several randomized controlled trials have confirmed the relationship between tighter BP control and reduction in diabetic complications [12].

A subsequent UKPDS study (UKPDS 38) randomized patients with diabetes to either tight BP control, which was defined as BP < 150/85 mmHg, or less tight control, defined as BP < 180/105 mmHg. After 9 years of follow-up, the mean BP achieved in the tight control group was 144/82 mmHg compared with 154/87 mmHg in the group assigned to less tight control. Compared with the less tight control group, the patients in the tight control group experienced a relative risk reduction of 24% in diabetes-related end points, 32% in deaths related to diabetes, 44% in strokes, 37% in microvascular end points, and 47% in decreased visual acuity [13].

The Hypertension Optimal Treatment (HOT) study addressed the possibilities of lowering BP even further. This trial enrolled 18,790 adult patients from 26 countries, with hypertension defined as the diastolic BP (DBP) between 100 and 115 mmHg. The participants were randomly assigned a target DBP of 90, 85, or 80 mmHg. In the three target groups, the BP was reduced from a mean of 170/105 to a mean of 143/85, 141/83, and 140/81 mmHg, respectively. The results show a trend toward decreased cardiovascular risks in the group with reduced BP levels; however, the differences were not statistically significant. In the subgroup of 1501 patients with diabetes mellitus at baseline, there was more compelling advantage of lower target DBP. Among those with diabetes assigned to the group with a target DBP ≤ 90 mmHg, there were 45 major cardiovascular events compared with only 22 major cardiovascular events among the group with a target DBP ≤ 80 mmHg. Therefore, the risk was halved with more intense BP treatment. The relative risk of major cardiovascular events in the group with target DBP ≤ 90 mmHg compared with the group with target DBP ≤ 80 mmHg was 2.06 (1.24, 3.44). The risk of cardiovascular mortality was also significantly reduced. Among the group with target DBP ≤ 90 mmHg, there were 22 events compared with seven events in the group with target DBP ≤ 80 mmHg. The relative risk of cardiovascular mortality in the group with target DBP ≤ 90 mmHg compared with the group with target DBP ≤ 80 mmHg was 3.0 (1.28, 7.08). There was a trend toward reduction in strokes, with 17 events in the group with target DBP ≤ 90 mmHg compared with 12 events in the group with target DBP ≤ 80 mmHg. However, this was not statistically significant with a relative risk of 1.43 (0.68 and 2.99) [14].

11.5   EVIDENCE AGAINST AGGRESSIVE BP REDUCTION IN PATIENTS WITH DIABETES

The results from the UKPDS [13] and HOT [14] trials demonstrate a clear benefit of tighter BP control in patients with diabetes. However, the average SBP achieved in the tight control groups was still in the hypertensive range, and the DBP was above what is currently considered "optimal" according to the "Seventh Report of the Joint National Committee on Prevention, Detection, Evaluation, and Treatment of High Blood Pressure" (JNC 7) [15] and American Diabetes Association (ADA) recommendations. Uncertainty remained as to whether lowering BP further would provide additional benefits in patients with both hypertension and diabetes.

Consequently, the Action to Control Cardiovascular Risk in Diabetes (ACCORD) BP trial tested the effect of treating to a lower target BP on major cardiovascular events in high-risk persons with type II diabetes. In this trial, 4733 participants were randomly assigned to either intensive therapy that targeted SBP < 120 mmHg or standard therapy that targeted SBP < 140 mmHg. After the first year of therapy, the average BP was 119/64 mmHg in the intensive-therapy group and 133/70 mmHg in the standard-therapy group. After an average of 5 years of follow-up, the rate of first occurrence of a major cardiovascular event was 1.87% per year in the intensive-therapy group compared with 2.09% per year in the standard-therapy group. Although there was a trend toward decreased risk with intensive therapy, the between-group difference was not statistically significant (hazard ratio with intensive therapy, 0.88; 95% CI, 0.73–1.06; $p = .20$). Furthermore, there were no statistically significant differences in many of the secondary outcomes including nonfatal MI, death from any cause, major coronary disease event, and fatal or nonfatal heart failure. There was a statistically significant difference in the rate of nonfatal stroke (0.30% per year in the intensive-therapy group vs. 0.47% per year in the standard-therapy group; hazard ratio, 0.63; 95% CI, 0.41–0.96; $p = .03$) and total stroke (0.32% per year in the intensive-therapy group vs. 0.53% per year in the standard-therapy group; hazard ratio, 0.59; 95% CI, 0.39–0.89; $p = .01$) [16]. There was no clear evidence of increased harm with intensive BP therapy. Nevertheless, this study also reported a possible detrimental effect of the intensive therapy on renal function. Mean serum creatinine in the intensive-therapy group was 1.1 mg/dL compared with 1.0 mg/dL in the standard-therapy group ($p < .001$). Mean estimated glomerular filtration rate in the intensive-therapy group was 74.8 mL/min/1.73 m^2 compared with 80.6 mL/min/1.73 m^2 in the standard-therapy group ($p < .001$). Further research is needed to confirm the potential detrimental effect of intensive BP therapy on renal function.

The absence of a statistically significant reduction in major cardiovascular events in the intensive-therapy group suggests a plateau effect to the benefit of BP reduction in diabetic patients. It also brings into question the benefit of intensive BP therapy in this group of patients. However, after taking into account the reduction in the rate of stroke within the intensive-therapy group coupled with the lack of evidence of increased harm within this group, it appears that intensive BP control is at least safe in this population and may add further benefit. Ultimately, the ideal goal for BP reduction for patients with diabetes remains uncertain.

11.6 RECOMMENDATIONS FOR NONPHARMACOLOGIC THERAPY FOR BP CONTROL IN PATIENTS WITH DIABETES

Despite this uncertainty, both the ADA Executive Summary for the "Standards of medical care in diabetes (2011)" [17] and the JNC 7 [15] recommend that BP in patients with diabetes should be controlled to levels of 130/80 mmHg or lower.

The ADA recommends that patients who have diabetes and a SBP between 130 and 139 mmHg or a DBP between 80 and 89 mmHg may initially be treated with lifestyle therapy including consuming a Dietary Approaches to Stop Hypertension (DASH) [17–19] diet (which emphasizes increased intake of fruits, vegetables, and low-fat dairy products; see Chapter 1), reducing sodium intake, moderating alcohol intake, losing weight if overweight, and increasing physical activity. If lifestyle modification fails to reduce BP to 130/80mmHg or less within 3 months, pharmacologic therapy should be considered [17]. Patients with severe hypertension (SBP ≥ 140 or DBP ≥ 90 mmHg) should receive pharmacologic therapy in addition to lifestyle therapy [17].

The remainder of this chapter presents the evidence for adoption of two specific nonpharmacologic therapies for treatment of hypertension in patients with diabetes: reduction of sodium and adoption of the DASH dietary pattern.

11.7   SODIUM RESTRICTION IN PATIENTS WITH DIABETES

There is ample evidence to suggest that decreasing dietary sodium intake results in a decrease in BP within the general population. Please refer to Chapter 2 for a review of this topic. Furthermore, there appears to be a subset of patients in whom BP is particularly sensitive to dietary salt intake. This phenomenon has been termed salt sensitivity. Although there is a lack of universal consensus on the definition of salt sensitivity, it is often defined as an increase in mean arterial pressure (MAP) of at least 10 mmHg in response to high-dietary salt intake or saline infusion [20]. The level of salt intake required to induce hypertension in salt-sensitive patients varies from patient to patient, with a range of 3–16 g/day [21]. Multiple studies have confirmed that the prevalence of salt sensitivity is higher among patients with diabetes than among patients without diabetes [20,22,23]. Strojek et al. [23] reported the prevalence of salt sensitivity among diabetic patients to be 43% compared with 17% in control subjects matched for age, gender, and body mass index ($p < .05$).

The high prevalence of salt sensitivity among patients with diabetes is important for several reasons. First, salt sensitivity is associated with increased rates of cardiovascular events and mortality. This association is present in normotensive individuals, but it appears to be greater in hypertensive individuals [24]. Second, the high prevalence of salt-sensitive hypertension in patients with diabetes might indicate that the patients with diabetes would benefit from salt restriction at least as much if not more than the general population.

The precise etiology underlying the correlation between diabetes and salt sensitivity remains unknown. However, evidence suggests that diabetes may predispose to salt sensitivity via alterations in vascular reactivity. Findings from a study by Tuck et al. [20] support this theory. This study evaluated the vascular response to angiotensin II infusion in patients with diabetes compared with patients without diabetes. The results showed that the patients with diabetes exhibited increased vascular response to angiotensin II. That is, the incremental increase in MAP induced by angiotensin II infusion was greater in patients with diabetes compared with patients without diabetes. This was true regardless of whether the patients with diabetes were hypertensive at baseline. Furthermore, this study reported a difference in the effect of dietary sodium on vascular response among patients with diabetes compared with patients without diabetes. Among patients without diabetes, the pressor sensitivity to angiotensin II was highly dependent on sodium balance. Patients without diabetes and who were on a sodium-restricted diet (20 mEq/day) had an average increase in MAP of around 5 mmHg in response to angiotensin II infusion at a rate of 3 ng/kg/min. When the same patients were then loaded with a high-sodium diet (250 mEq/day), their average increase in MAP increased to around 13 mmHg in response to the same infusion rate of angiotensin II. In contrast, the patients with diabetes exhibited an average increase in MAP of around 15 mmHg in response to angiotensin II infusion regardless of dietary sodium intake [20]. Thus, in patients with diabetes, the vascular response to angiotensin II in a low-sodium balance state is exaggerated and mirrors the response one would see in a patient in a high-sodium balance state who does not have diabetes.

There are several mechanisms by which diabetes may alter vascular reactivity. Hyperinsulinemia and insulin resistance (IR) have been shown to increase sodium retention, activate the sympathetic nervous system, and have direct effects on blood vessels [25].

Another possible explanation for the association between diabetes and salt sensitivity is that salt sensitivity predisposes to diabetes. This concept has been a topic of debate. Several studies have demonstrated that among lean patients with essential hypertension and no history of diabetes, those with salt-sensitive hypertension exhibit IR and impaired glucose tolerance. This phenomenon was not seen in subjects with salt-resistant hypertension [26–28]. A study by Fuenmayor et al. [28] also demonstrated that the degree of IR identified in salt-sensitive patients was correlated with the amount of dietary salt intake. IR was present during periods of salt restriction (60–70 mEq/day) but was exacerbated when salt intake increased (300 mEq/day) [28]. However, Iwaoka et al. [29] demonstrated the opposite effect, that is, *reduced* sodium intake increased IR and sodium loading reversed this effect. Ames et al. [30] also demonstrated that patients with diabetes and hypertension exhibited reduced glycemic and insulinemic responses to oral glucose tolerance testing after a 2-g oral sodium load, thus suggesting that sodium restriction in patients with diabetes may have an adverse effect on glucose metabolism. It should be noted that the glycemic and insulinemic responses to glucose loading are surrogate markers for overall diabetes control. There have been no studies evaluating the effect of dietary sodium on long-term glucose control, that is, hemoglobin A1c (HbA1c), or clinical outcomes in patients with diabetes.

In summary, there is strong evidence that dietary sodium restriction reduces BP in all individuals. The effect of dietary sodium on glycemic control and IR is not clear. Patients with diabetes are more likely to exhibit salt sensitivity, and therefore, to experience a greater increase in BP following a high-sodium meal. Such individuals with salt-sensitive hypertension tend to have the largest BP reductions during salt restriction [24,31]. Although we do not recommend screening for salt sensitivity, it stands to reason that patients with diabetes may experience enhanced BP control with dietary sodium restriction compared with individuals without diabetes, based on the increased incidence of salt sensitivity in this population. Therefore, we recommend that patients with diabetes and hypertension follow a sodium-restricted diet defined as no more than 1.5 g sodium per day. This is in concordance with the ADA clinical practice recommendations for 2011 [17].

11.8   IMPLEMENTATION OF THE DASH DIETARY PATTERN IN PATIENTS WITH DIABETES

The DASH dietary pattern emphasizes intake of fruits, vegetables, low-fat dairy foods, whole grains, poultry, fish, and nuts, and reduced levels of fats, red meat, sweets, and sugar-containing beverages to lower BP [18]. It is effective in lowering BP in patients in all age groups, in those with prehypertension as well as stage I hypertension, in patients without diabetes, and in Caucasians and African Americans [18,19]. DASH is also consistent with the current ADA dietary recommendations for treatment of hypertension [17].

Although very few studies have evaluated the effect of the DASH dietary pattern on BP or glucose in patients with diabetes, a few studies have looked at the effect of the DASH dietary pattern on insulin sensitivity, fasting glucose, and the risk for development of diabetes in patients without diabetes. In a substudy of the PREMIER trial, Ard et al. [32] determined the effect on insulin sensitivity of a comprehensive behavioral intervention alone versus the same behavioral intervention combined with the DASH dietary pattern. Fifty-five of the 810 participants who were randomized in PREMIER [33] had baseline intravenous glucose tolerance tests and were included in the substudy. The behavioral intervention focused on weight loss, reduced sodium intake, increased physical activity, and moderate alcohol intake. The behavioral intervention group and the intervention plus DASH group lost similar amounts of weight (5.69 vs. 6.56 kg, respectively). Both intervention groups showed improvement in glucose and insulin as compared to the control group. After adjusting for baseline differences, the intervention group that instituted the behavioral intervention and DASH had a suggestive 35% increase in insulin sensitivity as compared to the intervention only group ($p = .616$) [32].

In an effort to look specifically at the effect of the DASH dietary pattern alone versus DASH plus weight loss and exercise on insulin sensitivity, Blumenthal et al. [34] conducted a substudy of the ENCORE trial. In a group of 144 overweight hypertensive adults, the DASH diet paired with weight loss and exercise resulted in improvement in insulin sensitivity and glucose response as compared to the group exposed to the DASH diet alone ($p = .031$ and $p = .011$, respectively) [34]. One of the limitations of the study design is the lack of a group focused on weight loss and exercise only without adopting the DASH diet. Without this comparison group, one cannot definitively draw conclusions regarding the effect on insulin sensitivity of the DASH diet alone.

A third study by Azadbakht et al. [35] compared the effects of the DASH dietary pattern versus a weight-reducing diet on features of the metabolic syndrome. This investigation is essential in that improvement of features of the metabolic syndrome has the potential to lead to reduction in the incidence of type II diabetes. A total of 116 adults were randomized to one of three groups (control, weight-reducing diet, or the DASH dietary pattern with reduced calories). The reduction, net of control, in fasting blood glucose (−4 and −6 mg/dL) and weight (−16 and 15 kg) among men and women was higher in the DASH group (all $p < .05$ compared with the control group). After controlling for weight loss in the two intervention groups, the DASH dietary pattern continued to have a significant effect on reducing metabolic risk [35]. It is conceivable, then, that the reduction in metabolic risk seen in the context of the DASH diet could lead to a reduction in the incidence of type II diabetes.

Liese et al. [36] evaluated the association of the DASH diet with the incidence of type II diabetes in 862 participants in the Insulin Resistance Atherosclerosis Study (IRAS). A total of 148 participants developed type II diabetes after 5 years of follow-up. Type II diabetes odds ratios (ORs) were estimated at tertiles of the DASH adherence score. No association was observed in blacks or Hispanics (tertile 2 vs. tertile 1, 1.16 [95% CI, 0.61–2.18]; tertile 3 vs. tertile 1, 1.34 [95% CI, 0.70–2.58]). An inverse association was observed in whites (tertile 2 vs. tertile 1, OR 0.66 [95% CI, 0.29–1.48]). The association became significant for the most extreme contrast (tertile 3 vs. tertile 1, 0.31 [95% CI, 0.13–0.75]), with adjustment for covariates. Although no association was seen in blacks and Hispanics, the results should be taken in the context that there were a limited number of blacks and Hispanics in the study. These results, although not overwhelmingly convincing, do demonstrate that strict adherence to the DASH diet has the potential to lead to a reduction in the incidence of type II diabetes. Additional studies with a more diverse population are needed to further clarify the true association of the DASH dietary pattern with incidence of diabetes in blacks and Hispanics.

Much of the research regarding the DASH dietary pattern has focused on the relationship of DASH to precursors of type II diabetes (IR and metabolic syndrome) and to the development of diabetes. However, little is known about the effect of the DASH dietary pattern on cardiovascular risks (hypertension [HTN], glucose, lipids) in patients with type II diabetes. Azadbakht et al. [37] attempted to answer this question within the context of a randomized crossover clinical trial. Forty-four participants with type II diabetes were enrolled, and after a run-in period of 3 weeks, they were assigned to a control diet or the DASH eating pattern. Thirty-one participants completed the 8-week randomized phase. Caloric intake was not significantly different between the control group and the DASH group (2165 ± 29 vs. 2189 ± 35 Kcal/day, respectively; $p = .62$). The participants who followed the DASH eating pattern had significant reduction in body weight ($-5.0 ± 0.9$ kg; $p = .006$), waist circumference ($-6.7 ± 1.2$ cm; $p = .002$), fasting blood glucose levels ($-29.4 ± 6.3$ mg/dL; $p = .04$), HbA1c ($-1.7 ± 0.1\%$; $p = .04$), HDL cholesterol levels ($4.3 ± 0.9$ mg/dL; $p = .001$), and LDL cholesterol ($-17.2 ± 3.5$ mg/dL; $p = .02$). Additionally, the DASH diet had beneficial effects on SBP ($-13.6 ± 3.5$ vs. $-3.1 ± 2.7$ mmHg; $p = .02$) and DBP ($-9.5 ± 2.6$ vs. $-0.7 ± 3.3$ mmHg; $p = .04$). These results demonstrate that the DASH dietary pattern when associated with weight loss leads to a clinically significant reduction in glucose and HbA1c and can lead to reduction of other major cardiovascular risk factors. However, the effect of the DASH dietary pattern independent of weight loss on the same parameters is not clear.

In summary, there is evidence that the DASH dietary pattern can (1) reduce IR, (2) change features of the metabolic syndrome, (3) lead to decreased incidence of type II diabetes, and (4) decrease glucose, HbA1c, and lipids in patients with diabetes. Although most of the impact seen is in the context of weight loss, the change that occurs is statistically significant and is not accompanied by negative outcomes (i.e., hypoglycemia, hypotension). As such, the DASH dietary pattern, in conjunction with weight loss, increased physical activity (for patients with no contraindications), and sodium restriction, is recommended by the ADA for first-line treatment of prehypertension (SBP 130–139 and DBP 80–89 mmHg) in patients with type II diabetes.

11.9 CONCLUSION

The increase in prevalence of diabetes mellitus in the United States and worldwide is directly related to the epidemic increase in overweight and obesity. Hypertension is a common comorbidity seen in patients with diabetes, and the presence of the two conditions increases the risk for cardiovascular morbidity and mortality. There are very few trials that utilize the DASH dietary pattern in patients with diabetes, but the data available demonstrate a beneficial effect on glucose, BP, and lipids. Thus, the use of the DASH dietary pattern, in conjunction with weight loss, increased physical activity (for patients with no contraindications), and reduced sodium intake, is part of the current recommendations for nonpharmacologic treatment of prehypertension in patients with diabetes. These lifestyle guidelines are compatible with the ADA and JNC guidelines for individuals without diabetes. Once the BP is outside the prehypertension range or the BP is not improved after 3 months of lifestyle therapy, the recommendation of both the JNC 7 and ADA is to pair these same lifestyle recommendations with pharmacologic therapy (Table 11.1).

It should be noted, however, that until further studies are conducted to assess the safety of the DASH dietary pattern in patients with diabetes and chronic kidney disease, the above recommendations should be adopted with caution as those individuals may benefit from a diet lower in potassium content than that in the DASH dietary pattern.

TABLE 11.1
Summary: Take-Home Messages

Key Evidences	Recommendations for Health Care Practitioners

• Reduction of BP in patients with diabetes leads to reduced risk of cardiovascular morbidity and mortality, stroke, and microvascular end points
• Salt sensitivity is common in patients with diabetes
• Salt restriction can lead to reduction in BP in patients with diabetes
• The DASH dietary pattern may
  • Decrease IR
  • Decrease the incidence of type II diabetes
  • Decrease glucose, HbA1c, and lipids in patients with diabetes
	• JNC 7 suggests goal BP to be <130/80 mmHg
	• Patients with diabetes should limit salt intake to < 1.5 g sodium/day
	• Patients should be encouraged to adopt the DASH dietary pattern, to lose weight if overweight, and to increase physical activity if no contraindications are found (heart disease, retinopathy, neuropathy, etc.)
	• Pharmacologic therapy should be initiated in conjunction with lifestyle therapy if BP remains >130/80 mmHg after 3 months of lifestyle intervention

REFERENCES

1. Centers for Disease Control and Prevention. National diabetes fact sheet: General information and national estimates on diabetes in the United States, 2007. Atlanta, GA: U.S. Department of Health and Human Services, Centers for Disease Control and Prevention, 2008.

2. Sowers JR, Haffner S. Treatment of cardiovascular and renal risk factors in the diabetic hypertensive. *Hypertension.* 2002;40:781–788.

3. Lehto S, Rönnemaa T, Pyörälä K, Laakso M. Predictors of stroke in middle-aged patients with non–insulin-dependent diabetes. *Stroke.* 1996;27:63–68.

4. Miettinen H, Lehto S, Salomaa V et al. Impact of diabetes on mortality after the first myocardial infarction. *Diabetes Care.* 1998;21:69–75.

5. Bakris GL, Williams M, Dworkin L et al. Preserving renal function in adults with hypertension and diabetes: A consensus approach: National Kidney Foundation Hypertension and Diabetes Executive Committees Working Group. *Am J Kidney Dis.* 2000;36:646–661.

6. The National High Blood Pressure Education Program Working Group. National high blood pressure education program working group report on hypertension in diabetes. *Hypertension.* 1994;23:145–158.

7. Gress TW, Nieto FJ, Shahar E, Wofford MR, Brancati FL. Hypertension and antihypertensive therapy as risk factors for type 2 diabetes mellitus: Atherosclerosis Risk in Communities Study. *N Engl J Med.* 2000;342:905–912.

8. Mehler PS, Jeffers BW, Estacio R, Schrier RW. Association of hypertension and complications in non-insulin-dependent diabetes mellitus. *Am J Hypertens.* 1997;10:152–161.

9. Wang JG, Staessen JA, Gong L, Liu L. Chinese trial on isolated systolic hypertension in the elderly. Systolic Hypertension in China (Syst-China) Collaborative Group. *Arch Intern Med.* 2000;160:211–220.

10. Gasowski J, Birkenhäger WH, Staessen JA, de Leeuw PW. Benefit of antihypertensive treatment in the diabetic patients enrolled in the Systolic Hypertension in Europe (Syst-Eur) trial. *Cardiovasc Drugs Ther.* 2000;14:49–53.

11. Curb JD, Pressel SL, Cutler JA et al. Effect of diuretic-based antihypertensive treatment on cardiovascular disease risk in older diabetic patients with isolated systolic hypertension. Systolic Hypertension in the Elderly Program Cooperative Research Group. *JAMA.* 1996;276:1886–1892.

12. Adler AI, Stratton IM, Neil HA et al. Association of systolic blood pressure with macrovascular and microvascular complications of type 2 diabetes (UKPDS 36): Prospective observational study. *BMJ.* 2000;321:412–419.

13. UKPDS 38. Tight blood pressure control and risk of macrovascular and microvascular complications in type 2 diabetes: UKPDS 38. UK Prospective Diabetes Study Group. *BMJ.* 1998;317:703–713.

14. Hansson L, Zanchetti A, Carruthers SG et al. Effects of intensive blood pressure lowering and low-dose aspirin in patients with hypertension: Principal results of the Hypertension Optimal Treatment (HOT) randomized trial. *Lancet.* 1998;351:1755–1762.

15. Chobanian AV, Bakris GL, Black HR et al. Seventh Report of the Joint National Committee on Prevention, Detection, Evaluation and Treatment of High Blood Pressure. *Hypertension.* 2003;42:1206–1252.

16. The ACCORD Study Group. Effects of intensive blood-pressure control in type 2 diabetes mellitus. *N Engl J Med.* 2010;362:1575–1585.

17. American Diabetes Association. Standards of medical care in diabetes—2011. *Diabetes Care.* 2011;34:S11–S61.

18. Appel LJ, Moore TJ, Obarzanek E et al. A clinical trial of the effects of dietary patterns on blood pressure. *NEJM.* 1997;336:1117–1124.

19. Svetkey LP, Simons-Morton D, Vollmer WM et al. Effects of dietary patterns on blood pressure: Subgroup analysis of the Dietary Approaches to Stop Hypertension (DASH) randomized clinical trial. *Arch Intern Med.* 1999;159:285–293.

20. Tuck M, Corry D, Trujillo A. Salt-sensitive blood pressure and exaggerated vascular reactivity in the hypertension of diabetes mellitus. *Am J Med.* 1990;88:210–216.

21. Espinel CH. The Salt Step Test: Its usage in the diagnosis of salt-sensitive hypertension and in the detection of the salt hypertension threshold. *J Am Coll Nutr.* 1992;11:526–531.

22. Uzu T, Sakaguchi M, Yokomaku Y et al. Effects of high sodium intake and diuretics on the circadian rhythm of blood pressure in type 2 diabetic patients treated with an angiotensin II receptor blocker. *Clin Exp Nephrol.* 2009;13:300–306.

23. Strojek K, Grzeszczak W, Lacka B, Gorska J, Keller CK, Ritz E. Increased prevalence of salt sensitivity of blood pressure in IDDM with and without microalbuminuria. *Diabetologia.* 1995;38:1443–1448.

24. Weinberger MH. Salt sensitivity is associated with an increased mortality in both normal and hypertensive humans. *J Clin Hypertens.* 2002;4:274–276.

25. Feldstein CA. Salt intake, hypertension and diabetes mellitus. *J Hum Hypertens.* 2002;16 (Suppl 1):S48–S51.

26. Yatabe MS, Yatabe J, Yoneda M et al. Salt sensitivity is associated with insulin resistance, sympathetic over activity, and decreased suppression of circulating renin activity in lean patients with essential hypertension. *Am J Clin Nutr.* 2010;92:77–82.

27. Sharma AM, Ruland K, Spies KP, Distler A. Salt-sensitivity in young normotensive subjects is associated with a hyperinsulinemic response to oral glucose. *J Hypertension.* 1991;9:329–335.

28. Fuenmayor N, Moreira E, Cubeddu LX. Salt sensitivity is associated with insulin resistance in essential hypertension. *Am J Hypertens.* 1998;11:397–402.

29. Iwaoka T, Umeda T, Inoue J et al. Dietary NaCl restriction deteriorates oral glucose tolerance in hypertension subjects with impairment of glucose tolerance. *Am J Hypertens.* 1994;7:460–463.

30. Ames RP. The effect of sodium supplementation on glucose tolerance and insulin concentrations in patients with hypertension and diabetes mellitus. *Am J Hypertens.* 2001;14:653–659.

31. Chrysant SG, Weir MR, Weder AB et al. There are no racial, age, sex, or weight differences in the effect of salt on blood pressure in salt-sensitive hypertensive patients. *Arch Intern Med.* 1997;157:2489–2494.

32. Ard JD, Grambow SC, Liu D, Slentz CA, Kraus WE, Svetkey LP. The effect of the PREMIER interventions on insulin sensitivity. *Diabetes Care.* 2004;27:340–347.

33. Writing group of the PREMIER collaborative research group. Effects of comprehensive lifestyle modification on blood pressure control: Main results of the PREMIER clinical trial. *JAMA.* 2003;289:2083–2093.

34. Blumenthal JA, Babyak MA, Sherwood A et al. Effects of the dietary approaches to stop hypertension diet alone and in combination with exercise and caloric restriction on insulin sensitivity and lipids. *Hypertension.* 2010;55:1199–1205.

35. Azadbakht L, Mirmiran P, Esmaillzadeh A, Azizi T, Azizi F. Beneficial effects of a dietary approaches to stop hypertension eating plan on features of the metabolic syndrome. *Diabetes Care.* 2005;28:2823–2831.

36. Liese AD, Nichols M, Xuezheng S, D'Agostino RB, Haffner SM. Adherence to the DASH diet is inversely associated with incidence of type 2 diabetes: The Insulin Resistance Atherosclerosis Study. *Diabetes Care.* 2009;32:1434–1436.

37. Azadbakht L, Fard NR, Karimi M et al. Effects of the Dietary Approaches to Stop Hypertension (DASH) eating plan on cardiovascular risks among type 2 diabetic patients. *Diabetes Care.* 2011;34:55–57.

12 Lifestyle and Blood Pressure Control in Ethnic and Racial Minorities

Jessica Bartfield
Loyola University Gottlieb Memorial Hospital

Jamy D. Ard
University of Alabama at Birmingham

CONTENTS

12.1 BACKGROUND

Hypertension is highly prevalent in the U.S. population, affecting approximately one-third of all adults [1]. However, the prevalence, awareness, and severity of hypertension do vary by race/ethnicity. African Americans, for example, face more grim statistics, as hypertension tends to develop more frequently, at younger ages, and with greater severity among African Americans than among whites or Hispanic Americans [2]. According to the Centers for Disease Control (CDC), 44% and 42% of African American women and men, respectively, suffer from hypertension, compared with 31% and 28% of white men and women, respectively [1]. Although the larger Hispanic American population may not be as severely affected by hypertension as African Americans, the Hispanic population should not be considered as monolithic. There is a notable variation in hypertension risk among groups that comprise Hispanic Americans. For example, Puerto Rican Americans have the highest rates of hypertension-related morbidity compared with all other Hispanic groups and Caucasians. Some Hispanic groups, such as Mexican Americans, have a lower prevalence of hypertension (22%) compared with non-Hispanic whites (28%) [3]. The rates of awareness of hypertension are relatively high in all groups. For example, in the National Health and Nutrition Examination Surveys (NHANES 2005–2006) of African Americans with hypertension, approximately 81% had awareness of the diagnosis, which was comparable with the awareness of hypertension among non-Hispanic whites. On the other hand, Mexican Americans were less likely than African Americans to be aware of the presence of hypertension [3]. Furthermore, although the rates of blood pressure (BP) control have improved across all racial groups, more non-Hispanic whites demonstrate greater BP control (60%) than African Americans (49%) or Mexican Americans (54%) [4,5].

As a result of an earlier age of onset, greater disease severity, higher prevalence, and perhaps unique target-organ susceptibility, African Americans have an 80% higher stroke mortality rate, a 50% higher heart disease mortality rate, and a 320% higher rate of hypertension-related end-stage renal disease compared with non-Hispanic whites [6–8]. Despite being equally aware of their disease as whites, and even having similar levels of BP control (65% whites vs. 58% African Americans), African Americans display a much higher propensity for target end-organ damage as a result of hypertension. Even though African Americans have similar rates of BP control as whites, they bear a disproportionate population risk of target-organ damage, suggesting that greater emphasis be placed on higher rates of control and prevention of hypertension among African Americans. This disparity has spurred public health officials and clinical investigators to look for ways to improve the clinical translation of key recommendations for lifestyle modifications to control BP specifically in African American adult populations. The majority of lifestyle modification trials that have tested the recommended nonpharmacological BP control interventions have typically included small numbers of ethnic minority groups other than African Americans. Given the disparity for African Americans in hypertension prevalence, control, and sequelae, combined with the paucity of intervention data for other ethnic minority groups, this chapter primarily focuses on African Americans. However, the general concepts and approaches presented for consideration may have some applicability to other minority groups.

It remains unclear why hypertension affects African Americans so adversely compared with other ethnic or racial groups. Some theories suggest genetic mutations of epithelial sodium channels, enhanced intrarenal activation of the renin–angiotensin system, sympathetic overactivity, impaired vasodilatation and/or nitric oxide deficiency, and an attenuated nocturnal decline as explanations [9,10]. In addition, increase in body weight has been linked to an increase in the incidence of hypertension, and more African Americans carry excess weight, with a staggering 70% of men and 77% of women being overweight (body mass index [BMI] ≥ 25 kg/m^2) [11].

The rates of incidence of hypertension vary between sub-Saharan Africans and African Americans although they have similar genetic predispositions. Therefore, multiple factors such as genetics, environment, and culture are likely to influence this disparity. Hopefully, future studies dedicated to this topic will result in a better understanding.

For now, it is imperative that clinicians recognize and appropriately treat hypertension among African Americans. It is generally accepted that African Americans respond differently to pharmacological therapy for hypertension [9]. Similarly, lifestyle factors such as dietary compositions and patterns, alcohol intake, smoking, stress levels, body weight, and physical activity likely influence BP differently for African Americans when compared with other ethnic or racial groups. Furthermore, behavioral changes and lifestyle modifications may have to be approached and implemented differently among African Americans in order to have a significant and lasting effect on BP control. In this chapter, we review several key psychosocial and lifestyle factors that may play a role in the etiology of the disparity in hypertension prevalence, control, and sequelae and, therefore, may have particular relevance when one is trying to implement a lifestyle modification strategy for controlling BP in African Americans. We have provided two case examples to help guide the discussion of these issues.

12.2   CASE STUDIES

12.2.1   CASE 1

Mrs. S is a 55-year-old black woman with a history of increasing BP for the past 2 years. Her BP was previously documented as follows: systolic BP (SBP) = 126–135 mmHg and diastolic BP (DBP) = 85–88 mmHg. However, for the last two visits, she has an average BP of 144/90 mmHg. She has a family history of hypertension and an early incidence of coronary heart disease in her maternal grandmother. She does not smoke, consumes 1–2 alcoholic beverages annually, and her medical history is notable for obesity (BMI = 35 kg/m^2) and impaired fasting glucose on last examination of lab work before 6 months. She is generally sedentary, lives with her husband, and has two adolescent grandchildren. She works full time and is active in her community. She is under a significant amount of stress related to the caretaker role for the grandchildren and some of her volunteer work at the church. Her examination is normal, but it is noted that she has gained 10 lb in the past 6 months (current BMI = 36.5 kg/^{2}). She is concerned about her BP; however, she lets you know that she is not excited about the idea of using medication to control it. When you enquire about her usual food intake, she says that her eating has been pretty irregular with regard to the amount of time between meals, especially over the past 6 months. She usually has coffee in the morning, up to two cups, followed by a pastry or peanut butter crackers mid-morning. Lunch is typically purchased at a local restaurant or the workplace cafeteria and includes a sandwich, accompanied with chips, fries, or soup and a regular soda. She will have a snack from the vending machine or a piece of fruit from the cafeteria in the afternoons on rare occasions. She eats dinner at home with her family after her volunteer work or after returning home after the grandchildren's extracurricular activities. This is typically after 7 PM. If her husband has not cooked, she will typically pick up food from a restaurant as a carryout for the family to eat. If her husband cooks, he will prepare baked or fried meat, including poultry, fish, beef, or pork, 1–2 starchy items, one vegetable, and one bread item. She finds that she has been eating larger portions over the last year because she is so hungry in the evenings. She is also snacking about 2 h after dinner, preferring to have salty and sweet snacks.

12.2.2   CASE 2

Mr. F is a 46-year-old black man who presents for routine follow-up examination. He states that he has been without any complaints and is generally doing well. He does not have any significant medical history; his family history is notable for early onset of hypertension, with his mother and father who developed hypertension in their late 30s. His younger sister was recently diagnosed with hypertension. He was told at a recent screening at his place of employment that his BP was "mildly" elevated and that he should have it checked by his health care provider. He does not smoke and he takes one drink per day on an average, but this goes up during the summer and football season when he may have 4–5 beers in the weekend. He lives with his wife and works full time. He has a BMI of 29 kg/m^2 with a waist circumference of 38 in. His weight has been stable for 5 years. His BP in the office was 152/89 mmHg (average of two measures); 1 week later at a nurse visit to repeat his BP, the average was 148/92 mmHg. He is concerned that high BP medications will affect his sexual function and wants to avoid them if possible. When you inquire about some of his lifestyle behaviors, he reports that he usually has breakfast from the local fast food restaurant that is near his home, which typically includes a sausage biscuit, hash browns, and a cup of coffee or juice. He often skips lunch because of his work schedule, but he snacks throughout the day on baked goods that are available at his worksite. His wife usually prepares dinner at home. He is careful to watch his portion sizes and does not add salt to his food at the table, but he is unsure if his wife uses much salt when she cooks. A lot of the foods they eat regularly are frozen entrees like lasagna or casseroles, to which they add a salad or vegetable and bread. Most days of the week, he has a small dessert. He is physically active for approximately 150 min/week doing a variety of activities around the house, including yard and mechanical work, which he rates as moderate-intensity exercise.

12.3   EXISTING EVIDENCE

12.3.1   Stress

Stress derived from both psychosocial and environmental factors may contribute to the discrepancy in prevalence of hypertension between African Americans and other racial or ethnic groups. Factors such as high unemployment, higher rates of poverty, lower occupational status, and substandard living environments often result in harmful health behaviors and chronic diseases, with stress being a key mediating factor in the pathway [12]. Perceived racial discrimination is another stressor that has received

increasing attention toward research because of its potential to explain key disparities between non-Hispanic whites and ethnic minority groups. Racial discrimination has been associated with increased cardiovascular reactivity, inflammation, and
increased BP [13]. Many propose that cumulative exposure to such stressors leads
to chronic activation of both the sympathetic nervous system and autonomic activity
[14]. African Americans have been shown to typically respond to stress in an alpha
adrenergic pattern, which constricts the veins and arteries to the heart. This chronic
vasoconstriction African Americans experience as a result of persistent stress may
damage the vascular structure, causing high BP and its sequelae including heart disease and stroke [14]. Caucasians, however, primarily exhibit a more cardiac specific,
beta adrenergic pattern in response to stress, which acts mainly on cardiac muscles
to increase heart rate and cardiac output.

Earlier studies have also determined interesting associations between anger, or
other emotional manifestations of stress, and BP among African Americans. Several
investigators have hypothesized that suppression of anger, anxiety, and stress could
trigger increased sympathetic activity, including increased cardiac output and peripheral vascular resistance, and thus higher rates of hypertension. Indeed, multiple studies have found this positive relationship between anger suppression and high levels of
hypertension in both African American men and women, up to age 60, independent
of other risk factors [15,16]. Further, a common coping style of African Americans
exposed to stressors from social and environmental domains may be operant in
determining the response of BP to the stressor. The John Henryism trait as described
by James postulates that a strong behavioral predisposition to actively cope with
psychosocial stressors leads to a biological response that promotes elevated BP levels
[17]. This characteristic may lead to elevations in BP in the face of stressful circumstances, and individuals who do not actively seek to alter their environment, fight
discrimination, or increase their social standing may be less likely to have elevations
in BP despite the same type of exposure to the stressor [17].

Along with stress, the relationship between depression and hypertension among
African Americans has also been investigated. It remains unclear whether stress
triggers depression or vice versa, but both contribute to higher rates of hypertension.
African American women, for example, have the highest rates of hypertension, and
they had the greatest increase from 1988 to 2000 in the prevalence of hypertension,
compared with women and men of other ethnicities [1]. These women, particularly
those in caregiver roles, report higher levels of stress and more frequent symptoms of
depression. The combination of high stress and depressed mood may prompt behavioral changes such as increased food intake, weight gain, increased sodium intake,
and increased alcohol intake, which can all negatively influence BP [18].

Even if stress does not play a clear role in the etiology of hypertension, it cer-
tainly appears to play a central role in exacerbating hypertension [19]. In addition,
stress may impede proper treatment of hypertension. Stressors such as family health,
financial stability, lack of health insurance, and personal health consequences from
obesity can overwhelm a person and prevent one from seeking medical attention or
adhering to medical treatment.

Unfortunately, behavioral techniques, such as biofeedback relaxation, progressive muscle relaxation, yoga, and health promotion programs to reduce stress among

African Americans remain widely understudied, resulting in an extreme scarcity of data and thus no clinical guidelines for stress management in preventing or treating hypertension. One randomized controlled, single-blind study investigated the use of Transcendental Meditation in treating 127 elderly African Americans with hypertension [20]. This study compared a Transcendental Meditation program, including 20 min of quiet meditation twice a day, with a standard lifestyle modification education program and found a significantly greater reduction in BP with meditation, that is, SBP of 10.7 vs. 4.7 mmHg and DBP of 6.4 vs. 3.3 mmHg, respectively [20], in the group that underwent meditation versus the standard lifestyle modification group. The same research group also reported similar improvements in BP for a younger group of 150 African Americans randomly assigned to the same Transcendental Meditation program, progressive muscle relaxation, or conventional health education classes. However, when reviewing the broader literature on the association between stress reduction intervention and BP, the results of a meta-analysis of simple biofeedback techniques, relaxation-assisted biofeedback, progressive muscle relaxation, and stress management training did not show statistically significant improvements in BP [21]. In general, the authors note that many of the studies in the field were not of sufficient quality to be included in the meta-analysis, and more specific to this discussion, even fewer included sufficient numbers of African Americans to draw any conclusions regarding the effectiveness of the particular strategies for this subgroup. In the absence of more definitive evidence, we recommend that clinicians actively address stress reduction when treating hypertension in African Americans, as it has been clearly associated with higher BP levels and as stress reduction is unlikely to cause any harm; on the other hand, the direct impact of stress on BP may be low.

12.3.2 Physical Activity

As noted in earlier chapters, it is generally well accepted that increase in physical activity improves cardiovascular health and helps lower the heart rate, along with SBP and DBP. Likewise, inactivity and poor fitness lead to 30%–50% greater risk for developing hypertension [22]. Consequently, the majority of nonpharmacological interventions to lower BP incorporate regular physical activity. In 2008, the U.S. Department of Health and Human Services issued physical activity guidelines, recommending that adults do 2 h and 30 min a week (150 min in total) of moderate-intensity aerobic physical activity or 1 h and 15 min (75 min) a week of vigorous-intensity aerobic physical activity or an equivalent combination of moderate- and vigorous-intensity aerobic physical activity and dedicate two or more days per week to muscle-strengthening activities that involve all major muscle groups [23].

Although the benefits of physical activity are clear, achieving those benefits by maintaining a physically active lifestyle can be particularly challenging. This is true for all Americans and especially true for African Americans. In NHANES 2003–2004, Troiano et al. [24] used accelerometers to capture physical activity data among children and adults within the United States. Among all adults aged 20 or above, less than 5% did at least 30 min of moderate-intensity physical activity most days of the week. The levels of physical activity declined as age categories increased, and men generally had higher levels of activity compared with women. The total combined minutes of physical activity by age group is shown in Table 12.1. African American men, aged 20–59, had an average of only 11 min/day of sustained moderate-to-vigorous physical activity, whereas African American women of the same age group had only 6.8 min/day of moderate-to-vigorous physical activity. For both African American men and women, physical activity levels were generally higher in younger age categories compared with other ethnic groups, but as the age category increased, the levels of activity were similar to those of or significantly lower than those of either non-Hispanic whites or Mexican Americans [24].

The barriers to obtaining physical activity during leisure time have been researched the most in African American women as this race/sex group is among the lowest in terms of leisure-time physical activity while suffering the most from chronic diseases and risk factors, such as hypertension, that would benefit from higher levels of activity. A wide array of focus group and survey-based studies has examined African American women's perceived benefits and barriers to physical activity. It has generally been accepted that key demographic factors such as income, area of residence, education, and the number and the types of responsibilities have particular salience in determining the activity levels for African American women. However, Young and Voorhees [25] conducted a survey of 234 urban-dwelling African American women in Baltimore, Maryland and found few correlations between physical activity and sociodemographic or environmental factors, such as income, education, presence of sidewalks, perceived safety from crime, or presence of places to exercise. These findings may not be generalizable given the urban location. As an example, Sanderson et al. [26] also used the same survey among a sample of 567 rural Alabama women with lower income and education levels. In the rural sample, women with higher income (≥ $35,000 annual income) were approximately two times more likely to meet the recommendations for physical activity. Only 16.3% of women in the rural sample were in the highest income range, whereas in the urban sample, nearly 60% of the women had an annual income of $35,000 or more [26]. In this example, the context becomes especially relevant; the additional income and the potential resources that are associated with that income may be particularly important for an

TABLE 12.1
Total Daily Minutes of Physical Activity by Age and Race

Group (Years)	African American Men	African American Women	Mexican American Men	Mexican American Women	White Men	White Women
	Total Minutes of Physical Activity/Day					
6–11	114 (5.0)	87.4 (6.2)	97.0 (4.6)	70.8 (3.4)	92.3 (6.3)	73.1 (3.2)
12–15	54.1 (5.2)	26.4 (2.6)	50.6 (3.8)	26.9 (2.6)	41.0 (3.3)	22.4 (2.0)
16–19	42.5 (3.6)	18.1 (2.4)	41.0 (3.3)	25.7 (3.4)	29.3 (2.7)	19.1 (3.1)
20–59	37.9 (2.7)	20.0 (2.2)	45.7 (2.4)	22.1 (1.0)	34.6 (1.2)	19.7 (0.9)
60+	10.9 (1.0)	5.9 (0.8)	18.4 (2.2)	8.3 (1.2)	12.4 (0.8)	8.8 (0.6)

Source: Troiano, R.P. et al., *Med. Sci. Sports Exerc.*, 40, 181–188, 2008.

African American woman living in a community with limited resources available for physical activity.

Beyond the key demographic and environmental factors, other cultural norms have a significant influence on the beliefs, attitudes, and practices related to physical activity among African Americans. For some African Americans, the idea of leisure-time activity is counterintuitive given the manual nature of their daily jobs. Physical activity may be seen as "work," whereas being sedentary, or "resting," is the preferred way to relax after a long workday [27]. Additionally, African Americans may have very clear preferences for certain types of activities, perceiving that certain activities are not consistent with their self-identity as African Americans [28,29]. For example, blacks may view physical activities such as basketball and jump rope/double dutch as "mostly black" activities, whereas other activities such as hiking and skiing as being "mostly white" [29]. Going beyond the general preferences, some activities may be seen as less attractive because of the physical nature, exertion, or preparation required. This is especially true for water-related activities where hairstyle-related concerns are relevant [30,31].

Even beyond low levels of physical activity, the level of inactivity, or sedentary behavior specifically, appears to be linked to increasing health risk, including all-cause and cardiovascular disease mortality [32]. Sedentary behavior, defined as sitting or lying down and expending energy equivalent to 1.0–1.5 metabolic equivalents, is critical because it competes with *any* form of exercise, including light physical activity. In the Coronary Artery Risk Development in Young Adults (CARDIA) cohort, over one-third of African American men and women reported watching 4 or more hours of television per week compared with less than 10% of non-Hispanic whites; heavy television viewing was inversely associated with physical activity [33]. Some of the preferences for sedentary behaviors may be rooted in the cultural perceptions noted above (i.e., preference for "resting"). However, as access to the Internet increases and computer and television screens become more prevalent in homes across all racial groups, the opportunities for sedentary behaviors continue to increase. Matthews et al. [34] used the NHANES 2003–2004 accelerometry data to quantify the amount of time individuals spent in sedentary behaviors. White and African American women were equally spending about 7–8 h/day in sedentary behavior after the age of 12 years [34].

Given the variety of barriers and potential perceptions regarding physical activity, one may wonder if there is sufficient benefit for actively recommending physical activity as a part of lifestyle modification for African Americans with hypertension. A recent meta-analysis on the effect of aerobic exercise on BP cautioned that only 37 of 54 trials reported ethnic distribution, and only four of those trials focused on African Americans [35]. More recently, a small study of 19 African Americans with newly diagnosed hypertension showed that walking for 30 min/day, 5–7 days per week, improved SBP by 9% and DBP by 7% after 6 months [36]. Two other studies specifically enrolled African American women to establish the changes in BP with exercise, namely walking or other lifestyle physical activities such as stair climbing. One of the studies found that adhering to a cumulative 30 min of activity at least 5 days/week significantly reduced SBP by 6.4 mmHg after about 2 months [10]. Similarly, the other study illustrated how African American women who increased their mean number of steps per day from 3857 to 5281 (totaling close to 2.5 miles) lowered their SBP by 9% and DBP by 10% after 18 months [37].

Therefore, as part of the foundation of treatment, clinicians should recommend exercise as a part of the lifestyle modification for hypertensive African American patients. Although the current federal guidelines regarding exercise may seem overwhelming to many patients already strapped for time with work and family commitments, clinicians should reassure patients that helping to control BP with physical activity does not require a gym membership or fancy exercise equipment. Simply taking more steps throughout the day and/or doing a couple of 10-min bouts of activity have a significant impact on reducing high BP.

12.3.3 WEIGHT

As noted in earlier chapters, the relationship between body weight and BP has been well established. Particularly with short-term weight loss, each kilogram of weight loss typically translates into SBP and DBP reduction of 1 and 0.92 mmHg, respectively [38]. However, the relationship may not be the same for non-Hispanic whites and African Americans. In 1975, a large cardiovascular study including both non-Hispanic whites and African Americans found that both normal and overweight individuals who gained at least 10 lb over 7 years were 2.1 and 1.6 times more likely, respectively, to develop hypertension [39]. Later epidemiological studies found modest or inconsistent associations between increased BP and excess body weight specifically among African Americans [40]. The Pitt County Study published in 1998, analyzed data over 5 years and concluded that both baseline body weight and weight gain serve as independent predictors of increased BP, but not necessarily hypertension, among African Americans [41]. An analysis of indices of adiposity and their relationship to BP in a large sample of African American and non-Hispanic whites published in 2008 suggests that some of the observed variability in the associations may be related to different associations based on the hypertensive status and the measure of adiposity [42]. Although measures of overweight and obesity, such as BMI, waist circumference, or waist-to-hip ratios, were higher in hypertensive individuals, significant associations between these measures and BP were primarily seen in normotensive individuals. For African Americans, waist circumference—a surrogate marker of visceral adipose tissue— was the only marker independently associated with SBP in hypertensive individuals [42]. Although BMI is an important marker for overall excess adiposity, these data suggest that waist circumference may more accurately depict hypertensive risk in African Americans, likely as a result of differences in body composition and distribution of fat depots.

The variations in the relationship between excess adiposity and BP may be mediated by insulin resistance. Centrally located fat, usually distinguished by an abnormal waist circumference and independent of obesity, results in an increased insulin resistance. Insulin resistance likely contributes to further increased sympathetic nervous system activity and impaired vascular endothelial function, both underpinnings for hypertension [43]. One study found an association between insulin resistance and hypertension in African American men, but not women, which may imply that body composition serves as a better predictor for hypertension than obesity among African Americans [44].

For a given amount of weight loss, African Americans and non-Hispanic whites have been shown to improve insulin sensitivity proportionate to the weight loss achieved at equal rates [45]. However, the amount of weight loss that is typically achieved in weight loss interventions for African Americans is significantly lower than that for others, conferring smaller absolute benefit for improvements in insulin sensitivity, and thus BP. The ongoing challenge has been the development of effective weight loss strategies that produce equivalent amounts of weight loss for African Americans and non-Hispanic whites. For example, in the PREMIER trial, behavioral interventions designed to achieve moderate weight reduction resulted in an average weight loss of 3.5 kg in 6 months for African Americans compared with approximately 6-kg weight loss in non-African Americans (predominantly non-Hispanic whites) [46]. The associated BP reductions at 6 months were 1.2–2.1 mmHg in African American women and 4.6–6.0 mmHg in African American men, compared with 4.2–4.4 mmHg in non-African American women and 4.2–5.7 mmHg in non-African American men. Many of the largest, randomized controlled trials that have tested interventions designed to modify behavior and produce weight loss have also resulted in disparate outcomes for African Americans generally and African American women more specifically. At 12 months, the Diabetes Prevention Program resulted in weight loss of 7.1%–8.4% for most race/sex subgroups except for African American women who lost 4.5% [47].

The potential reasons for the disparate outcomes are relevant when considering the recommendations for an African American patient to lose weight for BP control. Potential physiological explanations exist to account for some of the differences in obesity and weight reduction outcomes between African Americans and non-African Americans. Included among these are differences in metabolic rates and insulin sensitivity. It has been well documented that in controlled settings, African American women have lower resting, sleeping, and activity energy expenditures than matched white women [48–51]. Weyer et al. [49] also noted that fat oxidation was lower for African American men compared with white men. Differences in insulin sensitivity may also contribute to the potential for obesity in African Americans. African Americans are more insulin resistant and have higher levels of fasting and postchallenge insulin [52–54]. Hyperinsulinemia may ultimately affect fat deposition by suppressing lipolysis [55,56], decreasing fat oxidation [49,51], and promoting the uptake of adipocyte triglyceride [57]. Therefore, it seems plausible to hypothesize that there is a direct link between these physiological factors and excess obesity in African Americans, resulting from efficient usage of energy, efficient storage of excess energy as fat, and preferential conservation of high-energy stores.

From a behavioral perspective, there are also key differences in weight-related behaviors and attitudes. For example, one could consider the differences in body image perception. African American women prefer larger body images and have less dissatisfaction with a larger body image as compared with white women [58–60]. This could potentially influence the desired body weight that is maintained or achieved through dieting [61]. Williamson et al. [62] found that African American women made a similar number of attempts to lose weight but set a weight loss goal that was 10 pounds more than the goal set by white women. These behavioral patterns affect energy intake and expenditure and appear to be prevalent in the African American community potentially as a function of culture [63].

When considering the available data, addressing overweight and obesity in an African American patient who may be prehypertensive or hypertensive is a complicated matter. However, the final decision to advocate for successful weight reduction or prevention of weight gain is likely to result in significant health benefits, even for lower amounts of weight loss. A Cochrane review of 18 randomized trials involving weight loss diets for hypertensive adults showed that losing 4%–8% of body weight correlated with 3 mmHg reduction in both SBP and DBP [64]. Weight reduction is also associated with other beneficial improvements in cardiometabolic risk factors, such as glycemic control and lipids. If the clinician can help the patient understand these benefits and maintain appreciation for the cultural perspective of the patient, the patient may be more accepting of the recommendation for behavioral change to promote weight loss.

To some extent, for African Americans, the changes in nutrient levels may regulate BP more effectively than the changes in body weight. There is clear evidence that dietary patterns can more strongly influence BP in African Americans when compared with Caucasians. The Dietary Approaches to Stop Hypertension (DASH) trial proved that adhering to a dietary pattern that includes high amounts of fruits and vegetables, low-fat dairy products, whole grains, and nuts but limited amounts of red meats, added sugars, and fats can lower BP within 2 weeks and leads to greater resolution of hypertension when compared with adhering to a typical American dietary pattern [65]. African Americans with hypertension experienced the greatest effect independent of any weight change, with a mean reduction of 13.2 mmHg (SBP) and 6.1 mmHg (DBP) [66]. Similar findings have been demonstrated with interventions that alter sodium intake. The DASH-Sodium Trial determined the effect of various levels of sodium intake on BP in persons eating a typical American diet or the DASH diet [67]. Overall, the total effect of reducing sodium intake from higher (142 mmol/day) to lower (65 mmol/day) was 6.7/3.5 mmHg in the control diet group and 3.0/1.6 mmHg in the DASH diet group. The combination of sodium reduction and the DASH dietary pattern was superior to the use of either intervention alone in reducing BP. Subgroup analysis revealed that the effects of sodium in lowering BP were more prominent in several key groups including patients with hypertension, African Americans, patients of age ≥ 45 years, and women on the DASH diet [68]. For a hypertensive, African American woman aged 45 or above, Vollmer et al. [68] estimated the effect of the lowest sodium DASH intervention to be a reduction in SBP of 15.1 mmHg.

12.4 PRACTICAL MESSAGE FOR PRACTITIONERS

12.4.1 APPROACH TO LIFESTYLE MODIFICATIONS—CULTURAL CONSIDERATIONS

Although all of the issues highlighted thus far have been discussed in the context of considering African American patients, it is clear that these issues have relevance to non-African American patients as well. All patients deal with psychosocial stress, choices related to physical activity and dietary intake, and body weight management. Individually, these factors are not unique to African Americans, and many of these issues are relevant collectively to other sociodemographic groups such as those who are from disadvantaged backgrounds due to limited resources or education. The uniqueness of the African American patient does become apparent, however, when one begins to consider the patient's social context and cultural norms that serve as a lens for interpreting and responding to the environment. This perspective provides some explanation for variable responses by racial/ethnic identity to the same stimulus or environment.

For many practitioners, the cultural perspective seems to be most distinct when it relates to food intake preferences. The traditional African American diet is based on the cultural traditions of "Soul Food," which is generally of less-than-optimal dietary quality, and these food preparation techniques and preferences have been passed down through several generations and are practiced by many African Americans even today [69]. Soul Food is often characterized as being high in added fat, sodium, and sugar; uses deep-fat frying prominently as a cooking technique; and features high-fat meats as main dishes and seasonings for vegetables. The traditional Soul Food diet does have some healthful components and focuses to a large extent on a number of fruits and vegetables, including a variety of greens, sweet potatoes, tomatoes, dried beans and peas, watermelon, blackberries, corn and okra; however, the traditional preparation techniques used for these fruit and vegetable items often leads to a significant increase in the associated number of calories and sodium. For African Americans, engaging in traditional cultural practices, such as preparing and eating Soul Food, is not necessarily a function of socioeconomic status (SES) [70]. African Americans with high levels of education and income may be just as likely to eat Soul Food as African Americans in lower education and income brackets; therefore, the practitioner cannot presume a particular preference based on income or educational attainment [69].

Although it is necessary to understand and respect the cultural perspective of each patient, some of the misperceptions or misinformation held by patients may be linked to cultural differences; in these instances, the practitioner should feel empowered to address the misinformation without fearing that the information will be a dismissal of the cultural perspective of the patient. For example, some African Americans may not understand the relationship between body weight and risk for chronic diseases [71]. When combined with the cultural preference for a larger body size, the lack of education and cultural preference may contribute to unnecessarily increased risk of chronic diseases. Without proper information, the individual may never reevaluate the preference for a larger body size in the context of potentially preventing a chronic disease. Providing this information to the patient may correct a knowledge deficit, thus prompting him or her to reconsider the preference for a larger body size and lead to weight loss efforts to reduce the risk for chronic diseases. The amount of weight reduction may still result in a higher than normal BMI (i.e., ≥ 25 kg/m^2); however, 5%–10% weight reduction would still be considered significant and effective for reduction in BP [72].

Another critical element of the cultural context related to adoption of lifestyle change recommendations is the family and social network. Increasingly, the importance of the interpersonal environment is being recognized in areas that are associated with lifestyle behaviors. The association between the increase in obesity prevalence and social networks was demonstrated based on data from the Framingham Heart Study [73]. The generalizability of this association with African Americans is unclear given that the minority population in the Framingham study is limited. Important differences in the social network for African Americans from mainstream culture may include the scope of family and the general type of support provided. Ard et al. [74] reported that African Americans often defined family in nontraditional ways and included other members of the surrounding community as sources of support. Therefore, efforts to engage the traditional "family members" alone may not produce the level of support desired. Further, when Kumanyika et al. [75] tested the effect of a culturally specific intervention designed to utilize the support of family and friends to promote weight loss for African Americans, there were no differences between those who participated both with family and friends compared with those who participated only with other study participants in assigned groups [75]. However, the authors did find that the participants were most successful at losing weight if their family and friends were more engaged in the intervention and they too lost more weight. Samuel-Hodge et al. [76] identified family cohesion (including the extent to which family members ask each other for help, feel close to each other, and value family togetherness) as an important predictor of weight loss in a sample of African American and white participants engaged in a weight loss intervention. However, the influence of family cohesion was different based on race. For African Americans, high family cohesion was associated with greater weight loss, whereas for whites, higher cohesion was associated with less weight loss. Based on these data, it appears that a broadly defined support network that can be effectively engaged may be predictive of adoption of behavioral change that can lead to weight reduction and, by extrapolation, potential reduction in BP.

It is difficult to consider the influence of culture and racial identity on lifestyle behaviors without acknowledging the influence of SES. Although not a foregone conclusion, minority race increases the probability of lower SES. Lower income households typically purchase fewer fruits and vegetables and spend less money per person on fruit and vegetable items [77]. These households are also often less likely to be near larger chain supermarkets, which have a wider variety of produce at better quality and lower prices; living near such food outlets has been associated with higher fruit and vegetable intake [78,79]. African Americans generally have higher levels of poverty and unemployment and lower levels of education. As a result, the implications of lower income and education on food-purchasing habits may be more relevant for a higher proportion of African Americans with hypertension compared with other racial/ethnic groups. Some studies have shown, however, that the availability of fruits and vegetables in the homes of African Americans is comparable with that in the homes of whites. In a study of Birmingham, Alabama, households, African Americans had similar availability of fruits and vegetables, and a significantly larger proportion of African Americans reported higher availability of items such as greens, sweet potatoes, okra, and other foods that are consistent with traditional African American dietary patterns, despite a higher cost per serving compared with other fruit and vegetable items [80]. This suggests that while cost concerns, income, and education are relevant factors for African Americans in making choices about food purchases, traditional preferences may be an overriding variable in predicting food-purchasing behaviors.

12.4.2 Approach to Case 1

Mrs. S has now been established with a diagnosis of stage I hypertension. She also has other risk factors that are important to consider in the formulation of a treatment plan, including impaired fasting glucose or prediabetes. Her modifiable risk factors associated with her BP include low physical activity/high sedentary behavior, obesity, and less-than-ideal diet quality/excess calorie intake. Based on these risk factors and comorbid conditions, the primary treatment goal would include implementing a lifestyle modification plan that results in weight reduction using a low-calorie, BP-lowering dietary pattern combined with increased physical activity. The use of the DASH dietary pattern with a reduced sodium intake would be a viable option. The choice of a dietary pattern is particularly important above and beyond the planned weight reduction as the dietary pattern can have effects independent of calorie restriction on the metabolic profile (i.e., improving her insulin resistance) [81,82]. Including physical activity as a component of the strategy promotes consistent weight reduction by combining calorie restriction with increased energy expenditure, leading to a larger energy deficit. Furthermore, the physical activity will have positive effects on BP and be critical to maintenance of weight loss.

There are several behavioral strategies that could be used to assist the patient with embracing the proposed strategy. A complete discussion of those strategies is outside the focus of this chapter. However, we focus on the considerations to make with regard to Mrs. S's race/ethnic identity. Understanding what she values as an African American woman can help you link motivations for behavioral change to something that is meaningful to her. For example, if she values being a leader in her church community, some of her motivation to make the suggested lifestyle changes may come from the idea that these changes will help her be more effective in her roles within the church. With her multiple responsibilities as a bread winner, caregiver, and volunteer, she may perceive that taking time for herself to exercise or do meal planning is not consistent with her roles as a grandmother, wife, or volunteer. In addition, it would be advisable to ask her to identify someone who might engage in these changes with her because social support could be important. Finally, helping her identify stressors and techniques for managing that stress more productively may be critical in helping her incorporate the lifestyle changes into her daily routine. Providing some specific resources and being open to nontraditional methods of stress management (e.g., prayer) will be important in validating the importance of stress management in the implementation of lifestyle changes.

12.3.3 Approach to Case 2

Mr. F has stage I hypertension now. Based on his family history, one might suppose that he has a strong genetic contribution to his risk of early onset hypertension. He is overweight (BMI = 29 kg/m^2) but thinks that others in his family would consider him "sickly" if he were to lose any significant amount of weight. When discussing treatment options with him, he reiterates that he would like to avoid medications if at all possible. Some of his family members seem to have significant side effects from the medications, which really concerns him. Because he is open to using nonpharmacological interventions to reduce his BP, you introduce him to the DASH dietary pattern combined with a reduced sodium intake. Based on the subgroup analysis of the DASH-Sodium trial, you might expect a patient that fits his profile (African American, male, hypertensive, age > 45) to reduce BP by 12.2/7.1 mmHg [68]. He is interested in this option but voices concerns about eating bland, "diet" food. He and his wife fry foods often and eat very few vegetables other than corn and peas (which are considered starches) and salad greens. Occasionally, they will prepare greens or green beans, but he is certain that their preparation techniques are not consistent with the DASH pattern as they typically include bacon, bacon grease, or fat back in their vegetables to add some "flavor." He feels fairly certain that he can increase his fruit intake because he likes to eat fruits. Finally, he has some concerns that adding more dairy to his diet will cause some gastrointestinal distress due to possible lactose intolerance. It is because of this concern that he currently does not drink milk or eat ice cream. He seems to "do ok" with cheeses.

The challenge of helping a patient initiate adoption of the DASH dietary pattern, particularly when the current pattern of eating is fairly different from the DASH pattern, requires patience and a measured approach. Helping the patient identify areas that are most easily modified as the first steps can be an ideal starting point. In addition, actively addressing concerns about the new dietary pattern (e.g., blandness, new foods, convenience, and cost) can help decrease the barriers to adoption. Identifying resources that can provide the patient with alternatives to current practices is a very valuable and practical way to further decrease the barriers. If a referral to a dietitian is required, provide specific instructions for the dietitian to guide the counseling. In this case, instructions for Mr. F to meet with a dietitian might include instruction on a low-sodium DASH dietary pattern with further instruction on alternatives to vegetable seasonings with high saturated fat and alternatives to frying. To accomplish the goals of the DASH dietary pattern, he will also need to restructure his eating pattern throughout the day, given the volume of food contained in the pattern. It would not be unexpected for him to lose some weight as he makes initial changes in his dietary intake because the increase in water- and fiber-containing foods increases overall bulk and decreases total energy density. The addition of these foods can often be associated with displacement of higher energy dense foods, especially when the goals of the plan are being met. In his case, it is likely that he may voluntarily discontinue the daily dessert because his level of satiety increases so consistently. Finally, to assist with adoption of the dairy component of the DASH pattern, you could consider testing for lactose malabsorption using a breath hydrogen test. However, based on data that suggest that 65%–75% of people of the African descent have lactose intolerance, it is a high likelihood that he has some level of lactose intolerance. The most efficient strategy may be use of low-lactose-containing dairy products such as cheese and yogurt to meet the dairy requirements or use of commercially available lactase supplements (Table 12.2).

TABLE 12.2

Summary: Take-Home Messages

Key Evidences	Recommendations for Health Care Practitioners
• Chronic exposure to psychosocial stressors in the form of perceived racial discrimination and adverse social conditions may play a role in vascular reactivity and contribute to the disparities in hypertension	• Despite lack of definitive evidence of benefit, actively address stress reduction when treating hypertension in African Americans, as it has been clearly associated with higher BP levels and as stress reduction is unlikely to cause any harm
• Physical activity may be seen as "work," whereas being sedentary, or "resting," is the preferred way to rejuvenate	• Clinicians should recommend exercise as a part of the lifestyle modifications for hypertensive African American patients. Increases in activity can be gradual, performed in 10-min bouts, and do not have to require significant expense
• African Americans may have very clear preferences for certain types of activities, perceiving that certain activities are not consistent with their self-identity as African Americans	• Clinicians should make the patient aware of the emerging risk of being sedentary and provide advice on ways to decrease the sedentary behaviors
• Because of increased screen time and more sedentary jobs, increase in sedentary behaviors may be as problematic as low levels of exercise	
• Moderate weight reduction leads to decreases in BP for African Americans who are prehypertensive or hypertensive	• Clinicians should help patients understand the relationship between body weight and BP
• African Americans may have different perceptions of body image that support maintenance of higher body weight	• If the clinician can help the patient understand the benefits of weight reduction and maintain appreciation for the cultural perspective of the patient, the patient may be more accepting of the recommendation for behavioral changes to promote weight loss
• Physiological and cultural differences may lead to less weight loss in a given intervention for African Americans when compared with non-African Americans	
• African Americans who follow the DASH diet (high fruits and vegetables, whole grains, low-fat dairy, limited red meats, added sugars and fats), particularly those with hypertension, experience greater reductions in SBP and DBP	• Clinicians should routinely counsel both prehypertensive and hypertensive patients about the benefits of following the DASH dietary pattern
• African Americans exhibit greater changes in BP with sodium intake	• Clinicians need to emphasize the effect of sodium intake and counsel patients on ways to reduce sodium in their diets

REFERENCES

1. National Center for Health Statistics (U.S.). *Health, United States, 2008*. Hyattsville, MD: National Center for Health Statistics, 2008.
2. Fray JCS, Douglas JG. *Pathophysiology of Hypertension in Blacks*. New York: Oxford University Press, 1993.
3. Ostchega Y, Yoon SS, Hughes J, Louis T. Hypertension awareness, treatment, and control—Continued disparities in adults: United States, 2005–2006. *NCHS Data Brief.* 2008(3):1–8.

4. Hertz RP, Unger AN, Cornell JA, Saunders E. Racial disparities in hypertension prevalence, awareness, and management. *Arch Intern Med.* 2005;165(18):2098–2104.

5. Bersamin A, Stafford RS, Winkleby MA. Predictors of hypertension awareness, treatment, and control among Mexican American women and men. *J Gen Intern Med.* 2009;24 Suppl 3:521–527.

6. Smith SR, Svetkey LP, Dennis VW. Racial differences in the incidence and progression of renal diseases. *Kidney Int.* 1991;40(5):815–822.

7. Owen WF, Jr. Racial differences in incidence, outcome, and quality of life for African–Americans on hemodialysis. *Blood Purif.* 1996;14(4):278–285.

8. Price DA, Owen WF, Jr. African–Americans on maintenance dialysis: A review of racial differences in incidence, treatment, and survival. *Adv Renal Replacement Ther.* 1997;4(1):3–12.

9. Gadegbeku CA, Lea JP, Jamerson KA. Update on disparities in the pathophysiology and management of hypertension: Focus on African Americans. *Med Clin North Am.* 2005;89(5):921–933, 930.

10. Staffileno BA, Minnick A, Coke LA, Hollenberg SM. Blood pressure responses to lifestyle physical activity among young, hypertension-prone African–American women. *J Cardiovasc Nurs.* 2007;22(2):107–117.

11. Flegal KM, Carroll MD, Ogden CL, Curtin LR. Prevalence and trends in obesity among US adults, 1999–2008. *JAMA.* 2010;303(3):235–241.

12. Neighbors HW, Braithwaite RL, Thompson E. Health promotion and African–Americans: From personal empowerment to community action. *Am J Health Promot.* 1995;9(4):281–287.

13. Williams DR, Mohammed SA. Discrimination and racial disparities in health: Evidence and needed research. *J Behav Med.* 2009;32(1):20–47.

14. Cohen S, Kessler RC, Gordon LU. *Measuring Stress: A Guide for Health and Social Scientists.* New York: Oxford University Press, 1995.

15. Harburg E, Blakelock EH, Jr., Roeper PR. Resentful and reflective coping with arbitrary authority and blood pressure: Detroit. *Psychosom Med.* 1979;41(3):189–202.

16. Johnson EH, Schork NJ, Spielberger CD. Emotional and familial determinants of elevated blood pressure in black and white adolescent females. *J Psychosom Res.* 1987;31(6):731–741.

17. James SA. John Henryism and the health of African–Americans. *Cult Med Psychiatry.* 1994;18(2):163–182.

18. Taylor JY, Washington OG, Artinian NT, Lichtenberg P. Relationship between depression and specific health indicators among hypertensive African American parents and grandparents. *Prog Cardiovasc Nurs.* 2008;23(2):68–78.

19. Anderson NB, McNeilly M, Myers H. Autonomic reactivity and hypertension in blacks: A review and proposed model. *Ethn Dis.* 1991;1(2):154–170.

20. Schneider RH, Staggers F, Alxander CN, et al. A randomised controlled trial of stress reduction for hypertension in older African Americans. *Hypertension.* 1995;26(5):820–827.

21. Rainforth MV, Schneider RH, Nidich SI, Gaylord-King C, Salerno JW, Anderson JW. Stress reduction programs in patients with elevated blood pressure: A systematic review and meta-analysis. *Curr Hypertens Rep.* 2007;9(6):520–528.

22. AHA. *Heart Disease and Stroke Statistics—2005 Update.* Dallas, TX: American Heart Association, 2005.

23. Physical Activity Guidelines Advisory Committee report, 2008. To the Secretary of Health and Human Services. Part A: Executive summary. *Nutr Rev.* 2009;67(2):114–120.

24. Troiano RP, Berrigan D, Dodd KW, Masse LC, Tilert T, McDowell M. Physical activity in the United States measured by accelerometer. *Med Sci Sports Exerc.* 2008;40(1):181–188.

25. Rohm Young D, Voorhees CC. Personal, social, and environmental correlates of physical activity in urban African–American women. *Am J Prev Med.* 2003;25(3):38.
26. Sanderson BK, Foushee HR, Bittner V, et al. Personal, social, and physical environmental correlates of physical activity in rural African–American women in Alabama. *Am J Prev Med.* 2003;25(3):30.
27. Airhihenbuwa CO, Kumanyika S, Agurs TD, Lowe A. Perceptions and beliefs about exercise, rest, and health among African–Americans. *Am J Health Prom.* 1995;9(6):426–429.
28. Hooker SP, Wilson DK, Griffin SF, Ainsworth BE. Perceptions of environmental supports for physical activity in African American and white adults in a rural county in South Carolina. *Prev Chronic Dis* [serial online] 2005 Oct [date cited]. *Prev. Chronic. Dis.* 2005;2(4):A11. Available from: http://www.cdc.gov/pcd/issues/2005/oct/05_0048.htm
29. Resnicow K, Jackson A, Braithwaite R, et al. Healthy body/healthy spirit: A church-based nutrition and physical activity intervention. *Health Educ Res.* 2002;17(5):562–573.
30. Barnes A, Goodrick G, Pavlik V, Markesino J, Laws D, Taylor W. Weight loss maintenance in African–American women: Focus Group Results and Questionnaire Development. *J Gen Intern Med.* 2007;22(7):915.
31. Baskin ML, Ahluwalia HK, Resnicow K. Obesity intervention among African–American children and adolescents. *Pediatr Clin North Am.* 2001;48(4):1027–1039.
32. Katzmarzyk PT, Church TS, Craig CL, Bouchard C. Sitting time and mortality from all causes, cardiovascular disease, and cancer. *Med Sci Sports Exerc.* 2009;41(5):998–1005.
33. Sidney S, Sternfeld B, Haskell WL, Jacobs DR, Jr., Chesney MA, Hulley SB. Television viewing and cardiovascular risk factors in young adults: The CARDIA study. *Ann Epidemiol.* 1996;6(2):154–159.
34. Matthews CE, Chen KY, Freedson PS, et al. Amount of time spent in sedentary behaviors in the United States, 2003–2004. *Am J Epidemiol.* 2008;167(7):875–881.
35. Whelton SP, Chin A, Xin X, He J. Effect of aerobic exercise on blood pressure: A meta-analysis of randomized, controlled trials. *Ann Intern Med.* 2002;136(7):493–503.
36. Sohn AJ, Hasnain M, Sinacore JM. Impact of exercise (walking) on blood pressure levels in African American adults with newly diagnosed hypertension. *Ethn Dis.* 2007;17(3):503–507.
37. Banks-Wallace J. Outcomes from Walk the Talk: A nursing intervention for black women. *ABNFJ.* 2007;18(1):19.
38. Neter JE, Stam BE, Kok FJ, Grobbee DE, Geleijnse JM. Influence of weight reduction on blood pressure: A meta-analysis of randomized controlled trials. *Hypertension.* 2003;42(5):878–884.
39. Paul O, Chicago Heart Association. *Epidemiology and Control of Hypertension: Papers and Discussions from the Second International Symposium on the Epidemiology of Hypertension Presented September 1974 by the Chicago Heart Association.* New York: Stratton Intercontinental Medical Book Corp, 1975.
40. Liu K, Ruth KJ, Flack JM, et al. Blood pressure in young blacks and whites: Relevance of obesity and lifestyle factors in determining differences. The CARDIA Study. Coronary Artery Risk Development in Young Adults. *Circulation.* 1996;93(1):60–66.
41. Curtis AB, Strogatz DS, James SA, Raghunathan TE. The contribution of baseline weight and weight gain to blood pressure change in African Americans: The Pitt County Study. *Ann Epidemiol.* 1998;8(8):497–503.
42. Kotchen TA, Grim CE, Kotchen JM, et al. Altered relationship of blood pressure to adiposity in hypertension. *Am J Hypertens.* 2008;21(3):284–289.
43. Kotchen TA. Obesity-related hypertension: Epidemiology, pathophysiology, and clinical management. *Am J Hypertens.* 2010;23(11):1170–1178.
44. Kidambi S, Kotchen JM, Krishnaswami S, Grim CE, Kotchen TA. Hypertension, insulin resistance, and aldosterone: Sex-specific relationships. *J Clin Hypertens (Greenwich).* 2009;11(3):130–137.

45. Gower BA, Weinsier RL, Jordan JM, Hunter GR, Desmond R. Effects of weight loss on changes in insulin sensitivity and lipid concentrations in premenopausal African American and white women. *Am J Clin Nutr.* 2002;76(5):923–927.

46. Appel LJ, Champagne CM, Harsha DW, et al. Effects of comprehensive lifestyle modification on blood pressure control: Main results of the PREMIER clinical trial. *JAMA.* 2003;289(16):2083–2093.

47. West DS, Prewitt TE, Bursac Z, Felix HC. Weight loss of black, white, and Hispanic men and women in the Diabetes Prevention Program. *Obesity.* 2008;16(6):1413.

48. Kimm SYS, Glynn NW, Aston CE, Poehlman ET, Daniels SR. Effects of race, cigarette smoking, and use of contraceptive medications on resting energy expenditure in young women. *Am. J. Epidemiol.* 2001;154(8):718–724.

49. Weyer C, Snitker S, Bogardus C, Ravussin E. Energy metabolism in African Americans: Potential risk factors for obesity. *Am J Clin Nutr.* 1999;70(1):13–20.

50. Hunter GR, Weinsier RL, Darnell BE, Zuckerman PA, Goran MI. Racial differences in energy expenditure and aerobic fitness in premenopausal women. *Am J Clin Nutr.* 2000;71(2):500–506.

51. Albu J, Shur M, Curi M, Murphy L, Heymsfield S, Pi-Sunyer F. Resting metabolic rate in obese, premenopausal black women. *Am J Clin Nutr.* 1997;66(3):531–538.

52. Goff DC, Jr, Zaccaro DJ, Haffner SM, Saad MF. Insulin sensitivity and the risk of incident hypertension: Insights from the Insulin Resistance Atherosclerosis Study. *Diabetes Care.* 2003;26(3):805–809.

53. Haffner SM. Epidemiology of insulin resistance and its relation to coronary artery disease. *Am J Cardiol.* 1999;84(1A):11J–14J.

54. Gower BA, Nagy TR, Goran MI. Visceral fat, insulin sensitivity, and lipids in prepubertal children. *Diabetes.* 1999;48(8):1515–1521.

55. Danadian K, Lewy V, Janosky JJ, Arslanian S. Lipolysis in African–American children: Is it a metabolic risk factor predisposing to obesity? *J Clin Endocrinol Metab.* 2001;86(7):3022–3026.

56. Albu JB, Curi M, Shur M, Murphy L, Matthews DE, Pi-Sunyer FX. Systemic resistance to the antilipolytic effect of insulin in black and white women with visceral obesity. *Am J Physiol.* 1999;277(3 Pt 1):E551–560.

57. Gower BA, Herd SL, Goran MI. Anti-lipolytic effects of insulin in African American and white prepubertal boys. *Obes Res.* 2001;9(3):224–228.

58. Melnyk MG, Weinstein E. Preventing obesity in black women by targeting adolescents: A literature review. *J Am Diet Assoc.* 1994;94(5):536–540.

59. Stevens J, Kumanyika SK, Keil JE. Attitudes toward body size and dieting: Differences between elderly black and white women. *Am J Public Health.* 1994;84(8):1322–1325.

60. Kumanyika S, Wilson JF, Guilford-Davenport M. Weight-related attitudes and behaviors of black women. *J Am Diet Assoc.* 1993;93(4):416–422.

61. Gordon-Larsen P. Obesity-related knowledge, attitudes, and behaviors in obese and non-obese urban Philadelphia female adolescents. *Obes Res.* 2001;9(2):112–118.

62. Williamson DF, Serdula MK, Anda RF, Levy A, Byers T. Weight loss attempts in adults: Goals, duration, and rate of weight loss. *Am J Public Health.* 1992;82(9):1251–1257.

63. Kumanyika SK, Morssink C, Agurs T. Models for dietary and weight change in African–American women: Identifying cultural components. *Ethn Dis.* 1992;2(2):166–175.

64. Mulrow CD, Chiquette E, Angel L, et al. Dieting to reduce body weight for controlling hypertension in adults. *Cochrane Database Syst Rev.* 2000(2):CD000484.

65. Conlin PR, Chow D, Miller ER, 3rd, et al. The effect of dietary patterns on blood pressure control in hypertensive patients: Results from the Dietary Approaches to Stop Hypertension (DASH) trial. *Am J Hypertens.* 2000;13(9):949–955.

66. Svetkey LP, Simons-Morton D, Vollmer WM, et al. Effects of dietary patterns on blood pressure: Subgroup analysis of the Dietary Approaches to Stop Hypertension (DASH) randomized clinical trial. *Arch Intern Med.* 1999;159(3):285–293.

67. Sacks FM, Svetkey LP, Vollmer WM, et al. Effects on blood pressure of reduced dietary sodium and the Dietary Approaches to Stop Hypertension (DASH) diet. DASH-Sodium Collaborative Research Group. *N Engl J Med.* 2001;344(1):3–10.

68. Vollmer WM, Sacks FM, Ard J, et al. Effects of diet and sodium intake on blood pressure: Subgroup analysis of the DASH-sodium trial. *Ann Intern Med.* 2001;135(12):1019–1028.

69. Jefferson WK, Zunker C, Feucht JC, et al. Use of the Nominal Group Technique (NGT) to understand the perceptions of the healthiness of foods associated with African Americans. *Eval Program Plann.* 2010;33(4):343–348.

70. James DC. Factors influencing food choices, dietary intake, and nutrition-related attitudes among African Americans: Application of a culturally sensitive model. *Ethn Health.* 2004;9(4):349–367.

71. Bennett G, Wolin K, Goodman M, et al. Attitudes regarding overweight, exercise, and health among blacks (United States). *Cancer Causes and Control.* 2006;17(1):95–101.

72. Chobanian AV, Bakris GL, Black HR, et al. The Seventh Report of the Joint National Committee on Prevention, Detection, Evaluation, and Treatment of High Blood Pressure: The JNC 7 report.[see comment][erratum appears in JAMA. 2003 Jul 9;290(2):197]. *JAMA.* 2003;289(19):2560–2572.

73. Christakis NA, Fowler JH. The spread of obesity in a large social network over 32 years. *N Engl J Med.* 2007;357(4):370–379.

74. Ard JD, Durant RW, Edwards LC, Svetkey LP. Perceptions of African-American culture and implications for clinical trial design. *Ethn Dis.* 2005;15(2):292–299.

75. Kumanyika SK, Wadden TA, Shults J, et al. Trial of family and friend support for weight loss in African American adults. *Arch Intern Med.* 2009;169(19):1795–1804.

76. Samuel-Hodge CD, Gizlice Z, Cai J, Brantley PJ, Ard JD, Svetkey LP. Family functioning and weight loss in a sample of African Americans and whites. *Ann Behav Med.* 2010;40(3):294–301.

77. French SA, Wall M, Mitchell NR. Household income differences in food sources and food items purchased. *Int J Behav Nutr Phys Act.* 2010;7:77.

78. Morland K, Wing S, Diez Roux A. The contextual effect of the local food environment on residents' diets: The atherosclerosis risk in communities study. *Am J Public Health.* 2002;92(11):1761–1767.

79. Morland K, Wing S, Diez Roux A, Poole C. Neighborhood characteristics associated with the location of food stores and food service places. *Am J Prev Med.* 2002;22(1):23–29.

80. Ard JD, Fitzpatrick S, Desmond RA, et al. The impact of cost on the availability of fruits and vegetables in the homes of schoolchildren in Birmingham, Alabama. *Am J Public Health.* 2007;97(2):367–372.

81. Lien LF, Brown AJ, Ard JD, et al. Effects of PREMIER lifestyle modifications on participants with and without the metabolic syndrome. *Hypertension.* 2007;50(4):609–616.

82. Ard JD, Grambow SC, Liu D, Slentz CA, Kraus WE, Svetkey LP. The effect of the PREMIER interventions on insulin sensitivity. *Diabetes Care.* 2004;27(2):340–347.

13 Biological Factors That Influence Blood Pressure Response to Lifestyle Modifications

Bei Sun and Jonathan S. Williams
Harvard Medical School

Paul R. Conlin
Harvard Medical School and VA Boston Healthcare System

CONTENTS

13.1 INTRODUCTION

Prevention and treatment of hypertension over the last 50 years have improved dramatically as a result of numerous therapeutic advances. But lifestyle modifications remain a cornerstone in the approach to patients with prehypertension or established hypertension. Nonpharmacologic interventions lower blood pressure (BP) and reduce the incidence of hypertension. Ample evidence affirms the favorable effects of dietary patterns, sodium restriction, exercise and weight loss, and other lifestyle changes on BP. However, the response of BP to lifestyle modifications may be influenced by unique biological factors. Many of these features are well studied and are easily identified in patients (e.g., age, race, body weight); others, such as genetic factors, are still evolving. Since the impact of lifestyle changes on BP is influenced by acceptance and adherence, a focus on biological factors may allow clinicians to target interventions on individuals who are most likely to benefit.

This chapter summarizes the BP-related effects of lifestyle modifications with a focus on the evidence that the biological factors such as race, age, and body weight and genetic factors influence the response of BP to various lifestyle changes.

13.2 RACE

African Americans (AAs) in general have a higher prevalence of hypertension, with earlier onset, greater severity, and more clinical sequelae than age-matched non-Hispanic whites and Mexican Americans [1,2]. Compared with other ethnic and racial groups, AAs have an 80% greater stroke mortality rate, 50% higher heart disease mortality rate, and 320% higher hypertension-related end-stage renal disease [3]. In general, AAs have higher dietary sodium and low dietary potassium intake [4], as well as higher prevalence of obesity and reduced physical activity [5].

A substantial body of evidence suggests that renal handling of salt tends to be different in AAs than in whites, resulting in a greater degree of sodium retention and volume expansion in AAs for a given salt intake. In a study of short-term intravenous sodium loading, AAs showed a delayed natriuretic response [6]. In an attempt to decipher the mechanisms of enhanced sodium transport in AAs, several theories have been proposed [6–11]. Based on the observation that AAs often have reduced urinary potassium excretion and the evidence that the diuretic furosemide considerably narrows the racial difference of urinary potassium excretion [7], it has been suggested that the increased activity of the renal Na–K–2Cl cotransporter may contribute to sodium sensitivity in AAs [12]. This is supported by animal models demonstrating that the increased activity of the renal Na–K–2Cl cotransporter is associated with salt-sensitive hypertension [13,14].

There is also a well-documented age- and BP-independent effect on plasma renin activity (PRA) in AAs, whereby low renin activity is frequently observed. Under normal physiologic conditions, the kidneys reabsorb and excrete excess sodium to maintain sodium balance. In comparison with non-AA individuals, AAs tend to have an impaired ability to excrete a sodium load with altered sodium kinetics [15,16]. This inappropriate sodium reabsorption may lead to suppression of PRA and aldosterone secretion and predisposition to salt-induced elevation of BP [15,16]. Thus, the low PRA may not be a primary abnormality but rather a consequence of defective sodium handling.

In addition, the suppressed PRA in AAs may be a consequence of increased activity of intrarenal renin–angiotensin system. By studying renal hemodynamics in normotensive AAs compared with whites, investigators found a blunted increase in renal plasma flow when individuals changed from a low-salt diet to a high-salt diet [17]. The vasoconstrictive response to angiotensin II was also blunted in AAs [18]. After receiving captopril (angiotensin-converting enzyme (ACE) inhibitor, a medication commonly used in hypertension treatment), AAs showed a marked renal vasodilation and an enhanced vasoconstrictive response to angiotensin II [19]. Collectively, the above findings suggest that the intrarenal renin–angiotensin system in AAs is important in their renal hemodynamic response to salt. Other hormonal abnormalities related to salt sensitivity, such as diminished kallikrein–kinin synthesis [12] and reduced nitric oxide production [20], also exist in AAs.

Besides greater responsiveness to reduced sodium intake, AAs have a greater response to the DASH diet in comparison to non-AA individuals (6.9/3.7 mmHg vs. 3.3/2.4 mmHg). The most significant effects of the DASH diet were observed in hypertensive AAs, with a reduction in BP of 13.2/6.1 mmHg [21,22]. When combined with sodium restriction, the DASH diet was again more effective in AAs [23,24]. Similarly, hypertensive AAs had greater effects on BP in comparison with non-AAs when the DASH diet was combined with angiotensin II receptor blockers [25]. One potential mechanism to explain these effects could be the commonly described salt sensitivity in hypertensive individuals and in AAs [16,26]. Pressure–natriuresis curve (arterial pressure–urinary sodium output relationship) is commonly used to assess the sodium sensitivity of BP by plotting the urinary sodium excretion rate against mean arterial pressure (MAP), in which the steeper is the slope, the less sensitive is BP to salt [27]. The DASH diet has been shown to increase the slope of the pressure–natriuresis curve in a manner that mimics a diuretic effect [28]. AAs and older individuals are known to be salt sensitive with a shallow slope in their pressure–natriuresis curves.

Another potential effect of the DASH diet on AAs may be through its enriched potassium content. The current recommendation for daily potassium intake is 4.7 g/day (120 mmol/day) [4]. Survey data indicate that a potassium-deficient diet is particularly common in AAs and has been associated with the high prevalence of hypertension and salt sensitivity [4,11]. Abundant evidence suggests that increased potassium may counteract the BP-raising effect of sodium chloride by promoting urinary sodium excretion [29]. Even mild potassium deficiency may induce sodium retention, BP elevation, and salt sensitivity [26,30,31]. Supplementing potassium to 120 mmol/day has been shown to suppress salt sensitivity in normotensive AA men to the levels found in normotensive white men [26]. Increasing dietary potassium intake induces a greater natriuresis in AAs than in whites [10,32].

13.3   AGE

All of the factors described above involving lifestyle modifications are an integral part of the treatment for hypertension in older individuals. A position paper from the American Society of Hypertension advocates a comprehensive lifestyle intervention, including reduced salt intake, higher potassium intake, and moderated alcohol consumption accompanied by increased physical activity and weight loss if overweight [33], to lower BP and improve BP control among elderly patients with hypertension.

Older individuals manifest greater changes in BP in response to reduced dietary sodium and the DASH diet. As noted above, the effects of the DASH diet on the pressure–natriuresis curve suggest that the DASH diet reduces the salt sensitivity of BP. This slope-changing effect of the DASH diet was more evident in older participants (>45 years) and hypertensive individuals [28]. Lowering dietary sodium intake by 100 mmol/day reduced systolic blood pressure by 7 mmHg in individuals over 45 years old versus 3.7 mmHg in younger persons ($p < .05$) [24].

The phenomenon of increased salt sensitivity in the elderly can be explained by several structural and functional alterations in the aging cardiovascular system and kidneys. Advancing age is accompanied by a progressive decrease in the number of functioning nephrons, resulting in compromised ability to excrete the sodium load [34]. With aging, there is also a progressive decline in the baseline PRA and its response to salt depletion and furosemide administration [35,36]. It is well known that the renin–angiotensin system plays a pivotal role in the regulation of sodium balance [37–39] and that the baseline PRA status could be a strong predictor of salt sensitivity: the BP of individuals with low PRA tends to have a greater response to salt depletion or repletion [40]. Results from a study of neurohumoral responses to short-term dietary salt loading followed by salt deprivation showed that the reduction in BP was inversely related to the increase in PRA and aldosterone secretion following salt restriction and suggested that the blunted activity of the renin–angiotensin system may contribute to salt sensitivity in humans [41].

There is also a marked increase in arterial stiffness with aging, especially with large elastic arteries such as the aorta [42]. These structural changes are mostly due to loss of vascular smooth muscle cells, increase in vessel wall collagen content and collagen cross-linking, calcium deposition, and disruption and thinning of the elastic fibers [43]. A stiff artery has decreased capacitance, thus any changes in intravascular volume will lead to greater changes in BP. Further, altered arterial baroreceptor function due to atherosclerosis or other senescence-related changes also contributes to the variability in salt sensitivity of BP in older patients [44,45]. Baroreceptor activity may play a critical role in buffering the increase in BP due to salt loading. As an example, the response of BP to increased dietary salt intake in rats showed minimal change when baroreceptors were intact but increased significantly (15 mmHg) in sinoaortic denervated rats [46].

13.4   BODY WEIGHT

Obesity is associated with many physiologic and metabolic changes that promote hypertension [47–49]. Substantial human and animal data link obesity-related hypertension to fluid retention. Insulin resistance is a key factor in the development of obesity-related salt sensitivity. Indeed, the prevalence of salt-sensitive hypertension is significantly higher in patients who have metabolic syndrome than those who do not have [50,51]. Higher levels of circulating insulin in obese individuals may enhance renal proximal tubule sodium reabsorption, leading to sodium retention and salt-sensitive hypertension [47,52].

Activation of the renin–angiotensin system is another key mechanism related to obesity-associated hypertension through its effects on both peripheral vasoconstriction and enhanced renal sodium reabsorption. Human studies have shown that the circulating level of all components of the renin–angiotensin system—angiotensinogen (AGT), PRA, aldosterone, and ACE—is elevated in obese individuals [53,54]. In addition, adipose tissue is metabolically active and releases many bioactive molecules, such as AGT, leptin, resistin, proinflammatory cytokines (e.g., tumor necrosis factor-α). Animal studies suggest an effect of these substances on aldosterone secretion, mineralocorticoid receptor (MR) activation [55], and sodium retention [56]. The important role of aldosterone secretion/MR activation in obesity-induced salt-sensitive hypertension has also been confirmed by the fact that MR blockade with eplerenone markedly attenuated sodium retention and hypertension due to chronic dietary-induced obesity [57]. Salt intake also has a greater impact on BP in obese than in nonobese people. In a study of adolescents, obese subjects showed a greater decline in BP with salt restriction than nonobese subjects. This enhanced pressure–natriuresis relationship normalized after weight loss [51].

In contrast to the adverse effects of obesity later in life, there is emerging evidence that children with low birth weight (LBW) are also at greater risk for developing hypertension later in life, particularly a salt-sensitive form of hypertension. LBW is defined by the World Health Organization as birth weight < 2500 g (5.5 lbs). It is likely a surrogate for intrauterine growth stress. LBW has been strongly associated with subsequent adult hypertension in many epidemiological studies in various populations [58–64].

An intuitively attractive hypothesis for the relationship between LBW and subsequent hypertension was proposed by Brenner and Chertow [65]. This hypothesis proposes that undernutrition *in utero* results in a congenital deficit in nephron number. The reduction in the nephron number predisposes to reduced renal sodium excretory capacity and resets the steepness of the pressure–natriuresis curve, rendering the kidney more salt sensitive in the setting of excess dietary sodium.

Ultimately, the kidney is the key organ in the development of salt-sensitive type of hypertension. Among many of the physiologic factors responding to increased salt intake, the most important relationship is that between renal salt handling and intravascular volume homeostasis [66]. According to the Borst–Guyton concept, hypertension can occur only when a factor impairs the excretory ability of the kidney and shifts the pressure–natriuresis relationship, resulting in an increased salt sensitivity of BP [66,67]. In humans, kidney development begins during the ninth week of gestation and progresses through the 36th week, with no new nephrons formed after birth [68]. Therefore, the number of glomeruli is influenced by both the intrauterine environment and the gestational stage. Studies of kidneys in preterm or growth-restricted infants showed significantly fewer nephrons than in infants in the control group, which persists postnatally [69,70].

Growing evidence suggests that people with a history of LBW are at risk for developing salt-sensitive hypertension. For such individuals, salt restriction may be particularly beneficial. For example, a study examining the relationship between the response of BP to salt intake and birth weight in 27 healthy adults showed a striking inverse correlation between changes in MAP and birth weight [71]. A similar relationship between LBW and salt sensitivity was shown in a study of 50 children [72]. Numerous animal models have also been developed to support the hypothesis of a close link between prenatal insult and postnatal disease [73–75].

13.5 GENETIC FACTORS

Essential hypertension is a polygenic, complex disease resulting from interactions of both environmental and genetic factors. Based on family studies, it is estimated that significant amounts of interindividual differences in BP are attributable to genetic variations [76–78]. The inheritance pattern for BP is clearly more complex than if it was merely a Mendelian trait. The susceptibility to hypertension can be explained by the synergistic efforts of many common genetic variants, each with minor effects. With advances in genomic discoveries and genotyping technology, genome-wide association studies (GWAS) have become the major method to dissect complex diseases and have successfully identified a few BP loci [79,80]. However, the single nucleotide polymorphisms identified in GWAS can only explain very small portions of the variability in BP, far less than the part explained by age and body mass index. One explanation is that the effects of genetic variants are conditional and are influenced by the differences in environmental factors (e.g., dietary intake) between populations.

The response of BP to specific lifestyle interventions also varies widely among individuals. In general, many nutritional and lifestyle interventions are more effective in AAs, older people, and hypertensive individuals [29,35]. Genetic variations could explain part of this variability [81,82] and may be useful to identify individuals who are likely to benefit most from these interventions. Genetic influences on the response of BP to lifestyle interventions have been studied in detail, especially in response to dietary sodium restriction and the DASH diet.

AGT is one of the earliest genes that have been studied with regard to salt sensitivity and hypertension. Linkage between essential hypertension and the *AGT* gene locus was initially documented in European sibling pairs (i.e., two or more siblings carrying the same phenotype). Subsequent screening showed that an *AGT* variant substituting methionine (M) for threonine (T) at codon 235 (235T) was more prevalent in hypertensive individuals than in normotensive individuals [83]. Individuals who are homozygous for 235T have approximately 20% higher plasma AGT levels than those who are homozygous for 235M. The 235T allele is in tight linkage disequilibrium with a promoter allele, -6A, and the latter was proved to have a higher basal transcription rate [84]. Several studies have indicated that this genetic variant may influence response of BP to nutritional and lifestyle interventions. The 235T allele has been reported as a genetic modifier of the salt-induced rise in BP [85]. Individuals with the 235T allele had approximately twice the increase in BP for every unit of increased sodium intake when compared with those with genotype MM [86]. With regard to the effects of the tightly linked -6A allele on salt sensitivity- and obesity-related hypertension, the AA genotype was associated with greater BP reduction than the GG genotype after dietary sodium reduction or weight loss, in the TOHP study phase II. Also, the incidence of hypertension was significantly lower after sodium reduction for persons with the AA genotype but not for persons with the GG genotype [87]. Similarly, the response of BP to the DASH diet was greatest in persons with the -6AA genotype and lowest in those with -6GG genotype [88]. Polymorphisms in the *AGT* gene are linked to the response of BP to weight loss, salt restriction, and the DASH diet.

The $\beta2$-adrenergic receptor ($\beta2$-AR) gene has also been extensively studied for its effects on the response of BP to lifestyle interventions. A linkage study showed that the $\beta2$-AR gene was associated with the response of BP to sodium loading and/ or volume depletion [89]. A missense mutation of the $\beta2$-AR (G46A) substituting glycine (Gly) for arginine (Arg) at position 16 (Gly16Arg) in the mature protein has been identified. This allele has been studied extensively and appears to be functional. For example, the Bergen Blood Pressure Study revealed a higher frequency of Arg16 in hypertensive offspring of hypertensive parents, and conversely the 16Gly variant was associated with lower BP in a dose-dependent fashion [90]. There is a growing body of evidence showing that homozygotes for $\beta2$-AR 46AA have blunted receptor function compared with 46GG.

Studies that investigated vascular hemodynamics by genotype showed that the individuals with the AA genotype have attenuated vasodilation in response to infusion of the β-agonist isoproterenol. This effect occurs through impaired agonist-mediated receptor downregulation and desensitization [91,92]. There also appears to be an association of the Arg16 genotype with salt sensitivity and regulation of PRA secretion. The Arg16 genotype was associated with a subset of hypertensive patients with low PRA and salt sensitivity [93]. In a substudy of the DASH-Sodium trial, participants carrying the $\beta2$-AR 46 A allele (both AA and AG) had blunted PRA and aldosterone responses after consuming the DASH diet. In addition, the response of BP to the DASH diet was greater in individuals with 46A allele when compared with those with 46GG [85,94]. Mechanistically, those with the GG genotype had significant increases in both PRA and aldosterone, but they also had the smallest responses of BP to the DASH diet. This activation of PRA and aldosterone observed in individuals with the GG genotype appears to be a counterregulatory maneuver affected by the DASH diet, resulting in a blunted response of BP. However, those individuals with the AA or AG genotype failed to increase PRA and aldosterone and had a greater reduction in BP in response to the DASH diet. Thus, it appears that the $\beta2$-AR genotype impacts the response of BP to DASH and sodium intake in part through its effects on PRA, with the presence of the A allele conferring an attenuated PRA response.

Unfortunately, the effects of other known genetic variants on the response of BP to lifestyle modifications are very limited and relatively minor. It is possible that high-throughput genetics with large-scale GWAS will allow future advances and thus is likely to identify additional genetic determinants associated with the responses of BP to lifestyle interventions.

13.6 SUMMARY

Hypertension results from the interplay of internal derangement and the external environment. Lifestyle or environmental interventions clearly reduce the incidence and prevalence of hypertension. However, ample evidence supports that the environmental influences on BP are largely due to the influence of biologically based dispositions and characteristics. Factors such as race, age, and body habitus are particularly important in predicting responses to nutrition and lifestyle interventions (Table 13.1). It should be noted that even though certain factors may predict a greater response to lifestyle interventions, for example, AAs and older individuals respond greater to the DASH dietary intervention, other individuals also respond favorably and significantly. Clinicians often overlook the benefits from such treatments and fail to incorporate them into their treatment regimen of patients with hypertension. In addition, efforts to encourage patients to make lifestyle changes are often met by low acceptance and adherence. Thus, identifying those patients whose clinical characteristics and/or demographics suggest that lifestyle modifications will have a great

TABLE 13.1
Summary of Evidence on Biological Factors Influencing BP Response to Lifestyle Modifications

Biologic Factor	Intervention with Enhanced Response of BP
Race	
African Americans	Salt restriction [16,26,95,96]
	DASH diet [21,22]
	DASH diet combined with salt restriction [23,24]
	DASH diet combined with losartan [25]
	Increasing dietary potassium intake [11,26]
Age	
Older people	Salt reduction [24]
	DASH diet [24,28]
Body Weight	
Obese people	Salt restriction [50,51]
People born with LBW	Salt restriction [71,72]
Genetic Factors	
AGT 235T carriers	Salt restriction [86]
AGT -6AA genotype	Sodium reduction [87]
	Weight loss [87]
	DASH diet [88]
β2AR 46A carriers	DASH diet [94]

DASH = Dietary Approaches to Stop Hypertension, *AGT* = angiotensinogen, *β2AR* = β2-adrenergic receptor gene.

impact can allow a more focused approach to individualizing lifestyle/nutritional interventions. Indeed, for some people, lifestyle interventions alone may be sufficient to control their hypertension. Clinicians should continue to counsel patients, particularly those likely to derive the most benefits, about the use of lifestyle/nutritional interventions. As a part of a comprehensive hypertension prevention and treatment strategy, lifestyle-modifying interventions are effective, involve minimal risk for most individuals, are often less expensive than antihypertensive medications, and favorably reduce cardiovascular disease risks.

REFERENCES

1. Cooper R, Rotimi C. Hypertension in blacks. *Am J Hypertens.* 1997;10(7 Pt 1):804–812.
2. Wang Y, Wang QJ. The prevalence of prehypertension and hypertension among US adults according to the new joint national committee guidelines: New challenges of the old problem. *Arch Intern Med.* 2004;164(19):2126–2134.
3. The sixth report of the Joint National Committee on prevention, detection, evaluation, and treatment of high blood pressure. *Arch Intern Med.* 1997;157(21):2413–2446.
4. Institute of Medicine. *Dietary Reference Intakes for Water, Potassium, Sodium Chloride, and Sulfate.* Washington, D.C.: The National Academies Press, 2005.

5. Flegal KM, Carroll MD, Ogden CL, Johnson CL. Prevalence and trends in obesity among US adults, 1999–2000. *JAMA*. 2002;288(14):1723–1727.
6. Luft FC, Grim CE, Higgins JT Jr., Weinberger MH. Differences in response to sodium administration in normotensive white and black subjects. *J Lab Clin Med*. 1977;90(3):555–562.
7. Luft FC, Grim CE, Fineberg N, Weinberger MC. Effects of volume expansion and contraction in normotensive whites, blacks, and subjects of different ages. *Circulation*. 1979;59(4):643–650.
8. Luft FC, Rankin LI, Bloch R, et al. Cardiovascular and humoral responses to extremes of sodium intake in normal black and white men. *Circulation*. 1979;60(3):697–706.
9. Pratt JH, Ambrosius WT, Agarwal R, Eckert GJ, Newman S. Racial difference in the activity of the amiloride-sensitive epithelial sodium channel. *Hypertension*. 2002;40(6):903–908.
10. Langford HG, Cushman WC, Hsu H. Chronic effect of KCl on black-white differences in plasma renin activity, aldosterone, and urinary electrolytes. *Am J Hypertens*. 1991;4(5 Pt 1):399–403.
11. Sagnella GA. Why is plasma renin activity lower in populations of African origin? *J Hum Hypertens*. 2001;15(1):17–25.
12. Aviv A, Hollenberg NK, Weder A. Urinary potassium excretion and sodium sensitivity in blacks. *Hypertension*. 2004;43(4):707–713.
13. Alvarez-Guerra M, Garay RP. Renal Na–K–Cl cotransporter NKCC2 in Dahl salt-sensitive rats. *J Hypertens*. 2002;20(4):721–727.
14. Ferrandi M, Salardi S, Parenti P, et al. Na+/K+/Cl(−)-cotransporter mediated Rb+ fluxes in membrane vesicles from kidneys of normotensive and hypertensive rats. *Biochim Biophys Acta*. 1990;1021(1):13–20.
15. Wedler B, Brier ME, Wiersbitzky M, et al. Sodium kinetics in salt-sensitive and salt-resistant normotensive and hypertensive subjects. *J Hypertens*. 1992;10(7):663–669.
16. Brier ME, Luft FC. Sodium kinetics in white and black normotensive subjects: Possible relevance to salt-sensitive hypertension. *Am J Med Sci*. 1994;307 Suppl 1:S38–42.
17. Price DA, Fisher ND, Lansang MC, Stevanovic R, Williams GH, Hollenberg NK. Renal perfusion in blacks: Alterations caused by insuppressibility of intrarenal renin with salt. *Hypertension*. 2002;40(2):186–189.
18. Price DA, Fisher ND, Osei SY, Lansang MC, Hollenberg NK. Renal perfusion and function in healthy African Americans. *Kidney Int*. 2001;59(3):1037–1043.
19. Forman JP, Price DA, Stevanovic R, Fisher ND. Racial differences in renal vascular response to angiotensin blockade with captopril or candesartan. *J Hypertens*. 2007;25(4):877–882.
20. Campese VM, Mozayeni P, Ye S, Gumbard M. High salt intake inhibits nitric oxide synthase expression and aggravates hypertension in rats with chronic renal failure. *J Nephrol*. 2002;15(4):407–413.
21. Appel LJ, Moore TJ, Obarzanek E, et al. A clinical trial of the effects of dietary patterns on blood pressure. DASH Collaborative Research Group. *N Engl J Med*. 1997;336(16):1117–1124.
22. Svetkey LP, Simons-Morton D, Vollmer WM, et al. Effects of dietary patterns on blood pressure: Subgroup analysis of the Dietary Approaches to Stop Hypertension (DASH) randomized clinical trial. *Arch Intern Med*. 1999;159(3):285–293.
23. Sacks FM, Svetkey LP, Vollmer WM, et al. Effects on blood pressure of reduced dietary sodium and the Dietary Approaches to Stop Hypertension (DASH) diet. DASH-Sodium Collaborative Research Group. *N Engl J Med*. 2001;344(1):3–10.
24. Vollmer WM, Sacks FM, Ard J, et al. Effects of diet and sodium intake on blood pressure: Subgroup analysis of the DASH-sodium trial. *Ann Intern Med*. 2001;135(12):1019–1028.

25. Conlin PR, Erlinger TP, Bohannon A, et al. The DASH diet enhances the blood pressure response to losartan in hypertensive patients. *Am J Hypertens.* 2003;16(5 Pt 1):337–342.

26. Morris RC, Jr., Sebastian A, Forman A, Tanaka M, Schmidlin O. Normotensive salt sensitivity: Effects of race and dietary potassium. *Hypertension.* 1999;33(1):18–23.

27. Kimura G, Brenner BM. Implications of the linear pressure-natriuresis relationship and importance of sodium sensitivity in hypertension. *J Hypertens.* 1997;15(10):1055–1061.

28. Akita S, Sacks FM, Svetkey LP, Conlin PR, Kimura G. Effects of the Dietary Approaches to Stop Hypertension (DASH) diet on the pressure-natriuresis relationship. *Hypertension.* 2003;42(1):8–13.

29. Barri YM, Wingo CS. The effects of potassium depletion and supplementation on blood pressure: A clinical review. *Am J Med Sci.* 1997;314(1):37–40.

30. Gallen IW, Rosa RM, Esparaz DY, et al. On the mechanism of the effects of potassium restriction on blood pressure and renal sodium retention. *Am J Kidney Dis.* 1998;31(1):19–27.

31. Krishna GG, Chusid P, Hoeldtke RD. Mild potassium depletion provokes renal sodium retention. *J Lab Clin Med.* 1987;109(6):724–730.

32. Pratt JH, Manatunga AK, Hanna MP, Ambrosius WT. Effect of administered potassium on the renin–aldosterone axis in young blacks compared with whites. *J Hypertens.* 1997;15(8):877–883.

33. Appel LJ. ASH position paper: Dietary approaches to lower blood pressure. *J Am Soc Hypertens.* 2009;3(5):321–331.

34. Epstein M, Hollenberg NK. Age as a determinant of renal sodium conservation in normal man. *J Lab Clin Med.* 1976;87(3):411–417.

35. Weidmann P, De Myttenaere-Bursztein S, Maxwell MH, de Lima J. Effect on aging on plasma renin and aldosterone in normal man. *Kidney Int.* 1975;8(5):325–333.

36. Wilson TW, McCaulay FA, Waslen TA. Effects of aging on responses to furosemide. *Prostaglandins.* 1989;38(6):675–687.

37. Graudal NA, Galloe AM, Garred P. Effects of sodium restriction on blood pressure, renin, aldosterone, catecholamines, cholesterols, and triglyceride: A meta-analysis. *JAMA.* 1998;279(17):1383–1391.

38. Rasmussen MS, Simonsen JA, Sandgaard NC, Hoilund-Carlsen PF, Bie P. Mechanisms of acute natriuresis in normal humans on low sodium diet. *J Physiol.* 2003;546(Pt 2):591–603.

39. Williams GH, Hollenberg NK. Sodium-sensitive essential hypertension: Emerging insights into an old entity. *J Am Coll Nutr.* 1989;8(6):490–494.

40. Weinberger MH. Salt sensitivity of blood pressure in humans. *Hypertension.* 1996;27(3 Pt 2):481–490.

41. He FJ, Markandu ND, MacGregor GA. Importance of the renin system for determining blood pressure fall with acute salt restriction in hypertensive and normotensive whites. *Hypertension.* 2001;38(3):321–325.

42. Mitchell GF, Parise H, Benjamin EJ, et al. Changes in arterial stiffness and wave reflection with advancing age in healthy men and women: The Framingham Heart Study. *Hypertension.* 2004;43(6):1239–1245.

43. Acelajado MC, Oparil S. Hypertension in the elderly. *Clin Geriatr Med.* 2009;25(3):391–412.

44. Shimada K, Kitazumi T, Sadakane N, Ogura H, Ozawa T. Age-related changes of baroreflex function, plasma norepinephrine, and blood pressure. *Hypertension.* 1985;7(1):113–117.

45. Sowers JR. Hypertension in the elderly. *Am J Med.* 1987;82(1B):1–8.

46. Osborn JW, Hornfeldt BJ. Arterial baroreceptor denervation impairs long-term regulation of arterial pressure during dietary salt loading. *Am J Physiol.* 1998;275(5 Pt 2): H1558–1566.

47. Fujita T. Aldosterone in salt-sensitive hypertension and metabolic syndrome. *J Mol Med.* 2008;86(6):729–734.
48. Sarzani R, Salvi F, Dessi-Fulgheri P, Rappelli A. Renin–angiotensin system, natriuretic peptides, obesity, metabolic syndrome, and hypertension: An integrated view in humans. *J Hypertens.* 2008;26(5):831–843.
49. Pausova Z. From big fat cells to high blood pressure: A pathway to obesity-associated hypertension. *Curr Opin Nephrol Hypertens.* 2006;15(2):173–178.
50. Uzu T, Kimura G, Yamauchi A, et al. Enhanced sodium sensitivity and disturbed circadian rhythm of blood pressure in essential hypertension. *J Hypertens.* 2006;24(8):1627–1632.
51. Rocchini AP, Key J, Bondie D, et al. The effect of weight loss on the sensitivity of blood pressure to sodium in obese adolescents. *N Engl J Med.* 1989;321(9):580–585.
52. Zheng Y, Yamada H, Sakamoto K, et al. Roles of insulin receptor substrates in insulin-induced stimulation of renal proximal bicarbonate absorption. *J Am Soc Nephrol.* 2005;16(8):2288–2295.
53. Cooper R, McFarlane-Anderson N, Bennett FI, et al. ACE, angiotensinogen and obesity: A potential pathway leading to hypertension. *J Hum Hypertens.* 1997;11(2):107–111.
54. Rossi GP, Belfiore A, Bernini G, et al. Body mass index predicts plasma aldosterone concentrations in overweight-obese primary hypertensive patients. *J Clin Endocrinol Metab.* 2008;93(7):2566–2571.
55. Hoppa MB, Collins S, Ramracheya R, et al. Chronic palmitate exposure inhibits insulin secretion by dissociation of Ca(2+) channels from secretory granules. *Cell metabolism.* 2009;10(6):455–465.
56. Fujita T. Aldosterone and CKD in metabolic syndrome. *Curr Hypertens Rep.* 2008;10(6):421–423.
57. de Paula RB, da Silva AA, Hall JE. Aldosterone antagonism attenuates obesity-induced hypertension and glomerular hyperfiltration. *Hypertension.* 2004;43(1):41–47.
58. Zandi-Nejad K, Luyckx VA, Brenner BM. Adult hypertension and kidney disease: The role of fetal programming. *Hypertension.* 2006;47(3):502–508.
59. Gamborg M, Byberg L, Rasmussen F, et al. Birth weight and systolic blood pressure in adolescence and adulthood: Meta-regression analysis of sex- and age-specific results from 20 Nordic studies. *Am J Epidemiol.* 2007;166(6):634–645.
60. Nuyt AM, Alexander BT. Developmental programming and hypertension. *Curr Opin Nephrol Hypertens.* 2009;18(2):144–152.
61. Sayers S, Singh G, Mott S, McDonnell J, Hoy W. Relationships between birth weight and biomarkers of chronic disease in childhood: Aboriginal Birth Cohort Study 1987–2001. *Paediatr Perinat Epidemiol.* 2009;23(6):548–556.
62. Tian JY, Cheng Q, Song XM, et al. Birth weight and risk of type 2 diabetes, abdominal obesity and hypertension among Chinese adults. *Eur J Endocrinol.* 2006;155(4):601–607.
63. Huxley RR, Shiell AW, Law CM. The role of size at birth and postnatal catch-up growth in determining systolic blood pressure: A systematic review of the literature. *J Hypertens.* 2000;18(7):815–831.
64. Whelton PK, He J, Cutler JA, et al. Effects of oral potassium on blood pressure. Meta-analysis of randomized controlled clinical trials. *JAMA.* 1997;277(20):1624–1632.
65. Brenner BM, Chertow GM. Congenital oligonephropathy and the etiology of adult hypertension and progressive renal injury. *Am J Kidney Dis.* 1994;23(2):171–175.
66. Guyton AC, Coleman TG, Young DB, Lohmeier TE, DeClue JW. Salt balance and long-term blood pressure control. *Ann Rev Med.* 1980;31:15–27.
67. Guyton AC, Coleman TG, Cowley AV, Jr., Scheel KW, Manning RD, Jr., Norman RA, Jr. Arterial pressure regulation. Overriding dominance of the kidneys in long-term regulation and in hypertension. *Am J Med.* 1972;52(5):584–594.
68. Hoy WE, Hughson MD, Bertram JF, Douglas-Denton R, Amann K. Nephron number, hypertension, renal disease, and renal failure. *J Am Soc Nephrol.* 2005;16(9):2557–2564.

69. Rodriguez MM, Gomez AH, Abitbol CL, Chandar JJ, Duara S, Zilleruelo GE. Histomorphometric analysis of postnatal glomerulogenesis in extremely preterm infants. *Pediatr Dev Pathol.* 2004;7(1):17–25.
70. Manalich R, Reyes L, Herrera M, Melendi C, Fundora I. Relationship between weight at birth and the number and size of renal glomeruli in humans: A histomorphometric study. *Kidney Int.* 2000;58(2):770–773.
71. de Boer MP, Ijzerman RG, de Jongh RT, et al. Birth weight relates to salt sensitivity of blood pressure in healthy adults. *Hypertension.* 2008;51(4):928–932.
72. Simonetti GD, Raio L, Surbek D, Nelle M, Frey FJ, Mohaupt MG. Salt sensitivity of children with low birth weight. *Hypertension.* 2008;52(4):625–630.
73. Woods LL, Weeks DA, Rasch R. Programming of adult blood pressure by maternal protein restriction: Role of nephrogenesis. *Kidney Int.* 2004;65(4):1339–1348.
74. Manning J, Vehaskari VM. Postnatal modulation of prenatally programmed hypertension by dietary Na and ACE inhibition. *Am J Physiol Regul Integr Comp Physiol.* 2005;288(1):R80–R84.
75. Salazar F, Reverte V, Saez F, Loria A, Llinas MT, Salazar FJ. Age- and sodium-sensitive hypertension and sex-dependent renal changes in rats with a reduced nephron number. *Hypertension.* 2008;51(4):1184–1189.
76. Ward R. Familial aggregation and genetic epidemiology of blood pressure. In Laragh JH, Brenner BM (eds.). *Hypertension: Pathophysiology, Diagnosis and Management.* Raven Press, NY, 1990:81–100.
77. Snieder H, Harshfield GA, Treiber FA. Heritability of blood pressure and hemodynamics in African– and European–American youth. *Hypertension.* 2003;41(6):1196–1201.
78. Hottenga JJ, Boomsma DI, Kupper N, et al. Heritability and stability of resting blood pressure. *Twin Res Hum Genet.* 2005;8(5):499–508.
79. Newton-Cheh C, Johnson T, Gateva V, et al. Genome-wide association study identifies eight loci associated with blood pressure. *Nat Genet.* 2009;41(6):666–676.
80. Levy D, Ehret GB, Rice K, et al. Genome-wide association study of blood pressure and hypertension. *Nat Genet.* 2009;41(6):677–687.
81. Luft FC, Miller JZ, Weinberger MH, Grim CE, Daugherty SA, Christian JC. Influence of genetic variance on sodium sensitivity of blood pressure. *Klin Wochenschr.* 1987;65(3):101–109.
82. Gu D, Rice T, Wang S, et al. Heritability of blood pressure responses to dietary sodium and potassium intake in a Chinese population. *Hypertension.* 2007;50(1):116–122.
83. Jeunemaitre X, Soubrier F, Kotelevtsev YV, et al. Molecular basis of human hypertension: Role of angiotensinogen. *Cell.* 1992;71(1):169–180.
84. Inoue I, Nakajima T, Williams CS, et al. A nucleotide substitution in the promoter of human angiotensinogen is associated with essential hypertension and affects basal transcription in vitro. *J Clin Invest.* 1997;99(7):1786–1797.
85. Svetkey LP, Harris EL, Martin E, et al. Modulation of the BP response to diet by genes in the renin–angiotensin system and the adrenergic nervous system. *Am J Hypertens.* 2011;24(2):209–217.
86. Norat T, Bowman R, Luben R, et al. Blood pressure and interactions between the angiotensin polymorphism AGT M235T and sodium intake: A cross-sectional population study. *Am J Clin Nutr.* 2008;88(2):392–397.
87. Hunt SC, Cook NR, Oberman A, et al. Angiotensinogen genotype, sodium reduction, weight loss, and prevention of hypertension: Trials of hypertension prevention, phase II. *Hypertension.* 1998;32(3):393–401.
88. Svetkey LP, Moore TJ, Simons-Morton DG, et al. Angiotensinogen genotype and blood pressure response in the Dietary Approaches to Stop Hypertension (DASH) study. *J Hypertens.* 2001;19(11):1949–1956.

89. Svetkey LP, Chen YT, McKeown SP, Preis L, Wilson AF. Preliminary evidence of linkage of salt sensitivity in black Americans at the beta 2-adrenergic receptor locus. *Hypertension.* 1997;29(4):918–922.

90. Timmermann B, Mo R, Luft FC, et al. Beta-2 adrenoceptor genetic variation is associated with genetic predisposition to essential hypertension: The Bergen Blood Pressure Study. *Kidney Int.* 1998;53(6):1455–1460.

91. Dishy V, Sofowora GG, Xie HG, et al. The effect of common polymorphisms of the beta2-adrenergic receptor on agonist-mediated vascular desensitization. *N Engl J Med.* 2001;345(14):1030–1035.

92. Cockcroft JR, Gazis AG, Cross DJ, et al. Beta(2)-adrenoceptor polymorphism determines vascular reactivity in humans. *Hypertension.* 2000;36(3):371–375.

93. Pojoga L, Kolatkar NS, Williams JS, et al. Beta-2 adrenergic receptor diplotype defines a subset of salt-sensitive hypertension. *Hypertension.* 2006;48(5):892–900.

94. Sun B, Williams JS, Svetkey LP, Kolatkar NS, Conlin PR. Beta2-adrenergic receptor genotype affects the renin-angiotensin-aldosterone system response to the Dietary Approaches to Stop Hypertension (DASH) dietary pattern. *Am J Clin Nutr.* 2010;92(2):444–449.

95. Luft FC, Miller JZ, Grim CE, et al. Salt sensitivity and resistance of blood pressure. Age and race as factors in physiological responses. *Hypertension.* 1991;17(1 Suppl):I102–108.

96. Sowers JR, Zemel MB, Zemel P, Beck FW, Walsh MF, Zawada ET. Salt sensitivity in blacks. Salt intake and natriuretic substances. *Hypertension.* 1988;12(5):485–490.

Section IV

Putting It All Together:
Practical Tools

14 Practical Application

Laura P. Svetkey
Duke University Medical Center

CONTENTS

In this book, we have attempted to be comprehensive in presenting evidence on the effect of nutrition and other lifestyle factors on blood pressure (BP). A broad discussion of this evidence is essential for understanding the current state of science. We have also attempted to frame the evidence into recommendations that are practical for those attempting to use it in a broad array of clinical roles, including physicians and other providers, dietitians, and health centers. In this section, we distill those recommendations into current national guidelines for prevention and control of high BP [1]. In addition, we translate key factors leading to successful lifestyle changes into practical tools for assessment and intervention that can be applied in a variety of settings. In doing so, we recognize that it may not be easy or even possible to apply these tools in the current health care system. In addition, we recognize the individual responsibility of the patient in making any behavior change. Nonetheless, we offer these tools as a blueprint, some or all of which can be adapted for use in your particular clinical setting.

The potential impact of lifestyle modifications is enormous. Based on a study on almost 43,000 men followed for 16 years, it has been found that an estimated 62% of cardiovascular events are preventable by adoption of lifestyle recommendations (Figure 14.1), most of which lower BP. Adopting even two recommendations during middle age lowers the cardiovascular risk by 27% [2]. Yet, most Americans do not adopt healthy lifestyle recommendations.

Based on a self-report (Figure 14.2), where respondents may be tempted to overstate their adherence to lifestyle guidelines, it was found that less than 25% reported adherence to any recommendations other than smoking cessation [3], about 18% reported adherence to none, and only 5% reported adherence to all these guidelines. These statistics highlight the challenge, but given the success of programs emphasizing lifestyle changes and providing specific tools for achieving them, we remain confident that the lifestyle goals can be achieved, with favorable effects on BP.

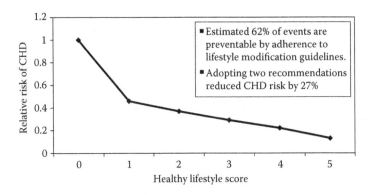

FIGURE 14.1 Potential impacts of lifestyle modifications. (From Chiuve, S. E. et al., *Circulation*, 114, 160–167, 2006.)

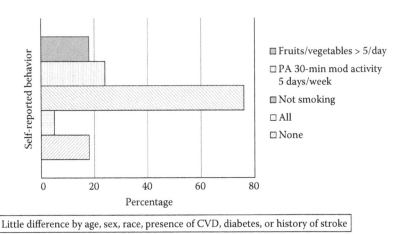

FIGURE 14.2 Adherence to lifestyle recommendations. (From Miller, R. R. et al., *Prev. Chronic. Dis.*, 2, 1–15, 2005.)

We propose adapting the 5A approach to client-centered counseling to help individuals achieve healthy lifestyle changes for lowering BP [4]. The 5 As are as follows: ask, advise, assess, assist, and arrange.

14.1 ASK

In the context of lifestyle changes for BP control, "ask" means inquiring about the patient's current lifestyle. Table 14.1 can be completed by the patient before the clinical encounter, and it allows the provider or the patient himself/herself to identify areas for improvement. Although not all areas can be addressed at each clinical encounter, the document serves as a resource that can be updated over time. Table 14.2 presents an alternative dietary assessment tool focusing on the Dietary

TABLE 14.1
Ask

Diet	In the last 24 h, what did you eat/drink for	List everything, with quantity (e.g., one McDonald's Big Mac)
	Breakfast	
	Lunch	
	Dinner	
	Alcoholic beverages (beer, wine, liquor)	
	Other beverages (indicate if diet or sugar-sweetened nondiet)	
	Snacks between meals or before bed	

Salt	Do you add salt to foods at the table?	Yes/No
	Do you add salt when cooking?	Yes/No
	Do you read food labels for salt content?	Yes/No
	Do you reduce salt intake in any other way?	Yes/No

Alcohol	In an average week, how many servings of alcoholic beverages do you have (include beer, wine, hard liquor, and mixed drinks). A serving is 12-oz beer, 5-oz wine, and 1.5-oz liquor			
	0	1–7	8–13	14 or more
	Note for clinician: Ok		Too high for women	Too high for everyone

Physical activity	**Do you:**	**Minutes each time**	**Number of times per week**
	Take a walk?		
	Go to a gym?		
	Play sports?		
	Get any other regular exercise? If yes, describe:		

Weight/height/BMI	What is your height?	
	What is your weight?	
	Calculate BMI; refer to http://www.nhlbisupport.com/bmi/	

Weight history	Do you consider your weight to be a problem?	Yes/No
	Have you ever tried to lose weight?	Yes/No
	If yes, what is the most you ever lost?	_____lb
	Did you regain any of it back?	Yes/No
	If yes, did you regain all the weight you lost?	Yes/No
	If yes, what led to the weight regain?	

Approaches to Stop Hypertension (DASH) dietary pattern, which has been shown to lower BP effectively (see Chapter 1).

14.2   ADVISE

Advising the patient involves both explaining what lifestyle changes are effective for lowering BP and providing the rationale for why it is important to adopt these lifestyle changes, that is, to improve BP control in those with hypertension treated with

TABLE 14.2

DASH Dietary Pattern Assessment

1. Write down your usual intakes of the following food groups using serving sizes defined below.
2. Compare your usual intakes to DASH recommendations and make goal/plans to move closer to DASH.

Food Group	DASH Recommendation	What Is a Serving?	Your Usual Intake	Goal
Fruits	4–6 servings/day	1 medium fruit, 1/2 cup canned fruit, 1/4 cup dried fruit, 6-oz fruit juice		
Vegetables	4–6 servings/day	1 cup raw leafy vegetable, 1/2 cup cooked vegetable, 6-oz vegetable juice		
Low fat or fat-free dairy	2–3 servings/day	8-oz milk, 1 cup yogurt, or 1.5-oz cheese		
Grains	7–8 servings/day	1 slice bread, 1/2 cup cooked rice, pasta, or cereal, preferably whole grain		
Meats, poultry, and fish	2 servings or less/day	3-oz cooked meats, poultry, or fish		
Nuts, seeds, and dried beans	4–5 servings/week or 0.5 servings/day	1/3 cup nuts, 2 tablespoon seeds, 1/2 cup cooked dried beans		
Sweets, sugared drinks	Less than 0.5 servings/day	8-oz sugared drink, 1 tablespoon sugar or syrup, 1 slice of cake or brownie or pie (~2–3 oz)		

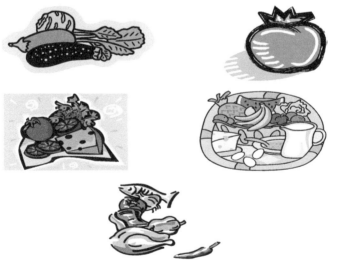

medication, to avoid medication in those with stage 1 hypertension, and to prevent hypertension in those with prehypertension. Table 14.3, which can be provided to patients as a resource, summarizes current recommendations, discussed in previous sections, with the rationale and clear goals for lowering BP and improving hypertension control.

TABLE 14.3
Advise and Assess

What Works	What It Means	What Is Recommended	Can I Do This? (0 = no way, 5 = no problem)
Weight loss	If you are overweight (BMI 25 or higher), even a small amount of weight loss can lower your BP. Check your BMI at http://www.nhlbisupport.com/bmi/	Lose 1–2 pounds/week by eating a healthy diet, reducing calories, and increasing physical activity.	0 1 2 3 4 5
DASH dietary pattern	DASH is a healthy dietary pattern that lowers BP by 5–15 points in most people	Each day, eat (men aim for the higher number and women aim for at least the lower number): 4–6 fruits 4–6 vegetables 2–3 low-fat dairy servings Reduce total and saturated fat Reduce sweets and sugar-sweetened beverages Select mostly whole grains More on DASH at www.nhlbi.nih.gov/health/public/heart/hbp/dash	0 1 2 3 4 5
Reduce salt intake	Limit sodium intake to no more than 2400 mg/day (about 6 g of salt)	Do not add salt at the table or to recipes Limit intake of prepared foods (e.g., frozen dinners) Limit intake of foods with very high salt (salted chips or nuts) Read food labels to see how much salt you are getting	0 1 2 3 4 5
Increase physical activity	Get moderate physical activity for 30 min most days of the week	Moderate physical activity is a brisk walk or some similar activity If you are already doing vigorous activity, keep it up If you are currently inactive, build up slowly	0 1 2 3 4 5
Keep alcohol intake at moderate levels	Too much alcohol (beer, wine, liquor) can keep BP high	For men, not more than 2 drinks/day For women, not more than 1 drink/day	0 1 2 3 4 5

14.3 ASSESS

Table 14.3 can also be used to provide an opportunity to assess the patient's perceived self-efficacy and their belief that they are capable of achieving the stated goal. Goals associated with low self-efficacy are unlikely to be achieved and are best reserved for future attention regardless of how important the provider may perceive them to be. Returning to Table 14.3 and reassessing, particularly after success with another goal, may reveal that self-efficacy has increased and that the goal can now be addressed.

14.4   ASSIST

When the provider and the patient have agreed on lifestyle goals, it is important to provide the patient with some practical tools for achieving behavior change. Behavior change interventions have generally been proven effective in the context of fairly intensive coaching. However, providing practical information on effective behavior change tools, such as self-monitoring and relapse prevention, may assist patients in achieving these goals on their own. These tools are summarized in Table 14.4, which

TABLE 14.4
Assist

Tip	How To Do It
Self-monitoring	Count calories
	Count food groups
	Count steps
	Weigh yourself at least weekly
	Check your BP
Goal setting	SMART goals:
	S—specific;
	M—measurable;
	A—action oriented, attainable;
	R—realistic;
	T—timely, relate to a time frame
Action planning	Specific
	Short-term
	Measurable
	Accountability
Relapse prevention	Identify "dangerous" situations and plan ahead
Social support	Ask for what you need
	Encouragement
	Exercise partner
	Do not nag
Reflect on motivation	Why is this important to me?
Resources	www.nhlbi.nih.gov/health/public/heart/hbp/dash
	Other online resources
	Resources in your community
	Walking routes
	YM/WCA
	Community organizations

can be provided to patients as a handout. In addition, Table 14.4 provides information on other resources to which local resources can be added by the patient or provider.

14.5   ARRANGE

Arranging follow-up, returning to the topic of lifestyle change at every clinical encounter, and following guidelines for monitoring and treating BP are all critical components of lifestyle treatment to prevent and manage high BP. In addition, there is evidence that patients are most successful with lifestyle changes when the recommendations are endorsed and reinforced by the provider. Providers should manage their own expectations: lifestyle change is often slow, incomplete, and relapsing. Like all other chronic conditions, adverse lifestyle changes require patience and persistence, both from the patient and the provider.

Arranging appropriate follow-up and taking every opportunity to reassess the motivation and the readiness to change, reinforce recommendations, and provide useful tools and information about resources constitute a practical strategy for helping patients achieve lifestyle changes that will prevent and treat high BP.

REFERENCES

1. Chobanian AV, Bakris GL, Black HR, et al. The Seventh Report of the Joint National Committee on Prevention, Detection, Evaluation, and Treatment of High Blood Pressure: The JNC 7 report. *Hypertension*. 2003;42:1206–1252.
2. Chiuve SE, McCullough ML, Sacks FM, Rimm EB. Healthy lifestyle factors in the primary prevention of coronary heart disease among men. *Circulation* 2006;114:160–167.
3. Miller RR, Sales AE, Kopjar B, Fihn SD, Bryson CL. Adherence to heart-healthy behaviors in a sample of the U.S. population. *Prev Chronic Dis* 2005;2:1–15.
4. Alexander SC, Cox ME, Turer CLB, et al. Do the five A's work when physicians counsel about weight loss? *Fam Med* 2011;43:179–184.

Index